Case Based Scenarios in
Pediatric Oncology

Case Based Scenarios in
Pediatric Oncology

Editors

Rachna Seth DNB
Professor and Chief
Division of Pediatric Oncology
Department of Pediatrics
All India Institute of Medical Sciences
New Delhi, India

Jagdish P Meena MD
Additional Professor
Division of Pediatric Oncology
Department of Pediatrics
All India Institute of Medical Sciences
New Delhi, India

Aditya Kumar Gupta MD FNB
Associate Professor
Division of Pediatric Oncology
Department of Pediatrics
All India Institute of Medical Sciences
New Delhi, India

Foreword
Shripad Banavali

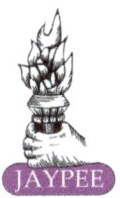

JAYPEE BROTHERS MEDICAL PUBLISHERS
The Health Sciences Publisher
New Delhi | London

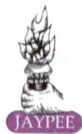 **Jaypee Brothers Medical Publishers (P) Ltd**

Headquarters
Jaypee Brothers Medical Publishers (P) Ltd
EMCA House, 23/23-B
Ansari Road, Daryaganj
New Delhi 110 002, India
Landline: +91-11-23272143, +91-11-23272703
+91-11-23282021, +91-11-23245672
Email: jaypee@jaypeebrothers.com

Corporate Office
Jaypee Brothers Medical Publishers (P) Ltd
4838/24, Ansari Road, Daryaganj
New Delhi 110 002, India
Phone: +91-11-43574357
Fax: +91-11-43574314
Email: jaypee@jaypeebrothers.com

Overseas Office
JP Medical Ltd
83 Victoria Street, London
SW1H 0HW (UK)
Phone: +44 20 3170 8910
Fax: +44 (0)20 3008 6180
Email: info@jpmedpub.com

Website: www.jaypeebrothers.com
Website: www.jaypeedigital.com

© 2023, Jaypee Brothers Medical Publishers

The views and opinions expressed in this book are solely those of the original contributor(s)/author(s) and do not necessarily represent those of editor(s) or publisher of the book.

All rights reserved. No part of this publication may be reproduced, stored or transmitted in any form or by any means, electronic, mechanical, photocopying, recording or otherwise, without the prior permission in writing of the publishers.

All brand names and product names used in this book are trade names, service marks, trademarks or registered trademarks of their respective owners. The publisher is not associated with any product or vendor mentioned in this book.

Medical knowledge and practice change constantly. This book is designed to provide accurate, authoritative information about the subject matter in question. However, readers are advised to check the most current information available on procedures included and check information from the manufacturer of each product to be administered, to verify the recommended dose, formula, method and duration of administration, adverse effects and contraindications. It is the responsibility of the practitioner to take all appropriate safety precautions. Neither the publisher nor the author(s)/editor(s) assume any liability for any injury and/or damage to persons or property arising from or related to use of material in this book.

This book is sold on the understanding that the publisher is not engaged in providing professional medical services. If such advice or services are required, the services of a competent medical professional should be sought.

Every effort has been made where necessary to contact holders of copyright to obtain permission to reproduce copyright material. If any have been inadvertently overlooked, the publisher will be pleased to make the necessary arrangements at the first opportunity.

Inquiries for bulk sales may be solicited at: jaypee@jaypeebrothers.com

Case Based Scenarios in Pediatric Oncology

First Edition: **2023**

ISBN: 978-93-5465-960-7

Dedicated to

Our Parents
Prof Anoop Saran Kapoor and Smt Shashi Kapoor
Shri HS Meena and Smt Lara Devi Meena
Shri Umashankar Prasad Gupta and Smt Bimala Devi
Who inculcated the values of hardwork and integrity in us.

Our Partners
Dr Sandeep Seth
Dr Anita Meena
Dr Nishtha Jaiswal
Who have always been patient and supporting during writing of the book.

Our Children
Ushmita and Udbhav Seth
Varenya Singh and Avanya Singh
Vandita and Viraj Gupta
Who were always there with us.

And also to
Our dedicated team of Pediatric Oncology residents, staff and patients
Without whose inspiration and support, this book would not have been possible.

Rachna Seth
Jagdish P Meena
Aditya Kumar Gupta

Contributors

Aditya Gupta MD
Senior Resident
Division of Pediatric Oncology
Department of Pediatrics
All India Institute of Medical Sciences
New Delhi, India

Aditya Kumar Gupta MD FNB
Associate Professor
Division of Pediatric Oncology
Department of Pediatrics
All India Institute of Medical Sciences
New Delhi, India

Debabrata Mohapatra MD
Senior Resident
Division of Pediatric Oncology
Department of Pediatrics
All India Institute of Medical Sciences
New Delhi, India

Debasish Sahoo MD DM
Assistant Professor
Department of Medical Oncology/Hematology
All India Institute of Medical Sciences
Bhubaneswar, Odisha, India

Gargi Das MD DM
Assistant Professor
Division of Pediatric Oncology
Department of Medical Oncology
Cancer Institute (WIA)
Chennai, Tamil Nadu, India

Himani Bhasin MD
Senior Resident
Division of Pediatric Oncology
Department of Pediatrics
All India Institute of Medical Sciences
New Delhi, India

Jagdish P Meena MD
Additional Professor
Division of Pediatric Oncology
Department of Pediatrics
All India Institute of Medical Sciences
New Delhi, India

Kanwaljeet Kaur Chopra DM
Senior Specialist
Department of Pediatrics
ESI PGIMSR, Basaidarapur
New Delhi, India

Kritika Setlur MD DNB
Senior Resident
Division of Pediatric Oncology
Department of Pediatrics
All India Institute of Medical Sciences
New Delhi, India

Meena H MD
Senior Resident
Division of Pediatric Oncology
Department of Pediatrics
All India Institute of Medical Sciences
New Delhi, India

Mohanaraj Ramachandran MD
Senior Resident
Division of Pediatric Oncology
Department of Pediatrics
All India Institute of Medical Sciences
New Delhi, India

Padma Sagarika Karri MD
Senior Resident
Division of Pediatric Oncology
Department of Pediatrics
All India Institute of Medical Sciences
New Delhi, India

Piali Mandal MD
Senior Resident
Division of Pediatric Oncology
Department of Pediatrics
All India Institute of Medical Sciences
New Delhi

Prasanth Srinivasan MD DM
Assistant Professor
Division of Pediatric Oncology
Department of Medical Oncology
Cancer Institute (WIA)
Chennai, Tamil Nadu, India

Prashant Prabhakar MD
Senior Resident
Division of Pediatric Oncology
Department of Pediatrics
All India Institute of Medical Sciences
New Delhi, India

Rachna Seth DNB
Professor and Chief
Division of Pediatric Oncology
Department of Pediatrics
All India Institute of Medical Sciences
New Delhi, India

Shilpa Khanna Arora MD
Senior Resident
Division of Pediatric Oncology
Department of Pediatrics
All India Institute of Medical Sciences
New Delhi, India

Foreword

It is a great honor that the 25th Annual Pediatric Hematology-Oncology Conference is being organized in India's Capital, by the Division of Pediatric Oncology at the AIIMS, New Delhi, that too in the year India is celebrating "Aazadi ka Amrit Mahotsav"!

The Organizing Team had the grand idea of taking out a book based on **"Case Based Scenarios in Pediatric Oncology"** to celebrate this occasion. Importantly, the book has been authored by Pediatric Oncology Superspecialty Students under the guidance of the Pediatric Oncology Faculty at the Department of Pediatrics, AIIMS, New Delhi. The organizers requested that I should write the foreword for this book and even forwarded me a few chapters for review.

There is no dearth of text-books giving us knowledge regarding Pediatric Oncology and at the same time there are many Reviews on the subject published from time to time. However, I found this format of starting with a case presentation and then raising various questions in regards to various practical and theoretical aspects of management of the case in a question-and-answer format very interesting. It makes it an interesting read and breaks away from the monotonous format of didactic reviews and book chapters. I hope the superspecialty students as well as the broad specialty students doing MD Pediatrics find this book very helpful. This way many practical aspects have been covered which will definitely help the students taking care of Hemato-Oncology patients to better take care of their patients in the clinics and the inpatients wards and at the same time gain knowledge.

The AIIMS team has covered most of the important aspects of management of Hemato-Oncology patients this year in Part I and I hope next year they will cover various solid tumors in Part II of this book. One practical advice that I would like to give to the team is that in addition to the book, the team may think of making 45 minutes to 1-hour video capsules of the same cases as is being done during "Panel Discussion" and put these on YouTube, so that more students who find it difficult to take out time to read, find it more easy to listen these video capsules.

Congratulations once again for converting this idea into a solid practical book which will be of immense help to our present and future students and wishing the team all the best for a very successful 25th Annual Conference of Pediatric Hemato-Oncology Chapter of IAP.

With warm regards,

Shripad Banavali MD
Director Academics
Tata Memorial Centre
Mumbai, Maharashtra, India
President Elect
Pediatric Hematology Oncology Chapter
Indian Academy of Pediatrics

Preface

Pediatric Oncology is a demanding specialty with varied and heterogeneous presentation of most childhood cancers. Case-based learning is a popular method of teaching and learning. The authors felt the need to publish a series of three books that would be dedicated to the presentation and discussion of a topic centered around a case. The first of the book series is dedicated to hematological emergencies, second to solid tumors and the third to survivorship and late effects. This is the first of the series which has discussed more than twenty cases in nineteen chapters.

The chapters of the book, written with a case-based discussion approach, have been authored by the Pediatric Oncology Superspecialty Resident doctors under the guidance of the faculty at AIIMS, New Delhi, India. The book is expected to benefit postgraduates and fellows pursuing a superspecialization course in Pediatric Oncology. Care has been taken to discuss the topic extensively and is likely to help the training students in both theory and practical examination. At the end of each chapter, opinion from another expert on how they would have approached this case, adding value to the scientific content of the chapter.

We hope that the book is well received.

Rachna Seth
Jagdish P Meena
Aditya Kumar Gupta

Acknowledgements

To all authors and experts who have contributed to the book.

Contents

1. **Acute Lymphoblastic Leukemia and Minimal Residual Disease** 1
   Gargi Das, Rachna Seth

2. **Acute Lymphoblastic Leukemia Relapse** 19
   Padma Sagarika Karri, Rachna Seth

3. **Acute Myeloid Leukemia** 40
   Kritika Setlur, Jagdish P Meena

4. **Acute Myeloid Leukemia Relapse** 58
   Kritika Setlur, Aditya Kumar Gupta

5. **Difficult Situations in Leukemia** 74

   5.1 **Infantile Leukemia**   74
   Gargi Das, Jagdish P Meena

   5.2 **Acute Leukemia in Down Syndrome**   86
   Gargi Das, Jagdish P Meena

   5.3 **Philadelphia-positive Acute Lymphoblastic Leukemia**   98
   Himani Bhasin, Rachna Seth

   5.4 **Acute Promyelocytic Leukemia**   124
   Debasish Sahoo, Jagdish P Meena

6. **Chronic Myeloid Leukemia** 138
   Prashant Prabhakar, Jagdish P Meena

7. **Juvenile Myelomonocytic Leukemia** 159
   Aditya Gupta, Aditya Kumar Gupta

8. **Anaplastic Large Cell Lymphoma** 171
   Prashant Prabhakar, Aditya Kumar Gupta

9. **Diffuse Large B Cell Lymphoma** 188
   Debabrata Mohapatra, Jagdish P Meena

10. **Burkitt Lymphoma** 205
    Meena H, Aditya Kumar Gupta

11. **Relapsed/Refractory Hodgkin Lymphoma** 219
   Piali Mandal, Rachna Seth

12. **Myelodysplastic Syndrome** 240
   Mohanaraj Ramachandran, Jagdish P Meena

13. **Langerhans Cell Histiocytosis** 251
   Shilpa Khanna Arora, Rachna Seth

14. **Non-Langerhans Cell Histiocytosis** 266
   Debasish Sahoo, Rachna Seth

15. **Autoimmune Lymphoproliferative Disorders** 280
   Kanwaljeet Kaur Chopra, Aditya Kumar Gupta

16. **Oncologic Emergencies** 292
   Prasanth Srinivasan, Rachna Seth

Index *339*

Abbreviations

2-CdA	Cladribine
2G	2nd Generation
6-MP	6 Mercaptopurine
ABC	ATP binding cassette
ABC	Activated B-Cell
ABG	Arterial blood gas
ABL	Abelson murine leukemia virus homolog
ACA	Additional chromosomal abnormalities
aCGH	Array comparative genomic hybridization
ADC	Antibody drug conjugate
AFP	Alpha fetoprotein
aGVHD	Acute graft versus host disease
AHA	American heart association
AHSCT	Autologous hematopoietic stem cell transplant
AIEOP	Associazione Italiana Ematologia Oncologia Pediatrica
AKI	Acute kidney injury
AKT	Ak strain transforming
ALCL	Anaplastic large cell lymphoma
ALK	Anaplastic lymphoma kinase
ALL	Acute lymphoblastic leukemia
ALP	Aspartate transaminase
ALPS	Autoimmune lymphoproliferative syndrome
ALT	Alanine transaminase
AMKL	Acute megakaryoblastic leukemia
AML	Acute myeloid leukemia
ANC	Absolute neutrophil count
AP	Accelerated phase
APML	Acute promyelocytic leukemia
APTT	Activated partial thromboplastin Time
Ara-C	Cytosine arabinoside
ASCO	American Society of Clinical Oncology
ATE	Arterial thrombotic events
ATO	Arsenic trioxide

ATP	Adenosine triphosphate	
ATRA	All trans retinoic acid	
ATT	Anti-tubercular therapy	
AYA	Adolescents and young adults	
beta-hCG	Beta subunit of human chorionic gonadotropin	
B/L	Bilateral	
B-ALL	B-cell acute lymphoblastic leukemia	
BAL	Bronco-alveolar lavage	
BC	Blast crisis	
BCL2	B cell lymphoma/Leukemia 2 protein	
BCL6	B cell lymphoma/leukemia 6 protein	
BCR-ABL	Breakpoint cluster Region - abelson proto-oncogene	
BCRP	Breast cancer resistance protein	
BEAM	BCNU, etoposide, Ara-C and melphalan	
BFM	Berlin Frankfurt Münster	
BL	Burkitt lymphoma	
BLNK	B cell linker protein	
BM	Bone marrow	
BMA	Bone marrow aspiration	
BMI	Body mass index	
BP	Blood pressure	
BV	Brentuximab vedotin	
C/S	Culture and sensitivity	
CART	Chimeric antigen receptor T cells	
CAVH	Continuous arterio-venous hemofiltration	
CBC	Complete Blood Count	
CBF	Core Binding Factor	
CCG	Children Cancer Group	
CCG	Center for cancer genomics	
CCyR	Complete cytogenetic response	
CD	Cluster of differentiation	
CDKN2A/B	Cyclin dependent kinase inhibitor 2A/B	
CECT	Contrast enhanced computed tomography	
CFT	Capillary filling time	
CHIPS	Childhood Hodgkin lymphoma international prognostic score	
CHR	Complete hematological response	
CI-TAD	Continuous infusion of 6 thioguanine + AraC + Daunorubicin	
CMA	Chormosomal microarray analysis	
CML	Chronic myeloid leukemia	
CMR	Complete metabolic response	
CMV	Cytomegalovirus	
CNS	Central nervous system	

COG	Children's oncology group
CP	Cysteine protease
CR	Complete response
CRT	Crania radiotherapy
CREBP	cAMP response element binding protein
CRi	Complete remission with incomplete recovery
CRLF2	Cytokine receptor like factor 2
CRP	C reactive protein
CSF	Cerebrospinal fluid
CsA	Cyclosporine A
CT	Computed tomography
CVD	Cardiovascular disease
CVL	Central venous line
CVS	Cardiovascular system
CVVH	Continuous venovenous hemofiltration
CXR	Chest X-Ray
ddPCR	Digital PCR
DEXA	Dual energy X-ray absorptiometry
DfN	Different from normal
DFS	Disease free survival
DHL	Double hit lymphoma
DIC	Disseminated intravascular coagulation
DLBCL	Diffuse large B cell lymphoma
DLC	Differential leucocyte count
DMR	Deep molecular response
DMRs	Differentially methylated regions
DNA	Deoxyribonucleic acid
DNMT	DNA methyl transferase
DNR	Daunorubicin
DOTIL	Disruptor of telomeric silencing
DS	Downs syndrome
DUSP-22	Dual specificity phosphatase-22
DxR, L DNR	Liposomal daunorubicin
EBF 1	Early B-cell factor 1
EBMT	European Society for Blood and Marrow Transplantation
EBV	Epstein-Barr Virus
EBV-LMP	Epstein-Barr Virus-latent membrane protein
ECD	Erdheim-Chester disease
ECG	Electrocardiogram
ECIL	European conference on infections in Leukemia
EFS	Event free survival
ELN	European leukemia net

ELTS	EUTOS Long term survival score
EMA	Epithelial membrane antigen
EM	Extramedullary
EMR	Early molecular response
EMT	Epithelial-Mesenchymal transition
ENT	Ear, Nose and Throat
EOC	End of consolidation
EOI	End of induction
EORTC	European Organization for Research and Treatment of Cancer
ER	Emergency room
ERK	Extracellular signal-regulated kinase
ERTL	Equally reactive to light
ESR	Erythrocyte sedimentation rate
ET	Extracellular Trap
EUTOS	European treatment and outcome study
EWS	Ewings sarcoma
EWOG	European working group
FAB	French-American-British
FCM	Flow cytometry
FDA	Food and drug administration
FDG	Fluorodeoxyglucose
FFP	Fresh frozen plasma
FFPE	Formalin fixed paraffin embedded
FiO_2	Fraction of inspired oxygen
FISH	Fluorescent in situ hybridization
FLAG	Fludrabine cytarabine GCSF
FLT3-ITD	FMS like tyrosine kinase, internal tandem duplication
FN	Febrile neutropenia
FNAC	Fine needle aspiration cytology
FPA	Fibrinopeptide A
G6PD	Glucose-6-phosphate dehydrogenase
GATA 3	GATA binding protein 3
GCB	Germinal center B-cell
GCS	Glasgow coma scale
GCSF	Granulocyte colony stimulating factor
GCT	Germ cell tumor
GEP	Gene expression profiling
GFR	Glomerular filtration rate
GI	Gastrointestinal
GM-CSF	Granulocyte macrophage colony-stimulating factor
GMALL	German multicenter ALL
GN	Ganglioneuroma

GNB	Ganglioneuroblastoma
GNB	Gram negative bacilli
GPE	General physical examination
GO	Gemtuzumab ozogamicin
GRB-2	Growth factor receptor-bound protein-2
GSK3β	Glycogen synthase kinase-3β
GTX	Granulocyte transfusion
GVHD	Graft versus host disease
Hb	Hemoglobin
HBsAg	Hepatitis B surface antigen
HCV	Hepatitis C virus
HDCT	High dose chemotherapy
HDU	High dependency unit
HES	Hydroxy ethyl starch
HiDAC	High dose cytarabine
HIV	Human immunodeficiency virus
HL	Hodgkin lymphoma
HLH	Hemophagocytic lymphohistiocytosis
HPE	Histopathological examination
HR	Heart rate
HR	High risk
HSCT	Hematopoietic stem cell transplant
IBMFS	Inherited bone marrow failure syndrome
ICE	Ifosfamide, carboplatin, etoposide
ICiCLe	Indian collaborative childhood leukemia group
ICT	Intracranial tension
Ida	Idarubicin
IDH	Isocitrate dehydrogenase
IDSA	Infectious Disease Society of America
IFD	Invasive fungal disease
Ig	Immunoglobulin
IGH	Immunoglobulin heavy chain
IHC	Immunohistochemistry
IHD	Intermittent hemodialysis
IKZF 1	IKAROS family zinc finger 1
IL	Interleukin
IMT	Inflammatory myofibroblastic tumor
INR	International normalized ratio
IPI	International prognostic index
IPS	International prognostic score
IR	Intermediate risk
IS	International standard

ISRT	Involved site radiotherapy
IT	Intrathecal
ITM	Intrathecal methotrexate
IV	Intravenous
IVF	Intravenous fluid
JAK-STAT	Janus kinase-signal transducers and activators of transcription
JMML	Juvenile myelomonocytic leukemia
JPLSG	Japanese leukemia/Lymphoma study group
KFT	Kidney function test
KMT2A	Histone-lysine N-methyltransferase 2A
LAIP	Leukemia Associated immunophenotype
LAP	Leucocyte alkaline phosphatase
LCH	Langerhans cell histiocytosis
LCM	Left costal margin
LDA	Low density array
LDH	Lactate dehydrogenase
LFA 1	Lymphocyte function-associated 1
LFT	Liver function test
LIC	Leukemia initiating cells
LL	Lymphoblastic lymphoma
LMIC	Low and middle income countries
LMB	Lymphoma malignancy B
LN	Lymph node
LTS	Life threatening symptoms/signs
LVEF	Left ventricular ejection fraction
LVSD	Left ventricular systolic dysfunction
mTOR	mammalian target of rapamycin
MAC	Myeloablative conditioning
MACE	Amsacrine cytarabine etoposide
MAPK	Mitogen activated protein kinase
MCFC	Multi-color flow cytometry
MCV	Mean corpuscular volume
MCyR	Major cytogenetic response
MDD	Minimal disseminated disease
MDR	Multi drug resistant
MDS	Myelodysplastic syndrome
MEK	Mitogen activated protein kinase
MiDAC	Mitoxantrone + Cytarabine
ML-DS	Myeloid Leukemia-Downs Syndrome
MMR	Major molecular response
6-MP	6 Mercaptopurine
MOA	Mechanism of action

MPAL	Mixed phenotypic acute leukemia
MPO	Myeloperoxidase
MPN	Myeloproliferative neoplasm
MPNST	Malignant peripheral nerve sheath tumor
MRP	Myeloid related protein
MRC	Medical research group
MRD	Minimal residual disease
MR	Medium risk
MRI	Magnetic resonance imaging
MRSA	Methicillin resistant *Staphylococcus aureus*
MS LCH	Multisystem Langerhans cell histiocytosis
MSD	Matched Sibling Donor
MSGERC	Mycoses Study Group Education and Research Consortium
MSH	MutS homolog
MUAC	Mid upper arm circumference
MUD	Matched unrelated donor
MUM 1	Multiple myeloma oncogene 1
MYC	Myelocytomatosis
NB	Nuclear body
NCCN	National comprehensive cancer network
NF1	Neurofibromatosis 1
NGS	Next generation sequencing
NHL	Non-Hodgkin lymphoma
NOPHO	Nordic Society of Paediatric Haematology and Oncology
NPM1	Nucleophosmin
NRC31	Nuclear receptor subfamily 3 group C member 1
NRM	Non relapse mortality
NRM	Non relapse mortality
NTKR3	Neurotrophic receptor tyrosine kinase
ORR	Overall response rate
OS	Overall survival
P/A	Per abdomen
PAI	Plasminogen activator inhibitor
pAML	Pediatric acute myeloid leukemia
PAX 5	Paired box protein 5
PB	Peripheral blood
PBCR	Population based cancer registry
PCR	Polymerase chain reaction
PCyR	Partial cytogenetic response
PD	Progressive disease
PD-L1	Programmed death ligand 1
PD1	Programmed cell death protein 1

PDGFRA	Platelet derived growth factor receptor alpha
PDGFRB	Platelet derived growth factor receptor beta
PEFR	Peak expiratory flow rate
PET	Positron emission tomography
PET/CT	Positron emission tomography/computed tomography
PFS	Progression free survival
PGP	P glycoprotein
Ph+	Philadelphia positive
PI3K	Phosphatidyl inositol 3 kinase
PICU	Pediatric intensive care unit
PLCγ	Phospholipase C gamma
PMBL	Primary mediastinal B-Cell lymphoma
PML	Promyelocytic leukemia protein
PNH	Paroxysmal nocturnal hemoglobinuria
POG	Pediatric oncology group
PR	Partial response
PRBC	Packed red blood cells
PRES	Posterior reversible encephalopathy
PT	Prothrombin time
PTH	Parathyroid hormone
PTEN	Phosphatase and tensin homologue
PTK2B	Protein tyrosine kinase 2 beta
PTPN11	Protein tyrosine phosphatase non receptor 11
qPCR	Quantitative real-time PCR
R/R	Relapsed or refractory
RAF	Rapidly accelerated fibrosarcoma
RARA	Retinoic acid receptor alpha
RARB	Retinoic acid receptor beta
RAS	Rat sarcoma
RB	Retinoblastoma
RBC	Red blood cell
RCC	Refractory cytopenia of childhood
RCM	Right costal margin
RCT	Randomized controlled trial
RDD	Rosai-Dorfman disease
RDP	Random donor platelet
RFT	Renal function test
RIC	Reduced intensity conditioning
RMS	Rhabdomyosarcoma
RNA	Ribonucleic acid
RO-	Risk organ negative
RO+	Risk organ positive

RQ-PCR	Quantitative real-time PCR
RR	Relative risk
RR	Respiratory rate
RRT	Renal replacement therapy
RS	Respiratory system
RT	Radiotherapy
RT-PCR	Reverse transcriptase polymerase chain reaction
RUNX	Runt related transcription factor
SCT	Stem cell transplant
SD	Stable disease
SDCT	Standard dose chemotherapy
SDS	Shwachman-Diamond syndrome
SEER	Surveillance, epidemiology, and end results
SGOT	Serum glutamic oxaloacetic transaminase
SGPT	**Serum glutamic pyruvic transaminase**
SIADH	Syndrome of inappropriate anti-diuretic hormone secretion
SLEDD	Sustained low efficiency daily diafiltration
SMN	Secondary malignant neoplasm
SMS	Superior mediastinal syndrome
SpO_2	Saturation
SR	Standard risk
SSC	Side scatter
SS LCH	Single system Langerhans cell histiocytosis
STAT	Signal transducer and activator of transcription
STLI	Subtotal lymph node irradiation
SVCS	Superior vena cava syndrome
T-ALL	T-cell acute lymphoblastic leukemia
t-PA	Tissue-plasminogen activator
TAM	Transient abnormal myelopoiesis
tAML	Therapy related acute myeloid leukemia
TAR	Thrombocytopenia with absent radii
TAT	Thrombin antithrombin complex
TB	Tuberculosis
TBI	Total body irradiation
TCR	T cell receptor
TCF3-PBX1	Transcription factor 3 - PBX Homeobox 1 fusion
TDM	Therapeutic drug monitoring
TF	Tissue factor
TGM2	Transglutaminase 2
TIT	Triple Intra thecal
TKD	Tyrosine kinase Domain
TKI	Tyrosine kinase inhibitor

TL-DS	Transient leukemia of DS
TLC	Total leucocyte count
TLI	Total lymphoid irradiation
TLS	Tumor lysis syndrome
TMD	Transient abnormal myelopoietic disorder
TMP-SMZ	Trimethoprim-sulfamethoxazole
TNF	Tumor necrosis factor
TP63	Tumor protein 63
TPGs	Translocator partner genes
TRM	Transplant Related Mortality/ Treatment related mortality
ULN	Upper limit of normal
u-PA	Urokinase-plasminogen activator
US	United states
USG	Ultrasonography
UTI	Urinary tract infection
VBL	Vinblastine
VCAM-1	Vascular cell adhesion molecule 1
VCR	Vincristine
VLA4	Very late antigen-4
VM-26	Teniposide
VRE	Vancomycin resistant Enterococcus
WBC	White blood cell
WHO	World Health Organization
WNL	Within normal limits
WT1	Wilms tumor protein

CHAPTER 1

Acute Lymphoblastic Leukemia and Minimal Residual Disease

Gargi Das, Rachna Seth

CASE VIGNETTE

A 7-year-old male child presented with fever, progressive pallor, cervical lymphadenopathy, and bony pains. On examination, he had wasting and stunting, multiple large cervical lymph nodes (largest 2 cm in size), with liver and spleen palpable 2 cm and 3 cm (nonbulky) below costal margin, respectively. Testis was normal in size and shape. Baseline complete blood count (CBC) revealed hemoglobin (Hb) of 10.7 g/dL, total leucocyte count (TLC) of 3,240/µL, and platelets of 100,000/µL. Peripheral smear examination revealed 15% blasts. We proceeded with a bone marrow (BM) aspirate examination, which revealed a near total replacement with blasts. BM flow cytometry (FCM) revealed 43% CD45 dim positive blasts which were CD34+ (heterogenous), HLA-DR+, CD19+ (heterogenous), cCD79a+, CD10+, CD81+ (dim), CD58+ (heterogenous), CD38+ (dim), and CD123+. Blasts were negative for CD20, cMPO, CD13, CD33, CD7, cCD3 and sCD3. He was diagnosed as a case of B-cell acute lymphoblastic leukemia (B-ALL) and started on a steroid prephase for 7 days (prednisolone at 60 mg/m^2/day). Day 8 cerebrospinal fluid (CSF) was negative for blasts (by morphology) and day 8 peripheral smear showed no blasts (good prednisolone response).

1. What is the risk stratification of this child?

As per the Indian Childhood Collaborative Leukemia (ICiCLe) group, the 7-year-old child has a nonbulky disease with TLC < 50,000/µL, no testicular and central nervous system (CNS) involvement, and a good prednisolone response, he was initially classified as a standard risk (SR) B-ALL.

2. What is important in the FCM in this child?

There are some markers that have been used for diagnosis (CD45, CD34, CD19, CD10, and cCD79a) along with some markers used to assist specifically for minimal residual disease (MRD) (CD58, CD81, CD38, and CD123, in this case). Each center may use their own set of markers, which are used to identify leukemia-associated immunophenotype (LAIP) during MRD assessment at end of induction/consolidation (EOI/EOC).

3. Is there anything else required for the risk stratification?

Patients of B-ALL should have a basic karyotype and FISH (fluorescence in situ hybridization) [with or without a polymerase chain reaction (PCR) analysis] prior to start of therapy. The main challenge is to decide the minimum/optimum molecular/cytogenetic analysis required in a low-income and middle-income country (LMIC), where cost is a constraint. A study done

Flowchart 1: Three-probe FISH (fluorescence in situ hybridization) approach to detect recurrent cytogenetic abnormalities in childhood acute lymphoblastic leukemia (ALL).

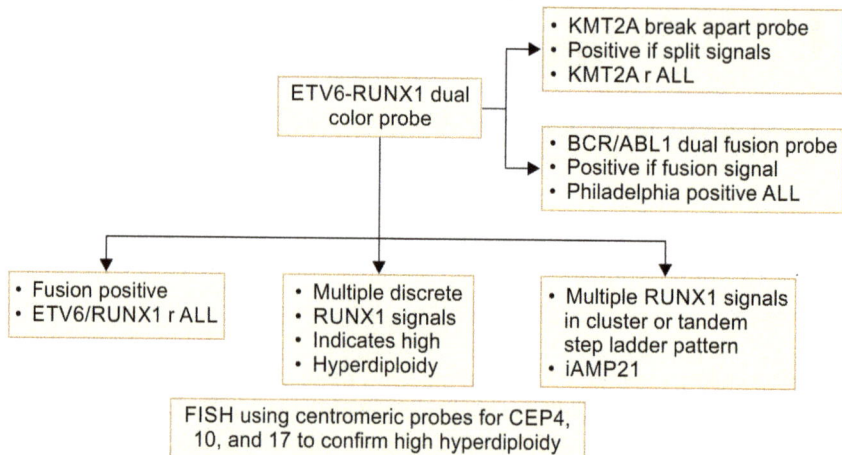

by Tata Medical Center, Kolkata, reported that a three-probe FISH approach could provide a practical approach for risk-stratified therapy in childhood ALL. **Flowchart 1** provides the approach. With this technique we can identify t(12;21), hyperdiploidy, iamp21, BCR/ABL1, and KMT2A rearrangements, which account for 60–70% of all known mutations in B-ALL.[1] A PCR may be performed when these tests are not available. It is noteworthy that a PCR will not identify aneuploidies and non-AF4 KMT2A translocations.

CASE *(Continued)*

At our center, we routinely get a karyotype, FISH to detect four rearrangements [t(12;21), BCR-ABL rearrangement, MLL rearrangement, and chromosome 19 rearrangement], and a PCR to confirm the findings. This child had a hyperdiploidy, with karyotype suggestive of 57 XY (+X, +7, +8, +15, +16, +16, +18, +19, +21, and +21). Child remained in SR and received a three-drug induction based on ICiCLe protocol (prednisolone, vincristine, and L-asparaginase).

Bone marrow aspirate at the EOI (day 35) revealed 2–3% blasts and MRD evaluation was as follows: 0.018% leukemic blasts which were CD45 dim positive, CD34+ (heterogenous), CD19+ (moderate), CD10+ (bright), CD38+ (moderate), CD81+ (dim), CD58+ (bright), HLADR+, negative for CD123, and CD20.

4. What is the interpretation of this MRD?

As the residual blasts share LAIP with baseline blasts, we may consider this to be detectable MRD. Detailed definition of MRD will be explained in the subsequent sections.

5. What is MRD?

Minimal residual disease describes disease that is present at a level below the sensitivity of morphological detection. As it is found in the absence of clinical signs or symptoms, it is termed as "minimal". With the advent of next-generation sequencing (NGS), a better term yet, would be "measurable residual disease". An MRD which is not detectable is potentially compatible with cure.[2]

In patients with ALL, the levels of MRD reflect the collective influence of leukemic cell genetics, microenvironment, host factors, and treatment efficacy on treatment response.

The goals for an MRD assessment would be:
- Providing prognostic information
- Assessing effectiveness of therapy
- Guidance for risk adjusted therapy
  - *MRD detected:* More or different therapy
  - *Not detected:* Less therapy needed, less toxicity
- Distinguish early recovery from persistent disease
  - The concept of hematogones
- Predicting early relapse.

Minimal residual disease can be assessed post induction, consolidation, prior to transplant, and any time when there is a doubt of relapse.[2]

Minimal residual disease assessment is typically performed on a BM specimen (first pull sample to avoid hemodilution). Peripheral blood affords a lower sensitivity for MRD detection as compared to BM (median 1.5 log lower sensitivity). This is mainly true for acute myeloid leukemia and B-ALL. For T-cell ALL (T-ALL), though the cell of origin comes from the BM, the maturation of T cells happens in the thymus, hence peripheral blood maybe used for T-ALL.[3]

6. What are the different methodologies to detect MRD? What is the ideal methodology for detection of MRD in a low–middle-income setting?

The various methods to detect MRD are described in **Table 1**.[4]

TABLE 1: Methods for minimal residual disease detection.

Method	Target	Applicability	Material	Sensitivity	Advantage	Disadvantage
MCFC	LAIPs/DfN	>90%	Cell suspension (PB, BM, FNAC)	6–8 Color: 10^{-4}	• Fast and easy to set up • Widely applicable	• Observer dependent • Less sensitive • Standardization may vary with each institute
RQ-PCR	Recurrent fusion genes: 12;21, BCR-ABL1, KMT2A-AF4	30–40%	RNA/DNA	$10^{-4}/10^{-5}$	• High sensitivity • Rapid and easy • Relatively easy • Stable throughout treatment	• Limited applicability (target-negative in >50% of patients) • Relatively expensive

Contd...

Contd...

Method	Target	Applicability	Material	Sensitivity	Advantage	Disadvantage
RQ-PCR	IG/TCR rearrangements	90–95%	RNA/DNA	$10^{-4}/10^{-5}$	• High sensitivity • Good applicability • Well standardized	• Dependent on ASO-primer • Laborious and time consuming • Affected by clonal evolution • Large amount of diagnostic DNA • Relatively expensive
Next-generation sequencing	IG/TCR gene rearrangements	>95%	DNA	$10^{-4}/10^{-6}$	• High sensitivity • High applicability • Clonal evolution identified • Not dependent on ASO-prime	• Not standardized • Complex bioinformatics analysis • Expensive

(ASO: allele-specific oligonucleotides; BM: bone marrow; DfN: different from normal; FNAC: fine needle aspiration cytology; IG: immunoglobulin; LIAPs: leukemia-associated immunophenotypes; MCFC: multicolor flow cytometry; PB: peripheral blood; RQ-PCR: real-time quantitative polymerase chain reaction; TCR: T-cell receptor)

Source: Adapted from the table by Starza ID et al. Minimal residual disease in acute lymphoblastic leukemia: Technical and clinical advances. Front Oncol. 2019.

Newer techniques have been developed including next-generation FCM and droplet digital PCR (ddPCR) which are advances of already available techniques, however not commonly used around the world.

7. What are the definitions related to MRD used commonly?[5]

a. *MRD negative:* Undetectable MRD
b. *MRD low positive:* Detectable MRD ≤ 10^{-4} [quantitative-PCR (qPCR)] or <0.01% [multicolor flow cytometry (MCFC)]
c. *MRD high positive:* Detectable MRD ≥ 10^{-4} to <10^{-3} (qPCR) or 0 > 0.01 to <0.1% (MCFC)
d. *MRD very high positive:* MRD ≥ 10^{-3} (qPCR) or >0.1% (MCFC).

8. Is there any evidence comparing MCFC with PCR for MRD detection in B-ALL?

In a study conducted by Bader et al. at all-time points, qPCR detected more MRD than MCFC. High/Very high MRD detection was equivalent using the two approaches (MCFC vs.

qPCR, 15 vs. 16%); however, low-level MRD (<0.01% by MFC, <10^{-4} by qPCR) was detected prehematopoietic stem cell transplantation (HSCT) in only 2% of MCFC patients versus 28% of qPCR patients. But it was also noted that low versus undetectable MRD pre-HSCT did not alter the outcome; hence, the clinical relevance of detecting such low levels of MRD is unknown.[6]

9. Is there any evidence comparing MCFC with NGS?

The higher analytic sensitivity and lower false-negative rate of NGS over flow cytometry for MRD detection in pediatric B-ALL is known and has been studied in the past. NGS and MCFC showed similar 5-year event-free survival (EFS) and overall survival (OS) for MRD-positive and -negative patients using an MRD threshold of 0.01%. However, NGS identified around 40% more patients with MRD positivity at this threshold who had worse outcomes than MCFC MRD-negative patients. In addition, NGS identified 20% of SR patients without MRD at any detectable level who had excellent 5-year EFS (98.1%) and OS (100%), who may benefit from deintensification of therapy.[7]

Though PCR and NGS are more sensitive, they are also more expensive and not universally present. MCFC have been around for a long time and is well standardized. Though definite training is required for MRD analysis by MCFC, it is the only method with extremely wide applicability and faster processing (turnaround time few hours in certain institutes).

Poisson statistics describe precision in rare event analysis. For an adequate sensitivity and precision, to detect an abnormal population at 0.01% of the mononuclear cells (1/10,000):
- Collect 250,000–1,000,000 events
- >500,000 events collected for all MRD studies usually.

CASE (Continued)

At our institute we use a 10–13 color MCFC for MRD analysis. We acquire 1,000,000 events and turnaround time is 12–24 hours and we have an established set of CD markers for MRD analysis. In B-ALL we routinely test for MRD at day 35 (after induction). We routinely do not assess for MRD before that.

10. What are the approaches for MRD detection by FCM?

There are two main approaches for MRD assessment different from normal (DfN) and LAIP approach.[8]
- *LAIP approach:* Defines certain CD markers at diagnosis and tracks these in subsequent samples as described in our case vignette. Each LAIP is present on both leukemic cells and normal nucleated BM cells (hematogones), but their pattern of expression vary. Maximum sensitivity is around 10^{-4}–10^{-5}. The major disadvantage is that if there is an instability of even one LAIP marker following treatment—MRD may be labeled as falsely "negative".
- *DfN approach:* This is based on the identification of aberrant differentiation/maturation profiles at follow-up and uses a fixed antibody panel. It is applied when:
  - Information from diagnosis is not available.
  - To detect new aberrancies, together with disappearance of diagnosis aberrancies, referred as "immunophenotype shifts".
    - Emerges from leukemia evolution or clonal selection.

The best method for detection of MRD is a "combination approach". This allows for detection of new aberrancies emerging at follow-up, and monitoring patients when there is an absence of diagnostic information. The term "LAIP-based DfN approach" has been coined by the European Leukemia Network for this combined strategy.

CASE (Continued)

As this child had a detectable MRD postinduction (MRD high positive), we retrospectively analyzed our case and had a few questions.

11. Do you think this child's initial risk stratification is correct?

a. Role of bulky disease in ALL.
The early studies of Berlin Frankfurt Munster (BFM) group, children's cancer group (CCG), and the pediatric oncology group (POG) used bulky disease in liver and spleen to define high-risk disease. But with advancements and more insight into the biology of ALL, molecular and cytogenetics, prednisolone response and MRD took over in the scheme of risk stratification. The ICiCLe group assigns children an intermediate risk if they present with bulky disease.

Our child had presence of liver and spleen (though not fulfilling definitions for bulky disease as per ICiCLe) and did not receive anthracycline during induction. Despite having a good prednisolone response, child had a persistent MRD. Is it possible that the presence of extramedullary (EM) disease should have warranted anthracyclines during induction?

b. Redefining high hyperdiploidy.
Children with B-ALL with high hyperdiploidy account for 25–30% of cases and have a favorable prognosis. It is defined by *"total chromosome number of 51–67 or by a DNA content ≥ 1.16, and by a characteristic karyotype pattern (gains of chromosomes X, 4, 6, 10, 14, 17, 18, and 21)."* However, around 10% of children with B-ALL and high hyperdiploidy relapse. Previous studies have reported the good prognostic value of trisomies of chromosomes 4, 10, 17, and 18. The poor risk group is identified either by *"the absence of both good-risk trisomies (+17, +18) or by the presence of only one of these good-risk trisomies and at least one of the poor-risk trisomies (+5, +20)."* There was a significant difference in relapse rate, EFS and OS, hence this group may benefit from intensification of therapy.[9]

The child in the vignette, had high hyperdiploidy, but the chromosomal involvement did not include the poor risk chromosome.

c. Role of Philadelphia-like (Ph-like) ALL.
The genomic landscape of ALL is ever expanding. Ph-like ALL is a unique subtype which has gained popularity over the last decade as they display a gene expression profile (GEP) like that of Ph-positive ALL, and frequently harbor IKZF1 alterations, but lacks the hallmark BCR-ABL1 oncoprotein. They are actually three times more common than Ph-positive ALL and comprise 10% of children with SR B-ALL and 15% of children with NCI high-risk B-ALL. It is seen more frequently in boys and are associated with adverse clinical features at presentation (initial TLC > 100,000/μL) and detectable MRD at the EOI therapy, notably due to the EBF1–PDGFRB fusion. Children with Ph-like ALL have an increased propensity to relapse and have outcomes which are inferior to KMT2A and BCR-ABL1 rearranged leukemias.[10]

Flowchart 2: Suggested approach for testing for Philadelphia-like (Ph-like) acute lymphoblastic leukemia (ALL) in low-income and middle-income countries (LMICs).

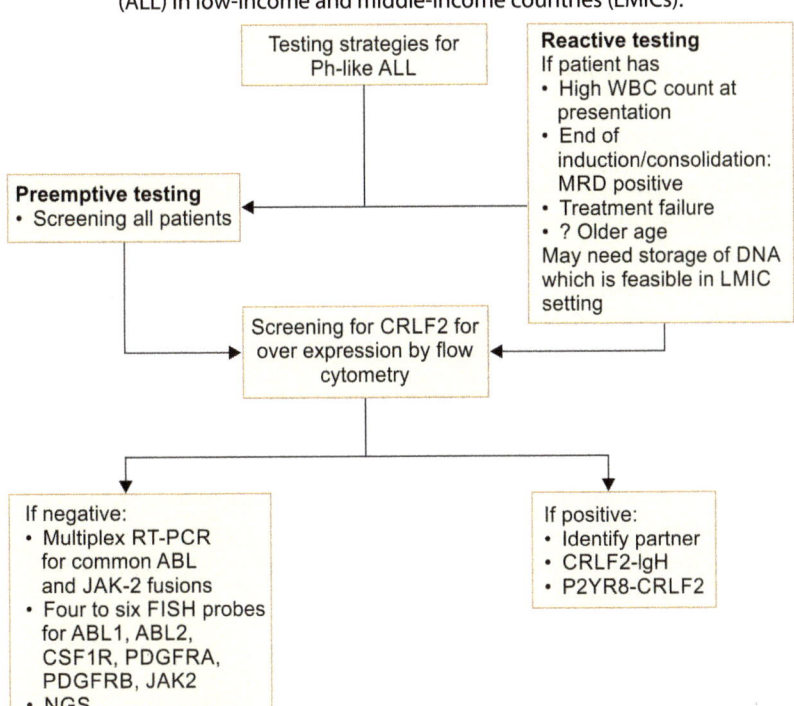

(FISH: fluorescence in situ hybridization; MRD: minimal residual disease; NGS: next-generation sequencing; RT-PCR: reverse transcription-polymerase chain reaction; WBC: white blood count)

i. **What are the Ph-like alterations?**
   For the purpose of this chapter, we have divided Ph-like alterations into five distinct subgroups based on the type of cytokine receptor or kinase fusion present.[10]
   1. *Rearrangements of CRLF2 (47%):* Most prevalent in all age groups.
   2. *ABL-class gene rearrangements (13%):* Including genes like ABL1, ABL2, PDGFRB, and CSF1R.
   3. *JAK2 and EPOR rearrangements (11%)*
   4. *Sequence mutations or deletions activating JAK-STAT or MAPK signaling pathways (13%):* IL7R, FLT3, and IL2RB, activating mutations of JAK-STAT pathway (JAK1 and JAK3) and deletion of genes that encode negative regulators of the JAK-STAT pathway (SH2B3).
   5. *Other rare kinase alterations:* RAS pathway mutations (NRAS, KRAS, PTPN11, NF)
   Similar to Ph-positive ALL, a unifying hallmark of Ph-like ALL is the high frequency of IKZF1 alterations relative to BCR-ABL negative non-Ph-like ALL (68 vs. 16%).
ii. **Who should we screen for Ph-like ALL?** A basic stepwise approach can be taken as described in **Flowchart 2**.
iii. **Any benefit for screening for Ph-like ALL?**

Yes, we can target these genes with certain drugs like ABL kinases (imatinib/dasatinib) for ABL rearrangements, JAK inhibitors (ruxolitinib) for JAK2/EPOR rearrangements and other mutations affecting JAK signaling pathway and drugs targeting JAK-STAT, PI3K, mTOR, and BCL2 for CRLF2-rearranged leukemias.[10]

CASE *(Continued)*

The child in the case vignette had a high hyperdiploidy, which portends a good risk, and still relapsed. It is unlikely that they harbored a Ph-like ALL mutation as well. Moreover, child had baseline nonbulky disease and low TLC, making Ph-like ALL unlikely.

At our institute, we do not store DNA at baseline, nor do we test for Ph-like ALL. Considering the morbidity of transplant and the relative ease to procure some inhibitors, it may be worthwhile to look for Ph-like ALL at initial diagnosis in low–middle-income countries.

12. How should we define complete remission (CR) in a child with B-ALL in the era of MRD?

Complete remission is traditionally defined as meeting all of the following response criteria:
- <5% blasts in the BM
- Normal maturation of all cellular components in the BM
- No EM disease (e.g., CNS, soft tissue disease)
- Absolute neutrophil count (ANC) ≥ 1,000/μL
- Platelets ≥ 100,000/μL
- Transfusion independent.

Complete remission with incomplete hematologic recovery (CRi) is defined as meeting all of the following response criteria:
- <5% blasts in the BM
- Normal maturation of all cellular components in the BM
- No EM disease (e.g., CNS, soft tissue disease)
- Transfusion independent (please note, if the physician documents transfusion dependence related to treatment and not the patient's underlying ALL, CR should be reported).

Primary induction failure: If a patient has never been in CR or CRi.

13. There is a significant variation in defining CR and time point to define CR. More importantly, the definition of induction failure differs between trial consortiums. With growing knowledge of MRD, should the definition of CR undergo modification? Even definitions for relapse do not include MRD, should there be a modification in the definition?

In an international consensus of the Ponte-di-Legno Consortium, the definitions of CR and treatment failure (TF) were given.[11]
- *Definition of CR:*
  - CR is to be assessed no earlier than EOI.
  - For CR, the following is required:
    - *BM:* M1 cytomorphology and/or MRD < 1%

- *CNS:* CNS1 status
- *Testes:* Normal on clinical examination, or a negative biopsy if clinical examination is not considered normal.
- *EM:* No evidence of leukemic infiltrates as evaluated clinically and by imaging; a preexisting leukemic mass (mediastinal mass included) must have decreased at least to one-third of the initial tumor volume.
- It is recommended that CR assessment of BM should be performed by cytomorphology, followed by a standardized MRD method. Complementary methods including genetic analysis may also be used to verify CR achievement.
- CNS status should be based on CSF cytomorphology (other methods such as MCFC or genetic analysis may be used in unclear cases), and clinical neurological examination, and CNS imaging in case of neurological clinical findings. Physical examination, imaging, or histologic examination of a tissue biopsy should be used for the evaluation of non-CNS EM disease.

- Definition of TF:
  - *"Failure to achieve CR at a clearly predefined time point (EOI and EOC or other time points during intensification) should be considered as a TF event."*
  - *"There was progress toward a consensus that a TF event is to be defined no earlier than the EOC, because this would allow a patient not achieving CR by EOI to be offered a consolidation therapy with agents not given during induction in an effort to overcome blast resistance and potentially achieve CR. If such a patient still does not achieve CR after this risk-adapted consolidation phase, this could reasonably define a TF event."*

14. Are there any risk factors for MRD to be detectable?

Minimal residual disease has been defined as the single most important factor to predict relapse in ALL. The Italian Association of Pediatric Hematology and Oncology (AIEOP)-BFM study, confirmed the prognostic value of PCR-MRD in its multivariate analysis but also found that WBC count, TEL/AML1 status, and DNA index retain independent significant impact on the hazard of relapse.[12] However, in most studies, MRD detectability overtakes the initial risk stratification and other prognostic factors in children with B-ALL. In a recent meta-analysis, it was shown that irrespective of the method used for detection, cutoff used (0.01 or 0.001%), the initial cytogenetics or phenotype of the child, or the time point of detection, a detectable MRD is associated with an increased risk of relapse.[13]

15. What are the options for a B-ALL with detectable MRD following induction?

The UK-ALL 2003 trial tested whether, clinical standard and intermediate-risk ALL who have persistent MRD at the EOI therapy benefit from augmented postremission therapy. They found a significantly improved EFS rate, though there were increased toxicity to methotrexate and L-asparaginase in the augmented arm. Though there was no significant improvement in OS, trends were toward improved survival.[14] The classification of high-risk patients using MRD assessment differs with different consortiums. The UK-ALL group defined MRD high risk as those with an MRD level of 0.01% or higher at day 29 of induction. This identifies almost 40–60% of the entire cohort with an intermediate prognosis compared with a smaller high-risk group (<10%) associated with a much higher risk of relapse identified by other study groups (MRD > 1% at day 42 in the St Jude study or >0.05% at week 12 in the AIEOP-BFM study).[14] Hence, in low–middle-income countries, where chances of cure following relapse are low, it is probably better to augment chemotherapy postinduction, along with providing good supportive care for the toxicities.

CASE *(Continued)*

As his MRD was detectable following induction, he was switched to the high-risk consolidation arm of the ICiCLe protocol. This includes cyclophosphamide, cytarabine, 6MP, dexamethasone, L-asparaginase, and vincristine (similar to augmented BFM consolidation block). Postconsolidation, BM aspirate revealed 2% blasts, while FCM revealed 2.6% blasts which were CD34+, Cd10+, CD19+, CD81+ (dim), CD58+, and negative for CD38, CD20, HLA DR, CD123, CD73, CD44, and CD304. This was like the LAIP at the beginning of treatment.

16. What are the options for a B-ALL with detectable MRD after consolidation?

As defined in the AIEOP-BFM 2000 study, the incidence of relapse in patients with detectable MRD postinduction depends on MRD postconsolidation. Patients with high MRD levels after induction but no detectable MRD after consolidation had a 5-year cumulative incidence of relapse of 20.7%, compared with 40.7% in patients with MRD still positive but at a level <10^{-3} after consolidation.[12] Hence, it is reasonable to assume that patients with a poor MRD response after 2 months of therapy, despite rather favorable risk criteria may benefit from treatment intensification, like HSCT, to compensate for the MRD-derived high relapse risk. The UK-ALL group also found that persistent MRD following augmented consolidation therapy indicates a degree of chemotherapy refractoriness that might not overcome by further dose intensification of standard chemotherapy drugs. Therefore, in their current trial, UK-ALL 2011, patients who have persistent high-level MRD (>0.5%) after augmented consolidation therapy are candidates for treatment with novel agents followed by a first remission allogeneic transplant.[14]

17. Is there any utility of doing an MRD analysis earlier (day 15/day 19) in B-ALL?

The St Judes Total Therapy 15 study, conducted a day 19 MRD analysis and found that the 10-year EFS was significantly inferior for patients with MRD ≥ 1% on day 19 compared with that of patients having lower MRD levels: 69.2 versus 95.5% for the provisional low-risk group and 65.1 versus 82.9% for the provisional SR group. For the provisional low-risk patients, an MRD level of <1% on day 19 predicted a superior outcome, regardless of the MRD level on day 46, while in provisional SR patients with MRD < 1% on day 19, persistent MRD on day 46 tended to have an inferior 10-year EFS compared with those having a detectable MRD (72.7 vs. 84.0%, $p = 0.06$) after receiving the same postremission treatment for SR ALL.[15]

18. What is the utility of sequential MRD assessment?

It is debatable whether a patient who goes into MRD-negative status after induction requires sequential MRD assessment. The St Jude Total Therapy 15 study was the first clinical trial to use MRD levels prospectively during and after remission induction therapy to guide risk-directed treatment. MRD levels were measured on days 19 and 46 of induction, and on week 7 of continuation treatment. Additional MRD determinations were made on weeks 17, 48, and 120 (end of therapy). Among patients attaining MRD-negative status after remission induction, MRD reemerged in 4 of 382 studied on week 7, 1 of 448 on week 17, and 1 of 437 on week 48; all but 1 of these 6 patients died despite additional treatment. By contrast, relapse occurred in only 2 of the 11 patients who had decreasing MRD levels between the EOI and week 7 of continuation therapy and were treated with chemotherapy alone. Hence, sequential MRD monitoring after remission induction is warranted for patients with detectable MRD. In case of decreasing MRD, we may consider to treat these children with chemotherapy alone protocols (especially if MRD is detected at low levels).[15]

CASE (Continued)

As per ICiCLe, children who have MRD negativity following B-ALL induction, are not tested for MRD again. We also do not do an early assessment of MRD, though this is the first risk adapted multicenter trial for pediatric ALL in India and may undergo modifications subsequently.

19. If resource was not a constraint, is this child an ideal case for immunotherapy? What is the evidence for immunotherapy?

Immunotherapy (blinatumomab, inotuzumab, and tisagenlecleucel) has a well-established role in relapsed and refractory ALL. All three treatments are most effective in patients with relatively low burden of disease and hence there is growing interest in these strategies for preventing relapse in MRD-positive patients.

- *Blinatumomab:* This is a bispecific T-cell engager targeting CD 19 antigen on B cells. It is more effective in patients with lower burden of disease, making it a particularly promising agent for the treatment of MRD. Adult trials have proven an improvement in both EFS and OS in patients receiving blinatumomab for MRD eradication. MRD became a modifiable risk factor due to immunotherapy. The impact of immunotherapeutic clearance of MRD on survival is greatest when applied early in the disease course. Whether HSCT is required after blinatumomab is an open question as 25% of patients who achieved MRD negativity and did not receive any further therapy, remained in continuous CR after a median follow up of 24 months.[16] The risk of transplant needs to be carefully weighed when making this decision. The COG has tested blinatumomab in pediatric ALL at first relapse[17] and is currently using blinatumomab in frontline therapy of ALL.
- *Inotuzumab:* Its role in relapsed and refractory ALL has been studied, leading to MRD eradication in 25–100% of patients.[18] It is currently being studied as frontline treatment in the latest COG trials.
- *Chimeric antigen receptor (CAR) T cells:* It is a form of adoptive immunotherapy which relies on the transfer of genetically modified effector cells to elicit an antileukemic immune response and therefore have the potential to persist in vivo, offering long-term disease control. The impact of various CAR constructs on MRD has been studied (mostly in the relapsed and refractory setting), with MRD negativity being achieved in 60–100% of patients.[18]

Cytokine release syndrome (CRS) and neurologic events occur less frequently when immunotherapy is used for MRD than in patients with relapsed/refractory disease, likely due to the decreased disease burden.[18]

20. In the era of immunotherapy, what are the challenges in detection of MRD?

T-cell mediated anti-CD19 therapy depletes normal and abnormal CD19 expressing B cells. The pattern of recovery differs from recovery post more traditional cytotoxic therapy. Moreover, there may be a selection of CD19 negative/CD22 positive clones and patients can relapse with CD19 positive or CD19 negative disease. In era of targeted therapy, single gating reagent may not be sufficient to identify normal population. Pattern of normal may change. Hence, we may need to use alternate blast antigen like CD34 or CD10/SSC or use alternate expression of B cells also to find blasts.

CASE *(Continued)*

Child's parents belonged to a lower socioeconomic strata and could not afford immunotherapy at this stage. Through government aid and assistance with nongovernmental organizations we were able to generate enough funds for chemotherapy and a BM transplant.

21. What are factors to be kept in mind prior to transplant in a child with B-ALL?

1. Is it important to achieve an MRD-negative status prior to transplant? If yes, what salvage regimens should we use?

Presence of MRD prior to transplant predicts relapse and poor survival. It was shown that there is no impact on EFS if MRD is negative or low, but high/very high MRD pretransplant is associated with almost 40% risk of relapse. Post-transplant detectable MRD on day +180 and day +365 are associated with inferior survival rates as well and are considered to have a greater impact on survival than pretransplant MRD. If at all a patient has detectable MRD pretransplant and undergoes HSCT, it is important to see if these patients achieve a negative or low-MRD status post-transplant, otherwise survival is dismal.[6] Hence, all efforts should be made to bring MRD to a low/undetectable state (preferably prior to transplant).

2. What are the indications for transplant in pediatric ALL?

The indications for transplant in pediatric ALL have evolved over time. According to the European Bone Marrow Transplant (EBMT) group, none of the baseline cytogenetic abnormalities warrants transplant in CR1. But, indications for transplant in CR1 may be guided by MRD. There is an "in general consensus" that detectable MRD following consolidation warrants a BM transplant. All T-ALL patients, and very early/early relapse warrants a transplant in CR2, and all cases of CR3 warrant a transplant provided they go into CR and have good performance status.[19]

CASE *(Continued)*

As the MRD was detectable, and had in fact increased, we switched the child to the AIEOP-BFM high-risk protocol, starting from the methotrexate blocks. He received three blocks followed by two reinductions. MRD at the end of reinduction 2 was not detectable (<0.01%) and the child was taken up for a 6/6 matched sibling donor (MSD) transplant.

3. **Describe HSCT in ALL.**
i. **What is the preferred conditioning regimen?**
   Most children receive a myeloablative conditioning regimen. This consists of total body irradiation (TBI) with etoposide or cyclophosphamide. If <4 years, busulfan (or treosulfan) + fludarabine ± Thiotepa.[19] The famous FORUM trial compared TBI + etoposide with chemoconditioning using busulfan/treosulfan + fludarabine + thiotepa. They found an improvement in OS and EFS with decreased relapse rates in patients receiving TBI. They also found an increase in TRM with chemoconditioning regimens with similar rates of acute graft versus host disease (aGVHD).[20]
ii. **What is the donor preference?**
   An MSD is the best donor available for transplant as they lead to quicker engraftment, faster immune reconstitution, less severe infections, and less GVHD. A matched unrelated donor (MUD) has similar outcomes to MSD. But it is not clearly proven if a mismatched cord blood or a haploidentical donor (T-cell depleted or with use of post-transplant cyclophosphamide), can result in good outcomes in children with ALL.[19] Younger donors are preferred with similar cytomegalovirus (CMV) status. If the recipient is a male, the EBMT recommends a male donor as compared to a female donor and as for source of stem cell, BM is preferred, however peripheral blood is more convenient and is also a safe option.[19]

CASE *(Continued)*

We used TBI (12 Gy/6# with cranial boost of 2 Gy) and etoposide as the conditioning regimen. He engrafted on day +10. His transplant was complicated by febrile neutropenia and mucositis. He was discharged on day +18. He is in remission 18 months following transplant. His post-transplant course was complicated by acute and chronic GVHD (cGVHD) (including skin and lung). He received steroids and ruxolitinib and is recovering from cGVHD.

■ REFERENCES

1. Parihar M, Singh MK, Islam R, Saha D, Mishra DK, Saha V, et al. A triple-probe FISH screening strategy for risk-stratified therapy of acute lymphoblastic leukaemia in low-resource settings. Pediatr Blood Cancer. 2018;65(12):e27366.
2. Campana D. Minimal residual disease in acute lymphoblastic leukemia. Semin Hematol. 2009;46(1):100-6.
3. Grimwade D, Freeman SD. Defining minimal residual disease in acute myeloid leukemia: Which platforms are ready for "prime time"? Blood. 2014;124(23):3345-55.
4. Starza ID, Chiaretti S, De Propris MS, Elia L, Cavalli M, De Novi LA, et al. Minimal residual disease in acute lymphoblastic leukemia: Technical and clinical advances. Front Oncol. 2019;9:726.
5. Kerst G, Kreyenberg H, Roth C, Well C, Dietz K, Coustan-Smith E, et al. Concurrent detection of minimal residual disease (MRD) in childhood acute lymphoblastic leukaemia by flow cytometry and real-time PCR. Br J Haematol. 2005;128(6):774-82.
6. Bader P, Salzmann-Manrique E, Balduzzi A, Dalle JH, Woolfrey AE, Bar M, et al. More precisely defining risk peri-HCT in pediatric ALL: Pre- vs post-MRD measures, serial positivity, and risk modeling. Blood Adv. 2019;3(21):3393-405.

7. Wood B, Wu D, Crossley B, Dai Y, Williamson D, Gawad C, et al. Measurable residual disease detection by high-throughput sequencing improves risk stratification for pediatric B-ALL. Blood. 2018;131(12):1350-9.
8. Döhner H, Estey E, Grimwade D, Amadori S, Appelbaum FR, Büchner T, et al. Diagnosis and management of AML in adults: 2017 ELN recommendations from an international expert panel. Blood. 2017;129(4):424-47.
9. Enshaei A, Vora A, Harrison CJ, Moppett J, Moorman AV. Defining low-risk high hyperdiploidy in patients with paediatric acute lymphoblastic leukaemia: a retrospective analysis of data from the UKALL97/99 and UKALL2003 clinical trials. Lancet Haematol. 2021;8(11):e828-39.
10. Tran TH, Loh ML. Ph-like acute lymphoblastic leukemia. Hematology. 2016;2016(1):561-6.
11. Buchmann S, Schrappe M, Baruchel A, Biondi A, Borowitz M, Campbell M, et al. Remission, treatment failure, and relapse in pediatric ALL: an international consensus of the Ponte-di-Legno Consortium. Blood. 2022;139(12):1785-93.
12. Conter V, Bartram CR, Valsecchi MG, Schrauder A, Panzer-Grümayer R, Möricke A, et al. Molecular response to treatment redefines all prognostic factors in children and adolescents with B-cell precursor acute lymphoblastic leukemia: results in 3184 patients of the AIEOP-BFM ALL 2000 study. Blood. 2010;115(16):3206-14.
13. Berry DA, Zhou S, Higley H, Mukundan L, Fu S, Reaman GH, et al. Association of minimal residual disease with clinical outcome in pediatric and adult acute lymphoblastic leukemia: a meta-analysis. JAMA Oncol. 2017;3(7):e170580.
14. Vora A, Goulden N, Mitchell C, Hancock J, Hough R, Rowntree C, et al. Augmented post-remission therapy for a minimal residual disease-defined high-risk subgroup of children and young people with clinical standard-risk and intermediate-risk acute lymphoblastic leukaemia (UKALL 2003): A randomised controlled trial. Lancet Oncol. 2014;15(8):809-18.
15. Pui CH, Pei D, Coustan-Smith E, Jeha S, Cheng C, Bowman WP, et al. Clinical utility of sequential minimal residual disease measurements in the context of risk-based therapy in childhood acute lymphoblastic leukaemia: a prospective study. Lancet Oncol. 2015;16(4):465-74.
16. Gökbuget N, Dombret H, Bonifacio M, Reichle A, Graux C, Faul C, et al. Blinatumomab for minimal residual disease in adults with B-cell precursor acute lymphoblastic leukemia. Blood. 2018;131(14):1522-31.
17. Brown PA, Ji L, Xu X, Devidas M, Hogan L, Borowitz MJ, et al. A randomized phase 3 trial of blinatumomab vs. chemotherapy as post-reinduction therapy in high and intermediate risk (HR/IR) first relapse of B-acute lymphoblastic leukemia (B-ALL) in children and adolescents/young adults (AYAs) demonstrates superior efficacy and tolerability of blinatumomab: a report from children's oncology group study AALL1331. Blood. 2019;134(Supplement_2):LBA-1.
18. Jasinski S, De Los Reyes FA, Yametti GC, Pierro J, Raetz E, Carroll WL. Immunotherapy in pediatric B-cell acute lymphoblastic leukemia: advances and ongoing challenges. Pediatr Drugs. 2020;22(5):485-99.
19. Carreras E, Dufour C, Mohty M, Kröger N (Eds). The EBMT Handbook: Hematopoietic Stem Cell Transplantation and Cellular Therapies, 7th edition. New York: Springer Cham; 2018.
20. Peters C, Dalle JH, Locatelli F, Poetschger U, Sedlacek P, Buechner J, et al. Total body irradiation or chemotherapy conditioning in childhood ALL: A multinational, randomized, noninferiority phase III study. J Clin Oncol. 2021;39(4):295-307.

EXPERT OPINION

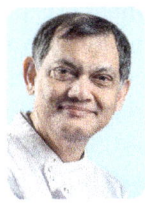

Vaskar Saha MBBS DCH MD FRCP FRCPath PhD
Head of Pediatric Hematology and Oncology at Tata Medical Center and
Director of the Tata Translational Cancer Research Centre, Kolkata
Professor of Pediatric Oncology at the University of Manchester, United Kingdom

1. Despite being a SR ALL, with hyperdiploidy (good risk cytogenetics), our child had persistent MRD positivity? What do you think were the causes for this?

High hyperdiploidy is defined as an increase in the modal chromosome number in leukemic blasts from 46 to between 51 and 67. The nonrandom gains most often affect X, 4, 6, 10, 14, 17, 18, and 21. In particular trisomies of +4, +6, +10, +17, and +18 are associated with good outcomes for children with B-cell precursor (BCP) ALL on current protocols. The best outcomes have been reported for patients with +17 and +18 or either +17 or +18 but no +5 or +20. Though this patient had an atypical high hyperdiploid karyotype, there were no additional poor risk features.

Depending on the induction protocol, around 40% of patients with high hyperdiploid BCP-ALL can have MRD levels of >0.01% at the EOI. The majority will clear MRD at the EOC. In this patient, the EOI MRD level was 0.018%, so just above the cutoff. This is not unusual. The EOC MRD was reported to be 2.6%. This sudden rise in MRD is quite unusual. At this level, the child has moved from being in CR to not in CR, bringing into question the reliability of the MRD. The report as presented simply states that the cells detected were CD34+, CD10+, CD19+, CD81+ (dim), and CD58+. FCM-based MRD is dependent on (1) the time of the aspirate—this should be ideally taken as the marrow is recovering prior to the flurry of regenerating hematogones, (2) obtaining sufficient cells, ideally over 4 million, and (3) operator expertise in distinguishing hematogones from malignant blasts.

Regenerating hematogones will express CD34, CD10, CD19, and CD58 as they progress from immaturity to maturity. Pre-B1 cells express dim CD45, CD34, CD19, and CD10 while pre-B2 cells have brighter CD45, CD19, and CD10 and partial CD20 but lack CD34. Pre-B1 and pre-B2 cells appear broadly distributed on CD20–CD10 and CD34–CD10 dot plots, while they form tight overlapping clusters. Mature B cells have negative to dim expression of CD10 and bright CD20. The most stable markers are reported to be CD73, CD44, and CD38, not included in this panel. CD58 is not considered to be a reliable marker for MRD evaluation. Normal hematogones do not have asynchronous expression of early and late antigens. To distinguish between these normal and the abnormal cells, one first needs to consider the comparative expression of these markers in normal and malignant cells. Evaluate the clusters of cells expressing the markers to identify and quantify the leukemic blast population.

In hindsight then, the EOI marrow aspirate was performed on time in an early regenerating marrow and the MRD report is possibly correct for this time point. With rapid disease clearance in consolidation, MRD assessment was possibly then done on a fully regenerated marrow and erroneously reported as positive. In such cases it is helpful to examine the marrow aspirate for cellularity and reconstitution. BFM high-risk blocks are intensively myelosuppressive with late marrow regeneration. The BFM recommends the use of granulocyte colony-stimulating factor (G-CSF) during these blocks, and this possibly could contribute to MRD negativity by FCM-based MRD.

2. Is it possible that the presence of EM disease should have warranted anthracyclines during induction?

As described in the report this child had multiple large cervical lymph nodes (largest 2 cm in size), with liver and spleen palpable 2 and 3 cm (nonbulky). All these are within expected presentations of BCP-ALL and are not considered independent risk factors requiring additional therapy.

3. How do you manage unusual sites/unusual presentations in ALL-like bony lesions, hypercalcemia, etc.?

These patients are usually managed on a case-by-case basis by the multidisciplinary team. Broadly, we do not consider electrolyte imbalances to be a risk factor. Unusual EM sites like bone or skin are rare. As there is no real consensus on how these patients should be treated, we usually treat these patients as high-risk, unless preexisting morbidity precludes this approach.

4. In a resource-limited setting, considering the morbidity of transplant and the relative ease to procure some inhibitors, should we test for Ph-like ALL in all cases of ALL upfront or should we restrict it to those patients with MRD positivity or other high-risk clinical features?

The cost of relapse is far more than the tests. High hyperdiploid ALL cells may rarely contain *TCF3::PBX1*, *BCR::ABL1*, *ETV6::RUNX1*, *KMT2A* rearrangements as well fusions typical of Ph-like ALL. Ph-like ALL can be identified in around 14% of SR ALL and associated with inferior EFS. Around 60% of Ph-like ALL have upregulated CRLF2, often because of a translocation and activation of the JAK-STAT pathway. At our center, all diagnostic samples are screened for CRLF2 expression by FCM. In patients whose blasts express CRLF2, we investigate for additional changes, e.g., *P2RY8::CRLF2* or *IGH::CRLF2* fusions. If present, we treat these patients as high risk. As these patients often have activation of the JAK-STAT pathway, they could potentially benefit as well from a JAK inhibitor, e.g., ruxolitinib. Ruxolitinib is expensive, toxic, and the benefits are as yet undetermined. For patients with a suboptimal response to treatment (EOI MRD > 1% or persistent MRD positivity at EOC), as in this case, we screen by FISH for *ABL1*, *ABL2*, and *PDGFR-α* rearrangements, as patients with fusions of these genes potentially benefit from adjuvant imatinib or dasatinib treatment. The proportion of Ph-like patients with ABL-class rearrangements though are fewer than those with aberrations in JAK-STAT signaling. Of late diagnostic samples from patients with suboptimal response are also being sequenced.

5. Is immunotherapy warranted upfront in children with MRD positivity postinduction/consolidation? Does the benefit outweigh cost?

At our center, we have a donor program with Amgen providing free access to blinatumomab. All BCP-ALL patients with suboptimal response to therapy are offered blinatumomab and an allogeneic stem cell transplant (allo-SCT). As illustrated in this case and previously reported by us, while almost half of the eligible patients cannot afford allo-SCT they can receive blinatumomab. Achieving low/negative MRD prior to allo-SCT significantly decreases relapse post-SCT. Blinatumomab has also been shown to more effective than chemotherapy in decreasing MRD levels as well as decreasing relapse. So, immunotherapy prior to allo-SCT is beneficial. Most patients at our center have demonstrated a decrease/negativity in MRD after receiving blinatumomab. Further follow-up will be required to see if those who were not transplanted maintain remission.

6. Does transplant in MRD-positive patients improve survival, or should we continue with chemotherapy?

This depends on whether the patient is being treated as frontline or relapse, the time of relapse, immunophenotype, and cytogenetics. In BCP-ALL, MRD of <10 after the first phase of therapy (induction) is associated with the best outcomes in both *de novo* and relapsed ALL. These patients do not normally require a transplant. In the preimmunotherapy era MRD of $\geq 10^{-1}$ at the EOI or persistent of MRD beyond consolidation are associated with higher recurrence rates. For T-ALL, those with detectable MRD at the EOI but negative at the EOC have excellent outcomes.

Does transplanting those with persistent MRD improve outcomes? Patients proceeding to allo-SCT, with MRD of 10^{-3} or lower prior to SCT have the best outcomes. This is perhaps best achieved in patients with persistent MRD with the aid of immunotherapy. The outcomes of patients with persistent or high MRD on frontline therapy who are transplanted does not differ significantly from patients who continue with chemotherapy. In the patients who were transplanted, high-risk relapse and EOI MRD $\geq 10^{-4}$, disease-free survival of 22% was reported; the numbers not transplanted were too few to comment. In very high-risk cytogenetic subtypes, e.g. Ph+ALL, potentially transplant in CR1 may be beneficial, though this benefit does not seem to translate to patients with a *KMT2A* rearrangement. Current evidence suggests a benefit for transplant in late medullary relapse BCP-ALL, but evidence of benefit of this strategy in other groups is equivocal.

7. Would you have managed this child differently?

At our center, we would have treated this patient as SR, based on the criteria provided. All patients who have a MRD of $\geq 10^{-4}$ are also tracked using PCR for Ig/TR rearrangements. We have previously reported the higher sensitivity and specificity of the PCR-based assay. Faced with a discordance between PCR and FCM, we would have proceeded to high-dose methotrexate and reassessed the marrow MRD again at this time point. Positivity by FCM but negative by PCR does occur and may indicate that the clones identified by the two techniques are different. In any case we would extend the FISH screen for such patients, and lately we also screen for *IKZF1* deletions and additional copy number changes that identify *IKZF1*^{plus}. Rarely a duplicated hypodiploid clone may mimic high hyperdiploidy. In such cases as this is due to duplication of a hypodiploid clone, two or four copies are seen of each chromosome and not trisomies as well as loss of heterozygosity. Most hypodiploid cases also have a mutated *TP53* gene. When we suspect such a case, we perform additional tests for copy number alterations, loss of heterozygosity, and *TP53* mutations.

The BFM high-risk arm is associated with TRM of around 10% in the west and have not shown better outcomes in high-risk patients compared to other less intensive protocols, so we do not use this in patients with persistent MRD. Increasingly we now perform drug profiling on banked diagnostic samples to identify drugs likely to be effective and treat patients accordingly. After this therapy patients are offered blinatumomab and allo-SCT.

CHAPTER 2

Acute Lymphoblastic Leukemia Relapse

Padma Sagarika Karri, Rachna Seth

CASE VIGNETTE

A 10-year-old boy, B-acute lymphoblastic leukemia (ALL) survivor, presents with complaints of right-sided painless scrotal swelling for 1 week, 4 months after the completion of treatment for his primary disease. He was diagnosed with standard-risk B-ALL at the age of 7 years, was treated on Indian Childhood Collaborative Leukemia (ICiCLE) standard risk B-ALL protocol, and bone marrow (BM) 1-month post-treatment completion was in morphological remission. He had no associated history of fever, progressive pallor, bleeding manifestations, headache, vomiting, seizures, or focal neurological deficits. On examination, right scrotal swelling was noted with no distinct increase in testis size. He had no significant lymphadenopathy or hepatosplenomegaly. Neurological examination did not reveal any focal neurological deficits. Ultrasound (USG) scrotum was done in suspicion of testicular relapse which showed mildly increased vascularity of the right testis with a small 6 mm hypoechoic focal lesion in the posterior half—possible testicular relapse of ALL. Cytology of fine needle aspirate from the right testis showed numerous blasts, consistent with leukemic infiltration **(Figs. 1A to F)**. Peripheral smear showed 2% blasts, and BM aspirate smear showed 40% blasts **(Figs. 2A to C)**. BM aspirate flow cytometry (FCM) showed 35% CD45 negative to dim positive blasts which are immunopositive for CD19, CD10, CD81, human leukocyte antigen (HLA)-DR, CD58, CD38 and negative for CD34 and CD20: B-ALL relapse. Cerebrospinal fluid (CSF) examination showed no blasts.

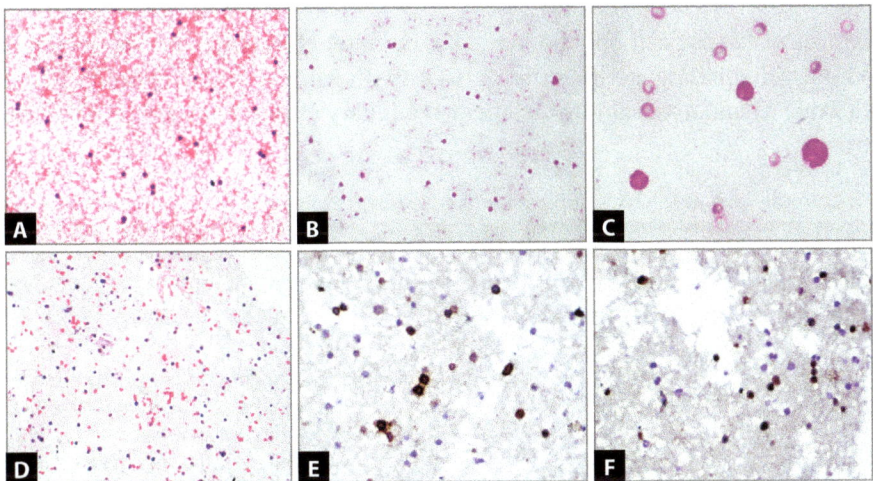

Figs. 1A to F: Ultrasound-guided testicular fine needle aspirate cytology (FNAC)—Papanicolaou and May-Grunwald Giemsa stained slides show scattered blasts (A and B, 20x), with opened-up chromatin and conspicuous nucleoli (C, 40x). Cell block shows similar cells (D, 20x) which are positive for CD79a (E, 40x) and Tdt (F, 40x).
Courtesy: Dr Anchal Kakkar, Department of Pathology, AIIMS, New Delhi.

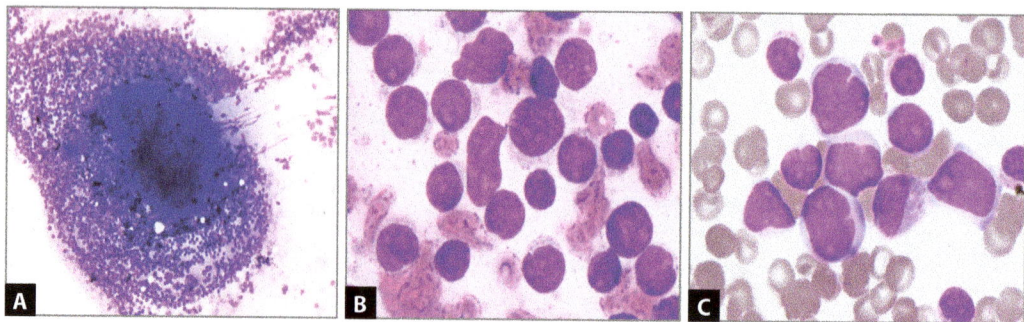

Figs. 2A to C: Bone marrow aspirate cytology shows infiltration by lymphoblasts (A, 20x) with high nuclear: cytoplasmic ratio, some with prominent nucleoli (B, 100x). Peripheral blood film shows lymphoblasts (C, 100x).
Courtesy: Dr Smeeta Gajendra, Department of Laboratory Oncology, BRA-IRCH, AIIMS, New Delhi.

1. What is the incidence of relapse in ALL? What features at the primary diagnosis of ALL are associated with a higher risk of relapse?

With current treatment strategies, the incidence of relapse in ALL ranges between 10 and 15%.[1] BM relapse is the principal form, central nervous system (CNS) relapse accounts for <10% and the incidence of testicular relapse has reduced to <2% with modern therapy. The majority of relapses occur while on treatment or within 2 years of treatment completion.[2] Age <1 year and ≥10 years, initial total leucocyte count ≥50,000/µL, poor prednisolone response, failure of induction therapy, end-of-induction minimal residual disease (MRD) ≥0.01%, high-risk cytogenetics, early precursor T-cell ALL are the features at primary diagnosis that are associated with a higher risk of relapse.

2. How is ALL relapse defined? What are the recent modifications as per the international consensus of the Ponte-di-Legno Consortium?

The diagnosis of relapse can only be made if complete remission (CR) has been previously achieved. Provided below are the criteria used to diagnose acute lymphoblastic leukemia relapse, **(Table 1)** and ascertain involvement-medullary **(Table 2)** as well as extramedullary **(Table 3)**.

TABLE 1: Currently used acute lymphoblastic leukemia relapse criteria.[3]

Localization	Definition/Threshold	Method
Isolated BM	≥25% blasts in BM without EM involvement	Cytomorphology of BM aspirate
Combined	≥5% blasts in BM and ≥1 EM site involvement	Cytomorphology of BM aspirate *and* Imaging and biopsy of the EM site (in the setting of combined relapse with BM involvement, biopsy of the EM site is not necessary if imaging features are compatible with leukemic infiltration)

Contd...

Contd...

Localization	Definition/Threshold	Method
Isolated CNS	>5/μL nucleated cells in CSF and evidence of blasts *or* Intracranial mass	Cytomorphology of CSF *or* Imaging *and* biopsy of the intracranial mass lesion
Isolated testicular	Uni- or bilateral testicular enlargement with leukemic infiltration confirmed by biopsy or fine needle aspiration cytology	Clinical examination *and* imaging *and* biopsy
Isolated EM site (others)		Imaging *and* biopsy

(BM: bone marrow; CNS: central nervous system; CSF: cerebrospinal fluid; EM: extramedullary)

Consensus criteria for ALL relapse developed by the Ponte-di-Legno Consortium.[4]

i. BM:

TABLE 2: Consensus criteria for bone marrow (BM) relapse definition in pediatric acute lymphoblastic leukemia.

MRD unavailable				MRD available			
BM1		BM2 (≥1 week later)		BM1		BM2 (≥1 week later)	
Cytomorphology	Others	Cytomorphology	MRD	Others	MRD
M3	Not necessary to define relapse	Not necessary to define relapse	≥25%	Not necessary to define relapse	Not necessary to define relapse
M2	One other test with ≥1% blasts	Not necessary to define relapse	5 to <25%	One other test with ≥1% blasts	Not necessary to define relapse
	None	M2		None	Two tests with ≥1% blasts
M1	Two other tests with ≥1% blasts	Not necessary to define relapse	1 to <5%	Two other tests with ≥1% blasts	Not necessary to define relapse
M3: ≥25% blasts M2: ≥5% and <25% blasts M1: <5% blasts				Zero or one other test with ≥1% blasts	Two tests with ≥1% blasts
Other tests—FISH/karyotype/PCR demonstrating leukemia-specific marker				Other tests—FCM/PCR/NGS-based MRD or FISH/karyotype/PCR demonstrating leukemia-specific marker or M2/M3 morphology	

(FISH: fluorescence in situ hybridization; FCM: flow cytometry; MRD: minimal residual disease; NGS: next-generation sequencing; PCR: polymerase chain reaction)

ii. *CNS and other extramedullary (EM) sites:*

TABLE 3: Consensus criteria for central nervous system (CNS) and other extramedullary (EM) relapse definition in pediatric acute lymphoblastic leukemia.

CNS relapse				
CSF1	CSF2 (≥1 week later)			
Cytomorphology	Cytomorphology	Others		Other EM sites
CNS3 (defined by cytomorphology, imaging, or biopsy)	Not necessary to define relapse	Not necessary to define relapse		• EM tumor burden confirmed by imaging and/or biopsy • Positive biopsy is needed to define relapse if it is the only potential relapse site • Imaging could be diagnostic if combined with other sites
CNS2	CNS2	One other positive test (FCM-MRD, FISH, indirect nuclear terminal deoxynucleotidyl transferase immunofluorescence assay)		
CNS2: <5 leucocytes/μL in CSF with detectable blasts in a centrifuged sample CNS3: ≥5 leucocytes/μL in CSF with identifiable blasts *or* Presence of intracranial mass/cranial nerve palsy with leukemic cells in CSF				
(CSF: cerebrospinal fluid; FCM: flow cytometry; FISH: fluorescence in situ hybridization; MRD: minimal residual disease)				

iii. *Combined relapse:*
Any BM relapse combined with any non-BM relapse (with each defined above).

3. What is the risk stratification scheme used for ALL relapses? What is the risk group of the ALL relapse in the aforementioned case?

The major risk factors for outcome following first relapse include (1) the time from primary diagnosis to relapse (lesser duration is worse) **(Table 4)**, (2) site of relapse [isolated BM is worse than combined or isolated extramedullary (IEM)], (3) immunophenotype (T cell is worse), and (4) MRD response to reinduction therapy. Based on these criteria, various groups have devised their risk stratification schemes **(Table 5)**.

TABLE 4: Definition of the time point of relapse.

Time point	After primary diagnosis		After completion of primary therapy
Late			≥6 months
	<18 months and ≥6 months (e.g., after discontinuation of therapy or after therapy B-NHL)		
Early	≥18 months	and	<6 months
Very early	<18 months	and	<6 months
(B-NHL: B-cell non-Hodgkin lymphoma)			

TABLE 5: Risk stratification scheme for first relapse.[1]

Risk status	Definition		
	BFM group, Western Europe[5]	Cancer Research UK Children's Cancer Group, United Kingdom[6]	Children's Oncology Group, North America[7]
Low/Standard	S1 • Late IEM relapse	• Late IEM relapse	• Late B-ALL marrow, end-block 1 MRD <0.1% • Late IEM, end-block 1 MRD <0.1%
Intermediate	S2 • Very early and early IEM relapses • Late B-ALL isolated marrow relapses • Early/late B-ALL combined relapses	• Early IEM relapse • Late isolated B-ALL marrow relapse • Early/late combined B-ALL marrow relapse	• Late B-ALL marrow, end-block 1 MRD ≥0.1% • Late IEM, end-block 1 MRD ≥0.1%
High	S3 and S4 • Very early and early B-ALL marrow relapses • Very early B-ALL combined relapses • T-ALL marrow relapses (regardless of timing)	• Very early IEM relapse • B-ALL early isolated marrow relapse • B-ALL very early marrow or combined relapse • T-ALL marrow or combined relapse, any timing	• Early B-ALL marrow • Early IEM • T-ALL relapse, any site and timing

(ALL: acute lymphoblastic leukemia; BFM: Berlin–Frankfurt–Münster; IEM: isolated extramedullary; MRD: minimal residual disease)
Source: Hunger SP, Raetz EA. How I treat relapsed acute lymphoblastic leukemia in the pediatric population. Blood. 2020;136(16):1803-12.

At our institute we use adapted UK ALL R3 **(Table 6 and Fig. 3)** and ALL REZ BFM 2002 **(Table 7 and Fig. 4)** protocols to treat first relapse of ALL. ALL REZ BFM 2002 is less preferred as the induction phase chemotherapy involves administration of high-dose methotrexate, which is not feasible timely due to resource constraints for in-patient care.

TABLE 6: Risk stratification according to UK ALL R3 trial.

	Non-T-cell			T-cell		
	Isolated extramedullary	Combined	Isolated marrow	Isolated extramedullary	Combined	Isolated marrow
Very early	High	High	High	High	High	High
Early	Intermediate	Intermediate	High	Intermediate	High	High
Late	Standard	Intermediate	Intermediate	Standard	High	High

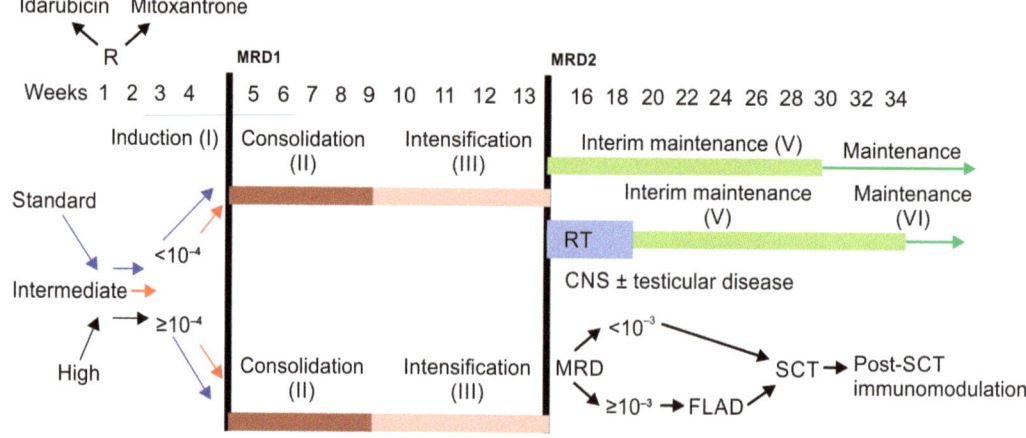

Fig. 3: Management scheme according to UK ALL R3 trial.
(CNS: central nervous system; FLAD: fludarabine, cytarabine and liposomal daunorubicin; MRD: minimal residual disease; SCT: stem cell transplant)
Adapted from: UK ALL R3 trial protocol.

TABLE 7: Risk groups (S1–S4) according to ALL REZ BFM 2002 trial.

	Non-T-cell			T-cell		
	Isolated extramedullary	Combined	Isolated marrow	Isolated extramedullary	Combined	Isolated marrow
Very early	S2	S4	S4	S2	S4	S4
Early	S2	S2	S3	S2	S4	S4
Late	S1	S2	S2	S1	S4	S4

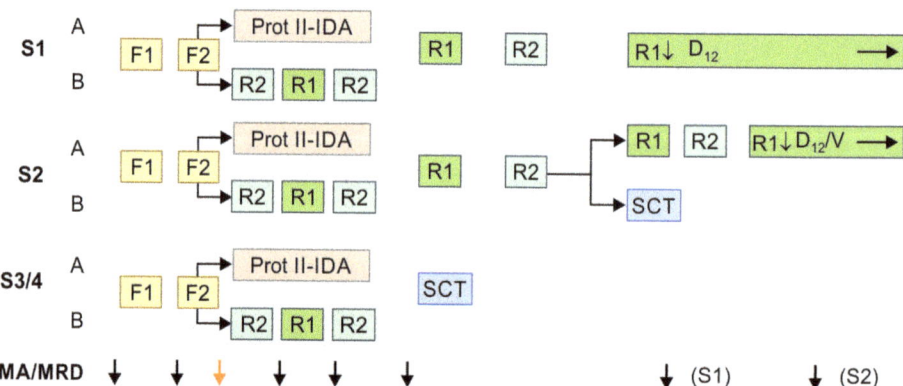

Fig. 4: Management scheme according to ALL REZ BFM 2002.
(BMA: bone marrow aspiration; IDA: idarubicin; MRD: minimal residual disease; SCT: stem cell transplant)
Adapted from: ALL REZ BFM 2002 trial protocol.

In the aforementioned case, the child presented with relapse in the BM and testis <6 months after the primary treatment completion and >18 months after primary diagnosis, therefore this is early combined BM and testicular relapse. He belongs to the intermediate-risk group according to the UK ALL R3 protocol and the S2 strategic group according to the ALL REZ BFM 2002 protocol.

4. What are the hypotheses postulated in relation to the biology of relapse?

Leukemic blasts at relapse are more drug-resistant than blasts at primary diagnosis.[8] Studies have concluded that in the majority of patients, the cells responsible for relapse are ancestral to the primary leukemia cells and the relapse clones are usually present as minor subpopulations at diagnosis, but expand during treatment.[9] It has been hypothesized that early relapses may be a result of the selection of a relatively resistant clone already present at primary diagnosis rather than the result of the emergence of a new clone by mutation.[2] Late relapses may be due to de novo development of second leukemia from a common premalignant clone.[2] Lineage switch at relapse is a rare phenomenon and is either due to relapse of the original clone with heterogeneity at the morphologic level or due to the generation of a novel clone. Patterns of recurring genomic alterations have helped in understanding the mechanisms of chemoresistance.[8] Mutations and deletions of tumor suppressor TP53, reduced expression of MSH6, deletions in the *NR3C1* gene, *CREBBP* mutations, and increased global promoter methylation were noted at relapse.[8]

Central nervous system relapse accounts for <10%. Blasts may (1) enter the CNS from the BM of the skull to the subarachnoid space via the bridging veins, or to CSF via the choroid plexus; (2) invade cerebral parenchyma via brain capillaries; (3) infiltrate the leptomeninges via bony lesions of the skull; (4) disseminate through nerve roots, then invading the subarachnoid space through the neural foramina; (5) chloromas can enter the extradural space by extension along the intervertebral foramina; and (6) be seeded either by CNS hemorrhage if the circulating blood contains blasts, or at the time of the diagnostic lumbar puncture, when traumatic.[2]

Testicular leukemia relapse is considered to occur because of insufficient exposure to chemotherapy: (1) chemotherapy concentration can be reduced in the interstitium; for example, methotrexate levels in the interstitium are lower than those in the serum by a factor of 2-4; (2) tight junctions between the myoid cells and the Sertoli cells prevent the entry of large molecules into the seminiferous tubule. Methotrexate levels in the seminiferous tubule are lower than those in the serum by a factor of 18-50; (3) the testes are 2.5°C colder than the body temperature, and this could decrease the efficacy of chemotherapy; (4) P-glycoprotein can export chemotherapy agents (e.g., doxorubicin) from the testes into capillaries; and (5) prostaglandin E2, anti-inflammatory cytokines, and complement inhibitors in the testes help to make the testes an immune-privileged site.[10]

5. What investigations are done at the time of diagnosis of relapse? What is the role of testing for somatic genetic alterations?

The initial investigations would be guided by the symptoms and signs at presentation, BM examination in the case of cytopenias, neuroimaging, and CSF analysis in the case of CNS signs, imaging and needle aspiration cytology/biopsy in the case of scrotal swelling. Irrespective of clinical presentation, testing should be done to evaluate disease status in both the BM and extramedullary sites (CNS and testes). BM aspiration morphology and FCM for immunophenotype, CSF morphology and FCM are done at our center. Further evaluation of testicular disease status using ultrasonography and fine-needle aspiration cytology is carried out only if abnormalities are noted on clinical examination.

Somatic genetic alterations are not used in the current ALL relapse risk stratification schemes. Current data suggests improved prognostication in relapsed B-ALL with the integration of genetics.[11] Unfavorable alterations influencing treatment decision-making have been identified. Tyrosine kinase inhibitors (TKIs) are used when Philadelphia chromosome or ABL-class fusion genes are detected. Ruxolitinib can be considered if JAK2 fusions are detected and the disease remains refractory. TP53 mutations are associated with extremely poor outcome and hence would be reasonable to consider hematopoietic stem cell transplant (HSCT) or CAR-T cells in second CR2.[12] Relapses with high-risk somatic genetic alterations [t(9;22), t(4;11), hypodiploidy] would need to be considered for HSCT in CR2.

At our center we use reverse transcriptase-polymerase chain reaction (RT-PCR) panel test for t(12; 21), t(9;22), t(17;19), and MLL rearrangements, in the relapse setting. TKIs (imatinib or dasatinib) are added to the treatment regimen in Philadelphia chromosome positive leukemias. Next-generation sequencing (NGS) for screening for mutations observed in the relapse setting is also routinely performed at our center.

6. **How would you counsel the family after the diagnosis of relapsed ALL?**

We use the six-step SPIKES protocol to deliver bad news **(Table 8)**.[13]

TABLE 8: SPIKES protocol for breaking bad news.

Step 1	S	SETTING UP the interview	• Arrange for some privacy—preferably a closed room • Involve family members if parents request • Sit down—avoid barriers in between • Make a connection with the parents—maintain eye contact • Manage time constraints and interruptions—mobile in silent mode
Step 2	P	Assessing the parents' PERCEPTION	Open-ended questions to understand the parents' perception of the medical condition. Correct misinformation and tailor the bad news to what they understand. Determine if they engage in any variation of illness denial—wishful thinking, omission of essential but unfavorable medical details of the illness, unrealistic expectations of treatment
Step 3	I	Obtaining the parents' INVITATION	• Ask parents' how much they want to know • Get permission to disclose bad news • Share intent to be open and honest
Step 4	K	Giving KNOWLEDGE and information to the parents	• Start at the level of comprehension and vocabulary of the parents • Try to use nontechnical words • Avoid excessive bluntness • Give information in small chunks and check periodically as to the parents' understanding • When prognosis is poor, avoid phrases as "there is nothing we can do for you," parents often have other important therapeutic goals as good pain control and symptom relief

Contd...

Contd...

Step 5	E	Addressing the parents' EMOTIONS with empathic responses	• Observe for any emotion on the part of the parent • Identify the emotion experienced by the parent by naming it to oneself • Identify the reason for the emotion • Give a brief period of time to express his/her feelings, make a connecting statement
Step 6	S	STRATEGY and SUMMARY	• Ensure parents are ready for discussing a treatment plan • Present treatment options, discuss, and make a plan for the future • Summarize the discussion checking the parents' understanding

Parents are counseled regarding the risk status at the diagnosis of relapse, the expected outcomes, the need for chemotherapy and HSCT and, the expected duration of treatment. Families would be counseled regarding the adverse effects of chemotherapy and radiation, the effects on fertility and option for fertility preservation shall be provided according to the age of the child. Emotional and social support would be provided by our social support team. We would guide them in registering under government health schemes for funding their treatment. Accommodation and basic needs support would be provided with the help of nongovernmental organizations (NGOs).

7. What are the principles used in the management of relapsed ALL?

We use a risk-stratified approach in the management of relapsed ALL, with response based on MRD. Submicroscopic involvement of the BM is a frequent finding in patients with isolated CNS relapse.[2] Using sensitive techniques like PCR, BM involvement can be demonstrated in up to 91% of patients with morphologically isolated testicular relapse.[2] This forms the rationale for the use of systemic chemotherapy along with site directed therapy for IEM relapsed ALL.

Low or standard-risk relapsed ALL is managed with chemotherapy (with intensive reinduction) and site-directed therapy for extramedullary involvement. High-risk relapsed ALL is managed with chemotherapy followed by HSCT. Intermediate-risk relapsed ALL is managed with chemotherapy alone or chemotherapy with HSCT based on MRD after reinduction chemotherapy. Adequate CNS control with cranial radiation for CNS relapses is essential. Novel therapies (immunotherapy and targeted agents) have been incorporated into relapsed ALL management protocols in recent times. Intensive supportive care is of paramount importance in the management of relapsed ALL.

8. The index child has been diagnosed as a case of early combined medullary and testicular B-ALL relapse. What reinduction regimen would you use in this child?

Reinduction with intensive chemotherapy is the current standard of care for first relapse of ALL. Although reinduction chemotherapy regimens differ significantly between various groups, the outcomes attained have been similar. We would use the four-drug induction [dexamethasone, polyethylene glycol (PEG) asparaginase, vincristine, anthracycline] regimen of UK ALL R3 **(Fig. 5)** at our center. Reinduction regimens for relapsed ALL are associated with high rates of toxicity and serious infections, thereby warranting in-patient administration of the regimen. At our center, we provide reinduction chemotherapy on out-patient basis due to resource constraints for admission of children.

We have adapted the regimen to our setting. We have shifted D1 anthracycline to D8, and spaced anthracycline dosing with a 1-week gap to avoid severe myelosuppression. Daunorubicin is used, as availability and affordability of mitoxantrone and idarubicin is a hurdle. We currently use intrathecal methotrexate as per UK ALL R3 protocol.

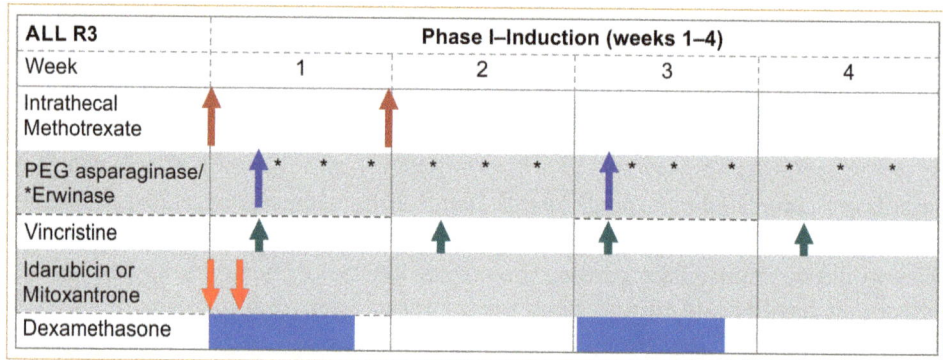

Fig. 5: UK ALL R3 protocol—Schematic representation of induction chemotherapy.
Adapted from: UK ALL R3 trial protocol.

9. What supportive care measures should be ensured while managing a child with relapsed ALL?

Antimicrobial prophylaxis is recommended since the infection risk is high with reinduction regimens.[14,15] At our center, we provide antifungal and anti-*Pneumocystis jirovecii* prophylaxis. We use voriconazole at 8 mg/kg/dose twice daily for antifungal prophylaxis as mold infections are prevalent. Sulfamethoxazole–trimethoprim (dosed at 5 mg/kg/dose of trimethoprim alternate day) is used for anti-*P. jirovecii* prophylaxis. Role of fluoroquinolone prophylaxis is currently under study at our center. Parents and children are counseled regarding general hygiene, oral and perianal region care. Frequent nutritional assessments are done during the treatment course and rehabilitation measures are ensured as required. Nasogastric tube feeding is encouraged in children whose dietary requirements are not met with oral feeding. We have established antimicrobial policies for therapy during episodes of febrile neutropenia and teams for daily monitoring of children with febrile neutropenia managed on outpatient department (OPD) basis.

10. The child received reinduction chemotherapy (four drug) according to the UK ALL R3 chemotherapy protocol. Postreinduction chemotherapy, BM was in morphological remission and MRD <0.01% (we use FCM-based MRD evaluation at our center). What would be the next step? What difference in management would be considered if he received reinduction chemotherapy according to the ALL REZ BFM 2002 chemotherapy protocol?

At our center, we use an MRD cutoff of <0.01% at the end of induction to decide on the need for HSCT postconsolidation therapy. If the end-of-induction MRD is <0.01%, we would proceed with the chemotherapy and site directed chemotherapy for extramedullary involvement **(Figs. 6A to E)**. We do not use prophylactic cranial irradiation for isolated BM relapses.

The end-of-induction MRD cutoff used in the ALL REZ BFM 2002 protocol is <0.1%, for the intermediate risk group to continue chemotherapy. It has been postulated that the anthracycline containing reinduction regimen of UK ALL R3 protocol is more intense than the F1/F2 blocks of ALL REZ BFM 2002 protocol and hence the need for deeper cutoff to continue chemotherapy.

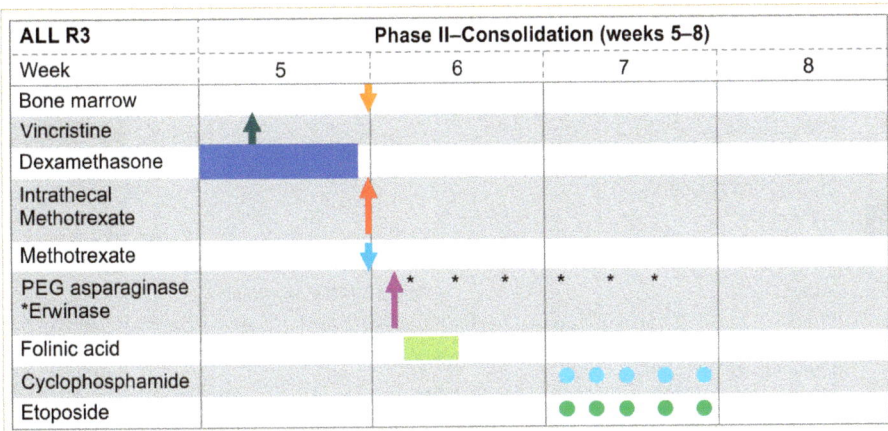

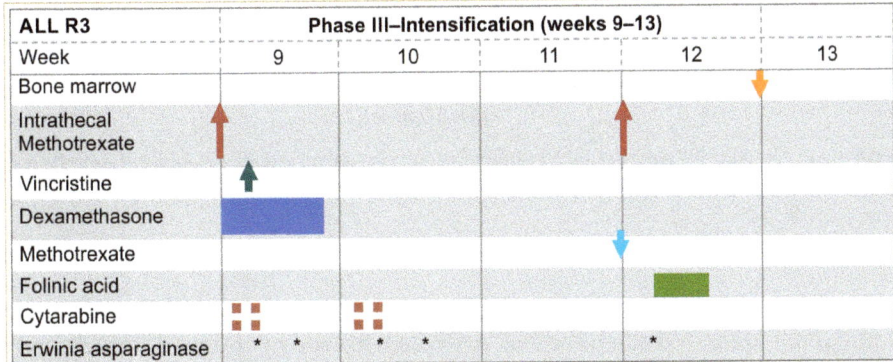

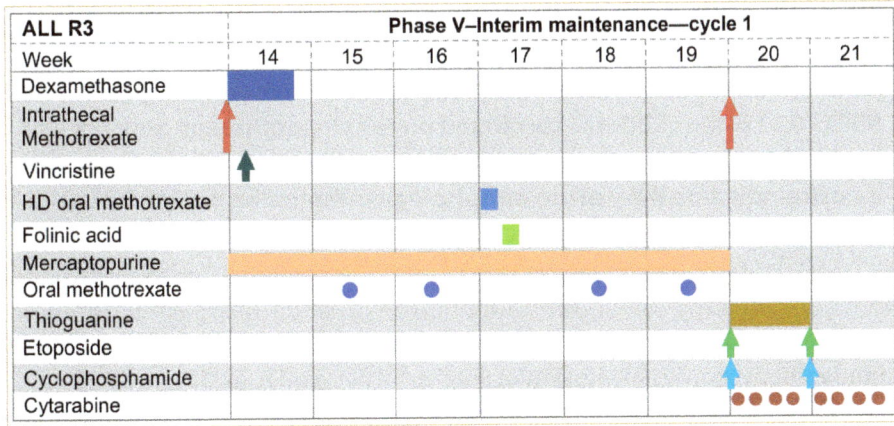

Figs. 6A to C

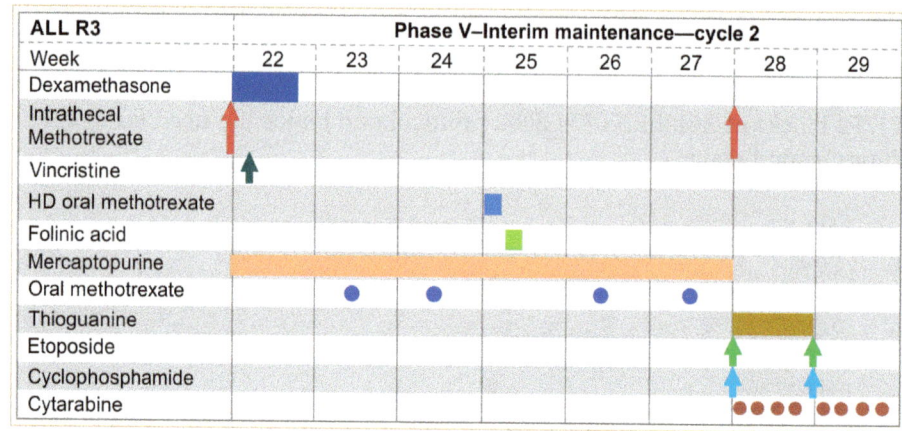

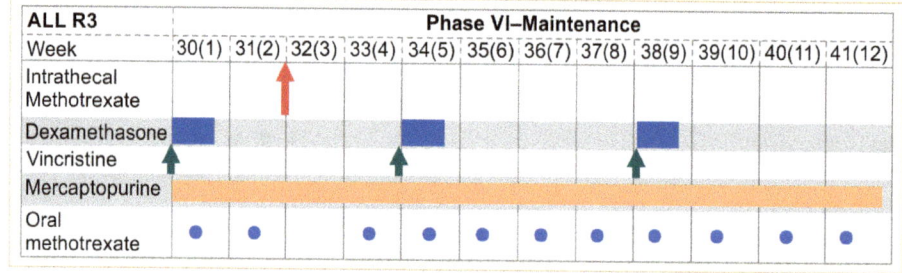

Figs. 6D and E

Figs. 6A to E: UK ALL R3 protocol: (A) Schematic representation of consolidation chemotherapy; (B) Intensification chemotherapy; (C and D) Interim maintenance chemotherapy; (E) Maintenance chemotherapy.
Adapted from: UK ALL R3 trial protocol.

According to the results of the ALL REZ BFM 2002 trial, the predictive value of MRD does not apply to the intermediate risk patients with early combined BM relapse and this subgroup of patients require HSCT irrespective of MRD status postinduction.[5] The results of intermediate risk patients on UK ALL R3 have not been published yet.

11. **As the postreinduction chemotherapy BM was in morphological remission and MRD <0.01% the child was continued on the chemotherapy arm. For this child on UK ALL R3 chemotherapy protocol, what would have been the management plan if postreinduction BM were in morphological remission but MRD >0.01%? What is the preferred postinduction therapy in the setting?**

In the scenario of postreinduction MRD ≥0.01%, HSCT is indicated. The current preferred postinduction therapy for end-of-induction poor MRD response is immunotherapy with blinatumomab. If MRD <0.01% is achieved after first 28-day cycle of blinatumomab [continuous intravenous (IV) infusion of 5 µg/m²/day from D1 to D7 and 15 µg/m²/day from D8 to D28], HSCT should be done immediately. If MRD post cycle one of blinatumomab is

≥0.01%, second cycle of blinatumomab needs to be administered to achieve MRD <0.01% prior to HSCT.

At our center, in children in CR2 with end-of-induction MRD ≥0.01%, we continue with the consolidation chemotherapy as per protocol for cases where affordability of blinatumomab is a limiting factor. Reassessment MRD is performed postconsolidation therapy, prior to HSCT. If MRD is <0.01% we would proceed with HSCT, or if MRD is ≥0.01% we would use alternative chemotherapy regimens (FLAG or FLAG-Ida) to achieve MRD <0.01% and then proceed with HSCT.

12. What would have been the management plan if postreinduction BM were not in morphological remission?

If the response to reinduction is an M3 marrow, inotuzumab and/or chimeric antigen receptor (CAR), T-cell therapy can be used.[1] If the response is an M2 marrow, blinatumomab can be used.[1]

At our center, we palliate reinduction failures due to inaccessibility to immunotherapy.

13. The aforementioned child, a case of early combined medullary and testicular relapse, postreinduction MRD negative, received consolidation and intensification chemotherapy according to the UK ALL R3 protocol. The child underwent right orchiectomy and simultaneous biopsy of the clinically uninvolved left testis showed no leukemic infiltration. What would be your next step? How would you provide site-directed therapy for extramedullary involvement in relapsed ALL?

We are currently following the site-directed therapy guidelines of the ALL REZ BFM 2002 protocol **(Table 9)**.

TABLE 9: Guidelines for site-directed therapy.

UK ALL R3	CNS relapse	Recommended dose of cranial irradiation		24 Gy in 15 fractions of 1.6 Gy starting from week 14
	Testicular relapse	Recommended dose of testicular radiation	Irrespective of laterality of involvement	24 Gy in 12 daily fractions to both testes starting week 14
ALL REZ BFM 2002	CNS relapse	Recommended dose of craniospinal/cranial irradiation		18 Gy
		If previous exposure to cranial irradiation	>15 Gy in children aged <2 years	15 Gy
			>18 Gy in children aged ≥2 years	15 Gy

Contd...

Contd...

		Interval to the first course of cranial radiation therapy <24 months and if previous dose	>12 Gy in children aged <2 years	15 Gy
			>15 Gy in children aged ≥2 years	15 Gy
	Testicular relapse	Clinically involved testes		Orchiectomy or 24 Gy irradiation
		If unilateral clinically involved testis, biopsy the contralateral testis	No involvement	15 Gy
			Involved or biopsy not done	18 Gy
		Clinically noninvolved testis, involvement detected by ultrasound—needs to be biopsied	No involvement	15 Gy
			Involved or biopsy not done	18 Gy

(CNS: central nervous system)

The child had clinical and tissue proven involvement of the right testis at diagnosis, and hence underwent right orchiectomy. Biopsy of the clinically uninvolved left testis during the surgery showed no leukemic infiltration, hence the left testis would be irradiated with 15 Gy. Following site-directed therapy he would be continued on interim maintenance and maintenance chemotherapy.

14. What are the indications for HSCT in the setting of first relapse of ALL?

The following are the indications for allogeneic HSCT in the setting of the first relapse of ALL, i.e., in CR2:
- High-risk ALL relapses (very early IEM ALL relapse, B-ALL early isolated marrow relapse, B-ALL very early marrow or combined relapse, T-ALL marrow or combined relapse, any timing)
- Intermediate risk ALL (early IEM ALL relapse, late isolated B-ALL marrow relapse, early/late combined B-ALL marrow relapse) with end-of-induction MRD ≥ 0.01%.
- Adverse cytogenetic/molecular profile at relapse—Philadelphia chromosome positive ALL relapse, MLL rearrangement ALL relapse, hypodiploid ALL relapse, TP53-positive ALL relapse.

15. What is the role of blinatumomab in the management of ALL relapse?

Blinatumomab is a CD3/CD19-directed bispecific T-cell engager molecule that engages T cells to lyse CD19-expressing B cells, approved for the treatment of pediatric relapsed/refractory B-ALL.[16,17] A recent study that compared two cycles of UK ALL R3 postinduction chemotherapy to two cycles of blinatumomab in intermediate and high-risk first-relapse of B-ALL, was stopped early because of improved disease-free survival, superior overall survival (OS), lower toxicity, and superior MRD clearance with blinatumomab.[7] This is the first randomized trial suggesting a survival benefit for immunotherapy in patients with B-ALL, likely derived from the percentage of patients who were able to undergo transplant.[7] Blinatumomab use postreinduction is associated with higher rates of MRD negativity and lesser adverse effects with increased proportion of patients able to continue till HSCT. Blinatumomab provides a bridge to HSCT which is essential to maintain durable remissions. Blinatumomab has also been used as a bridge to further chemostatic therapy in patients who experienced overwhelming toxicity during induction chemotherapy or at higher risk for chemotherapy related toxicity. High-blast percentage (BM not in morphological remission) is a risk factor for blinatumomab resistance and hence is not recommended in such settings. Cytokine release syndrome (CRS) and neurotoxicity (encephalopathy and seizures) are the most serious blinatumomab-specific adverse effects. The fraction of patients with higher grades of CRS and neurotoxicity requiring discontinuation of blinatumomab is very low.

16. What are the other immunotherapy agents used in the management of relapsed ALL?

Other immunotherapy agents used in the management of B-ALL relapses include:
- *Inotuzumab:* It is a CD22-directed antibody conjugated to calicheamicin approved for relapsed/refractory pediatric B-ALL. Phase II trials have shown that inotuzumab is effective and well-tolerated in pediatric relapsed/refractory B-ALL.[18-20] Inotuzumab is not curative, but acts as a bridge to potentially curative therapy. Unlike blinatumomab which requires a continuous infusion and tisagenlecleucel which requires extraction, modification, infusion of T cells; inotuzumab has the benefit of easier administration. Response rates with inotuzumab have been encouraging in heavily pretreated cases. Sinusoidal obstruction syndrome postallogeneic HSCT is a significant adverse effect of use of inotuzumab.
- *CAR T-cell therapy:* CAR T-cells are genetically modified polyclonal T or natural killer (NK) cells with fusion proteins to guide them toward a given molecule in the tumor cell surface.[21] Targeting moiety is presented in native form without the need for additional processing within the groove major histocompatibility complex (MHC) molecules, therefore CAR T cells identify target tumor cells regardless of a patient's MHC haplotype.[21] In the ELIANA trial, a single infusion of the anti-CD19 CAR T-cell therapy, tisagenlecleucel, provided durable remission with long-term persistence in pediatric and young adult patients with relapsed or refractory B-cell ALL, with transient high-grade toxic effects.[22] Compared to blinatumomab and inotuzumab, tisagenlecleucel is associated with higher survival outcomes in relapsed/refractory B-ALL, and has the potential for long-term cure without subsequent HSCT. As of now, CAR T-cell therapy is not used up front in the treatment of first relapse of B-ALL, it is used in refractory disease.

At our center, resource constraints limit the use of immunotherapy in relapsed B-ALL.

17. How do you manage Ph-positive B-ALL relapses at your center?

Tyrosine kinase inhibitor therapy and HSCT in CR2 are two important therapeutic considerations in the management of t(9;22) positive/bcr-ABL translocation positive/Philadelphia chromosome-positive B-ALL relapse. At our center, we perform baseline ABL kinase domain mutations testing for Ph-positive ALL relapses at diagnosis. We use the second-generation TKI, Dasatinib at a dose of 80 mg/m/day due to its superior CNS penetration, along with reinduction chemotherapy as per UK ALL R3 protocol.[23] Reinduction is followed by consolidation chemotherapy and HSCT once MRD is negative. Studies related to the use of blinatumomab as consolidation therapy in children with Ph-positive ALL are lacking. The ALACANTRA study has shown long-term durable responses to blinatumomab in adults with relapsed/refractory Ph ALL.[24] A retrospective study in children with relapsed/refractory B-ALL has shown relatively good outcomes for patients with Philadelphia chromosome-positive or Philadelphia chromosome-like ALL, with a 2-year progression-free survival (PFS) of 70%.[25] There have been no randomized control trials for the post-HSCT use of TKIs in Ph ALL. We follow the preemptive approach for TKI use, as current data do not support the use of prophylactic post-HSCT TKI. In the preemptive approach BM aspiration is done periodically to assess MRD at 1, 2, 3, 6, 9, and 12 months post-HSCT.[26] If MRD positivity is documented, ABL kinase domain mutation testing is done and TKI started. Imatinib is preferred as is least myelosuppressive, in case of mutation conferring resistance an alternative TKI is used. Post-HSCT TKI is continued for at least 1 year from MRD positivity and is discontinued when reassessment MRD is negative.[26] If MRD continues to remain positive after 1 month of TKI, alternate therapies like CAR T-cell therapy should be considered.[26]

18. How do you manage T-ALL relapses at your center?

Compared to B-ALL, relapses happen earlier, most within 2 years of diagnosis, for T-ALL.[1] Outcomes for T-ALL relapses are poor, with OS rates of <25%. Hence, HSCT is a preferred option for T-ALL relapses regardless of the site or timing of relapse.[1] The principle of management of T-ALL includes reinduction and HSCT as soon as a negative MRD is achieved. The reinduction regimens available are UK ALL R3 regimen, ALL REZ BFM 2002 regimen, NECTAR regimen (Nelarabine, cyclophosphamide, and etoposide), and COG AALL07P1 regimen (bortezomib added to a prednisone-based four drug induction).[27-29] If CNS involvement is present, NECTAR may be more practical to administer postinduction as concomitant administration of nelarabine and intrathecal chemotherapy increases the risk of neurotoxicity. Daratumumab, CD38-directed monoclonal antibody, has shown promising preclinical activity in T-ALL and is being tested with chemotherapy in relapsed/refractory T-ALL. CDK4/6 inhibitor palbociclib, venetoclax (selective BCL2 inhibitor), and navitoclax (BCL-2, BCL-XL, and BCL-W inhibitor) are currently under investigation in relapsed/refractory T-ALL.[1,30-32]

At our center, we palliate T-ALL relapses.

19. What are the outcomes of first relapse of ALL?

Current data suggests a 5-year OS rate of 50% for first relapse of acute leukemia.[27,28] Current trials show a long-term OS of 70% for late marrow relapse with good MRD response, with multiagent chemotherapy.[33-35] The 5-year OS of isolated CNS relapse is 65%, early isolated CNS relapses have inferior outcomes with 3-year OS of 52%.

■ REFERENCES

1. Hunger SP, Raetz EA. How I treat relapsed acute lymphoblastic leukemia in the pediatric population. Blood. 2020;136(16):1803-12.
2. Locatelli F, Schrappe M, Bernardo ME, Rutella S. How I treat relapsed childhood acute lymphoblastic leukemia. Blood. 2012;120(14):2807-16.

3. Buchmann S, Schrappe M, Baruchel A, Biondi A, Borowitz M, Campbell M, et al. Remission, treatment failure, and relapse in pediatric ALL: an international consensus of the Ponte-di-Legno Consortium. Blood. 2022;139(12 Suppl 1):1-5.
4. Buchmann S, Schrappe M, Baruchel A, Biondi A, Borowitz M, Campbell M, et al. Remission, treatment failure, and relapse in pediatric ALL: an international consensus of the Ponte-di-Legno Consortium. Blood. 2022;139(12):1785-93.
5. Eckert C, Henze G, Seeger K, Hagedorn N, Mann G, Panzer-Grümayer R, et al. Use of allogeneic hematopoietic stem-cell transplantation based on minimal residual disease response improves outcomes for children with relapsed acute lymphoblastic leukemia in the intermediate-risk group. J Clin Oncol. 2013;31(21):2736-42.
6. Parker C, Waters R, Leighton C, Hancock J, Sutton R, Moorman AV, et al. Effect of mitoxantrone on outcome of children with first relapse of acute lymphoblastic leukaemia (ALL R3): an open-label randomised trial. Lancet. 2010;376(9757):2009-17.
7. Brown PA, Ji L, Xu X, Devidas M, Hogan LE, Borowitz MJ, et al. Effect of postreinduction therapy consolidation with blinatumomab vs chemotherapy on disease-free survival in children, adolescents, and young adults with first relapse of B-cell acute lymphoblastic leukemia: a randomized clinical trial. JAMA. 2021;325(9):833-42.
8. Bhojwani D, Pui CH. Relapsed childhood acute lymphoblastic leukaemia. Lancet Oncol. 2013;14(6):e205-17.
9. Mullighan CG, Phillips LA, Su X, Ma J, Miller CB, Shurtleff SA, et al. Genomic analysis of the clonal origins of relapsed acute lymphoblastic leukemia. Science. 2008;322(5906):1377-80.
10. Nguyen HTK, Terao MA, Green DM, Pui CH, Inaba H. Testicular involvement of acute lymphoblastic leukemia in children and adolescents: Diagnosis, biology, and management. Cancer. 2021;127(17):3067-81.
11. Irving JA, Enshaei A, Parker CA, Sutton R, Kuiper RP, Erhorn A, et al. Integration of genetic and clinical risk factors improves prognostication in relapsed childhood B-cell precursor acute lymphoblastic leukemia. Blood. 2016;128(7):911-22.
12. Yu CH, Chang WT, Jou ST, Lin TK, Chang YH, Lin CY, et al. TP53 alterations in relapsed childhood acute lymphoblastic leukemia. Cancer Sci. 2020;111(1):229-38.
13. Baile WF, Buckman R, Lenzi R, Glober G, Beale EA, Kudelka AP. SPIKES-A six-step protocol for delivering bad news: application to the patient with cancer. Oncologist. 2000;5(4):302-11.
14. Alexander S, Fisher BT, Gaur AH, Dvorak CC, Villa Luna D, Dang H, et al. Effect of levofloxacin prophylaxis on bacteremia in children with acute leukemia or undergoing hematopoietic stem cell transplantation: a randomized clinical trial. JAMA. 2018;320(10):995-1004.
15. Science M, Robinson PD, MacDonald T, Rassekh SR, Dupuis LL, Sung L. Guideline for primary antifungal prophylaxis for pediatric patients with cancer or hematopoietic stem cell transplant recipients. Pediatr Blood Cancer. 2014;61(3):393-400.
16. Locatelli F, Zugmaier G, Rizzari C, Morris JD, Gruhn B, Klingebiel T, et al. Effect of blinatumomab vs chemotherapy on event-free survival among children with high-risk first-relapse B-cell acute lymphoblastic leukemia: a randomized clinical trial. JAMA. 2021;325(9):843-54.
17. Locatelli F, Zugmaier G, Mergen N, Bader P, Jeha S, Schlegel PG, et al. Blinatumomab in pediatric relapsed/refractory B-cell acute lymphoblastic leukemia: RIALTO expanded access study final analysis. Blood Adv. 2022;6(3):1004-14.
18. Bhojwani D, Sposto R, Shah NN, Rodriguez V, Yuan C, Stetler-Stevenson M, et al. Inotuzumab ozogamicin in pediatric patients with relapsed/refractory acute lymphoblastic leukemia. Leukemia. 2019;33(4):884-92.
19. O'Brien MM, Ji L, Shah NN, Rheingold SR, Bhojwani D, Yuan CM, et al. Phase II trial of inotuzumab ozogamicin in children and adolescents with relapsed or refractory B-cell acute lymphoblastic leukemia: Children's oncology group protocol AALL1621. J Clin Oncol. 2022;40(9):956-67.

20. Pennesi E, Michels N, Brivio E, van der Velden VHJ, Jiang Y, Thano A, et al. Inotuzumab ozogamicin as single agent in pediatric patients with relapsed and refractory acute lymphoblastic leukemia: Results from a phase II trial. Leukemia. 2022;36(6):1516-24.
21. Sheykhhasan M, Manoochehri H, Dama P. Use of CAR T-cell for acute lymphoblastic leukemia (ALL) treatment: A review study. Cancer Gene Ther. 2022;29(8-9):1080-96.
22. Maude SL, Laetsch TW, Buechner J, Rives S, Boyer M, Bittencourt H, et al. Tisagenlecleucel in children and young adults with B-cell lymphoblastic leukemia. N Engl J Med. 2018;378(5):439-48.
23. Shen S, Chen X, Cai J, Yu J, Gao J, Hu S, et al. Effect of dasatinib vs imatinib in the treatment of pediatric Philadelphia chromosome-positive acute lymphoblastic leukemia: a randomized clinical trial. JAMA Oncol. 2020;6(3):358-66.
24. Martinelli G, Boissel N, Chevallier P, Ottmann O, Gökbuget N, Rambaldi A, et al. Long-term follow-up of blinatumomab in patients with relapsed/refractory Philadelphia chromosome-positive B-cell precursor acute lymphoblastic leukaemia: final analysis of ALCANTARA study. Eur J Cancer. 2021;146:107-14.
25. Sutton R, Pozza LD, Khaw SL, Fraser C, Revesz T, Chamberlain J, et al. Outcomes for Australian children with relapsed/refractory acute lymphoblastic leukaemia treated with blinatumomab. Pediatr Blood Cancer. 2021;68(5):e28922.
26. Vettenranta K, Dobšinská V, Kertész G, Svec P, Buechner J, Schultz KR. What is the role of HSCT in Philadelphia-chromosome-positive and Philadelphia-chromosome-like ALL in the tyrosine kinase inhibitor era? Front Pediatr. 2022;9:807002.
27. Commander LA, Seif AE, Insogna IG, Rheingold SR. Salvage therapy with nelarabine, etoposide, and cyclophosphamide in relapsed/refractory paediatric T-cell lymphoblastic leukaemia and lymphoma. Br J Haematol. 2010;150(3):345-51.
28. Luskin MR, Ganetsky A, Landsburg DJ, Loren AW, Porter DL, Nasta SD, et al. Nelarabine, cyclophosphamide and etoposide for adults with relapsed T-cell acute lymphoblastic leukaemia and lymphoma. Br J Haematol. 2016;174(2):332-4.
29. Horton TM, Whitlock JA, Lu X, O'Brien MM, Borowitz MJ, Devidas M, et al. Bortezomib reinduction chemotherapy in high-risk ALL in first relapse: a report from the children's oncology group. Br J Haematol. 2019;186(2):274-85.
30. Bride KL, Vincent TL, Im SY, Aplenc R, Barrett DM, Carroll WL, et al. Preclinical efficacy of daratumumab in T-cell acute lymphoblastic leukemia. Blood. 2018;131(9):995-9.
31. Rheingold SR, Ji L, Xu X, Devidas M, Brown PA, Gore L, et al. Prognostic factors for survival after relapsed acute lymphoblastic leukemia (ALL): a children's oncology group (COG) study. In: 2019 ASCO Annual Meeting I. J Clin Oncol. 2019;37(15_suppl):10008.
32. Oskarsson T, Söderhäll S, Arvidson J, Forestier E, Montgomery S, Bottai M, et al. Relapsed childhood acute lymphoblastic leukemia in the Nordic countries: prognostic factors, treatment and outcome. Haematologica. 2016;101(1):68-76.
33. Lew G, Chen Y, Lu X, Rheingold SR, Whitlock JA, Devidas M, et al. Outcomes after late bone marrow and very early central nervous system relapse of childhood B-acute lymphoblastic leukemia: a report from the children's oncology group phase III study AALL0433. Haematologica. 2021;106(1):46-55.
34. Eckert C, Groeneveld-Krentz S, Kirschner-Schwabe R, Hagedorn N, Chen-Santel C, Bader P, et al. Improving stratification for children with late bone marrow B-cell acute lymphoblastic leukemia relapses with refined response classification and integration of genetics. J Clin Oncol. 2019;37(36):3493-506.
35. Parker C, Krishnan S, Hamadeh L, Irving JAE, Kuiper RP, Révész T, et al. Outcomes of patients with childhood B-cell precursor acute lymphoblastic leukaemia with late bone marrow relapses: long-term follow-up of the ALLR3 open-label randomised trial. Lancet Haematol. 2019;6(4):e204-e216.

EXPERT OPINION

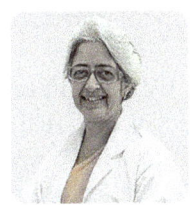

Gauri Kapoor MD PhD
Director, Department of Pediatric Hematology Oncology and BMT
Rajiv Gandhi Cancer Institute and Research Centre, New Delhi, India

Relapsed Acute Lymphoblastic Leukemia

Relapse ALL is the fourth most common oncological condition in children and its management is a challenge as treatment outcome is <50%. Therapeutic options vary based on the first-line protocol used and the risk factors. At our center we include the following risk factors: (1) time from diagnosis to relapse, (2) site of relapse (marrow worse than extramedullary), (3) immunophenotype (T worse than B), and (4) MRD response to reinduction therapy.

We do not routinely use somatic genetic alterations in risk assignment following relapse, however, several unfavorable alterations have been identified and could influence treatment decision-making. In selected subset of patients where NGS and RNA-based fusion gene testing is available: we would add imatinib or dasatinib to reinduction therapy for patients with Philadelphia chromosome or if an ABL-class gene fusion was detected. In case TP53 mutation is detected it is known to be associated with very poor outcome, hence we would recommend HSCT for all such cases. Although ruxolitinib is under investigation for those with CRLF2/JAK-STAT mutations we have not tried them.

Time from diagnosis to relapse is highly prognostic. Exact times and terminologies differ between groups. Berlin–Frankfurt–Münster (BFM) and UK definitions (Hunger 2020) are what we follow: very early (18 months from diagnosis), early (18 months from diagnosis but, 6 months after completion of treatment), and late (>6 months after completion of treatment). In the present case the child had National Cancer Institute (NCI) standard risk B-ALL, was treated on the standard risk arm of ICiCLE protocol for B-ALL, had an early (<6 months after completion of treatment) combined marrow and testicular relapse.

At our center we use ALL-BFM 95 as our front-line chemotherapy protocol which has a cumulative anthracycline dose of 240 mg/m^2. Hence, we follow ALL-BFM REZ 2002, as this relapse protocol has an anthracycline-free 4-week reinduction (F1/F2). Early combined marrow relapse of B-ALL would stratify the patient as intermediate risk ALL by BFM criteria and would be treated as strategic risk group S2. Patients in group S2 receive eight alternating blocks R1 and R2 after the induction blocks F1 and F2, followed by 6MP/MTX maintenance to complete 2 years of therapy. Triple intrathecal is used in this protocol for all relapse patients irrespective of site of relapse.

In the provided case: Patient achieved MRD <0.01% with a four-drug reinduction and was continued with chemotherapy as per UK ALL R3 protocol. We agree that MRD after induction is the strongest predictor of prognosis in intermediate risk relapsed ALL as shown by many groups including the BFM.[1]

The MRD cutoff we use is 0.01% (10^{-4}). We usually reserve HSCT for patients with poor MRD response after the first 4 weeks of reinduction, i.e., >0.01%. However, if MRD is between 0.1 and 0.01% we repeat after 2 R blocks and if it does not drop to <0.01% it remains a poor responder. In the provided case we would treat with chemotherapy alone as he is a good responder. However, we would do HLA typing for all cases and if match sibling donor is available option of HSCT would be offered. We would not recommend haplo or matched unrelated donor (MUD) HSCT in this situation.

Response assessment for IEM site relapse:
- *If CSF was positive at relapse:* CSF cytology (along with intrathecal) every week till it clears, and then serially as per protocol. If there were any parenchymal infiltrates on magnetic resonance imaging (MRI), then imaging would be repeated at the end of reinduction.
- *For patients with testicular disease at relapse:* We would assess testicular size clinically and use USG to look for resolution of changes at end of reinduction.

Refractory CNS/testicular disease—prognosis is poor, we individualize treatment on case to case basis taking family into confidence.

Ponte-de-Legno consortium consensus criteria for relapse—in our routine clinical practice when we carry out a BM evaluation for suspected medullary relapse and blast percentage is low—we would repeat a BM MRD by FCM after 1-2 weeks to confirm a marrow relapse.

Blinatumomab as consolidation for CNS disease—we have not used it in this scenario. In the paper by Aldoss I et al. (Cancer 2022)—a history of extramedullary disease predicted an inferior response to blinatumomab therapy with a higher risk for relapse/progression at extramedullary sites (particularly CNS). It has been shown that consolidation with allogenic transplantation in patients who primarily responded to blinatumomab did not abrogate the risk of extramedullary relapse.

Blinatumomab as consolidation for Ph positive relapse—we have not used it. A study in adults using "Propensity score analysis" showed benefit of blinatumomab consolidation compared to patients treated with standard chemotherapy and TKI (Cancer 2020).

For Ph positive ALL relapse—post-HSCT we continue TKI for 2 years.

Relapse T-ALL—relapses occur early with T-ALL as opposed to B-All and usually occur within 2 years of diagnosis. Early or very early marrow relapse is almost incurable in our experience and we would usually recommend palliation in these cases. The reinduction schedule that we have used has been quite variable, it includes: (1) NECTAR (nelarabine, cyclophosphamide, and etoposide) chemotherapy protocol, literature shows CR2 rates of 38% (PBC 2022); (2) FLAG: Idar; (3) Daratumomab for CD 38 positive leukemia; and (4) COG AALL07P1 regimen (bortezomib added to a prednisone-based four-drug reinduction), that is reported to give CR2 rates of 68% in 22 T-ALL patients, could also be considered (BJH 2019). Some investigators have reported venetoclax/navitoclax plus chemotherapy, while others use four-drug reinduction as per UK ALL R3, however, we have not used this combination. In our experience we have not been able to achieve CR2 in T-ALL with early marrow relapse. In view of overall poor outcome of relapsed T-ALL, if CR2 is achieved, HSCT is the preferred option, regardless of the site or timing of relapse. So we recommend reinduction chemotherapy followed by HSCT with the best available donor as soon as an MRD-negative CR is achieved.

In case of a testicular or CNS relapse the involved compartment is irradiated after the completion of intensive phase of treatment. Role of cranial/craniospinal radiation therapy (RT) in relapse ALL—we use cranial radiation therapy (CRT) (18 Gy) for all CNS relapse for children age >3 years. For patients with testicular relapse in remission, we use bilateral testicular RT dose 19.8 Gy in 11 fractions, for those with residual disease 25.2 Gy in 13 fractions.

To conclude, it is extremely important to correctly risk stratify patients and have a detailed counseling of family regarding details of treatment, likely outcomes and late effects of therapy.

REFERENCE

1. Eckert C, von Stackelberg A, Seeger K, Groeneveld TWL, Peters C, Klingebiel T, et al. Minimal residual disease after induction is the strongest predictor of prognosis in intermediate risk relapsed acute lymphoblastic leukaemia – Long-term results of trial ALL-REZ BFM P95/96. Eur J Cancer. 2013;49(6):1346-55.

CHAPTER 3

Acute Myeloid Leukemia

Kritika Setlur, Jagdish P Meena

CASE VIGNETTE

Patient L presented at 6 years of age with a 1-month history of progressive pallor, fever, and gum bleeding. His peripheral smear was suggestive of myeloid blasts, and bone marrow examination and flow cytometry confirmed a diagnosis of acute myeloid leukemia (AML). Further work-up revealed an 8:21 translocation on karyotyping.

1. How do we diagnose AML?

The international consensus classification of myeloid neoplasms and acute leukemia lays down diagnostic criteria for AML as 20% or more myeloid blasts in blood or bone marrow, *or* a blast count of 10% or more in the presence of certain recurrent genetic abnormalities, as listed below.

- Acute promyelocytic leukemia (APML) with t(15;17)(q24.1;q21.2)/PML::RARA
- APML with other RARA rearrangements
- t(8;21)(q22;q22.1)/RUNX1::RUNX1T1
- inv(16)(p13.1q22) or t(16;16)(p13.1;q22)/CBFB::MYH11
- t(9;11)(p21.3;q23.3)/MLLT3::KMT2A
- Other KMT2A rearrangements [e.g., t(10;11), t(4;11)]
- t(6;9)(p22.3;q34.1)/DEK::NUP214
- inv(3)(q21.3q26.2) or t(3;3)(q21.3;q26.2)/GATA2; MECOM(EVI1)
- Other MECOM rearrangements [e.g., t(2;3), t(3;8)]
- Mutated NPM1
- In frame bZIP, CEBPA mutations ≥10%.

As well as certain other rarer recurrent abnormalities such as AML with t(16;21)(q24.3;q22.1)/RUNX1::CBFA2T3, AML (megakaryoblastic) with t(1;22)(p13.3;q13.1)/RBM15::MRTF1, etc.[1]

ELN 2017 recommendations for the morphological diagnosis of AML states that for morphological diagnosis, we must count at least 200 leukocytes on blood smears and 500 nucleated cells on spiculated marrow smears. The blast count also includes so-called "blast equivalents," which in AML with monocytic or myelomonocytic differentiation include monoblasts and promonoblasts.[2]

Immunophenotyping is required for the diagnosis of AML M0 and AMKL, and plays a supportive role in the diagnosis of other subtypes as well. It is also useful for differentiating AML from mixed phenotypic acute leukemia (MPAL).

Useful markers for immunophenotyping are given in **Table 1**.

TABLE 1: Immunophenotyping markers.

AML diagnosis	
Precursors	CD34, CD117, CD133, HLA DR
Myelomonocytic	CD4, CD11b, CD11c, CD13, CD14, CD15, CD33, CD64, CD65, CD184, iMPO or lysozyme
Megakaryocytic	CD41, CD42, CD61
Erythroid	CD235a
Lineage aberrant	CD2, CD7, CD19, CD56
Pan leucocyte markers	CD11a, CD45
MPAL diagnosis	
Myeloid	MPO, monocytic differentiation (2 of lysozyme, CD11c, CD14, CD64)
B lineage	CD19 strong with one of OR CD19 weak with two of: CD79a, CD22, CD10
T lineage	cCD3 or sCD3

(AML: acute myeloid leukemia; cCD: cytoplasmic clusters of differentiation; CD: clusters of differentiation; iMPO: intracellular myeloperoxidase; MPAL: mixed-phenotype acute leukemia; sCD: surface clusters of differentiation)

Source: Creutzig U, van den Heuvel-Eibrink MM, Gibson B, Dworzak MN, Adachi S, de Bont E, et al. Diagnosis and management of acute myeloid leukemia in children and adolescents: recommendations from an international expert panel. Blood. 2012;120(16):3187-205.

The minimum panel recommended to use for diagnosis of AML to fulfil World Health Organization (WHO) and European Group for the Immunological Characterization of Leukemias (EGIL) criteria include: CD34, CD117, CD11b, CD11c, CD13, CD14, CD15, CD33, CD64, CD65, iMPO, lysozyme, CD41, and CD61.[3]

2. Are all AMLs the same? How do we risk stratify a new case of AML?

The treatment of AML has long remained a challenge to pediatric hematoncologists.

Retrospective analysis of the AML Berlin-Frankfurt-Munster (BFM) trials found that the 5 years probability of overall survival (OS) has increased from 49 (years 1987–1992) to 76% (years 2010–2012) without much change in the rate of relapse and nonresponse. On further analysis, three main factors were identified by this group as contributing to improved outcomes, the first being *intensification of first-line therapy*, the second being *better supportive care*, and the third *salvage therapies in nonresponders and relapsed AML*. Of the three, the last factor was found to have contributed most significantly and consistently to improved outcomes.[4] This observation emphasizes the importance of early identification of patients that are likely to be at high risk for nonresponse/relapse in order to institute salvage therapies early.

3. How do we identify these so-called "high-risk AMLs"?

Risk stratification of pediatric acute myeloid leukemia (pAML) at baseline is guided by the identification of certain known "favorable risk" and "adverse risk" genetic alterations. Since these have a prognostic and therapeutic significance, the International BFM Study Group

AML Committee recommends cytogenetics and molecular studies as a part of the baseline diagnostic workup in AML.

At the time of initial bone marrow studies, the following are recommended:[3]
- Cytogenetics/FISH (fluorescence in situ hybridization) with AT LEAST the following:
  - t(8;21)(q22;q22)/RUNX1-RUNX1T1
  - inv(16)(p13.1q22) or t(16;16)(p13.1;q22)/CBFB-MYH11
  - t(15;17)(q22;q21)/PML-RARA
  - MLL
- Molecular genetics reverse transcription-polymerase chain reaction/next-generation sequencing (RT-PCR/NGS) to identify AT LEAST the following:
  - FLT3-ITD
  - WT1
  - C-KIT
  - CEBPA (double mutation)
  - NPM1
  - Specific MLL-abnormalities with favorable or very poor prognosis (e.g., MLL-AF1Q, AF6, AF10)

On the basis of the above, AML may be classified at baseline into standard risk (i.e., presence of a favorable risk genetic alteration), high risk (i.e., presence of an adverse risk genetic alteration), and intermediate risk (i.e., presence of neither known favorable nor known adverse risk genetics).

4. What is the role of NGS in initial workup of a case of AML?

The role of NGS in the initial workup of a case of AML lies in the following four areas:
1. *Risk stratification:* Genetic alterations form an important part of initial risk stratification for AML. The latest ELN 2022 risk categorization includes a variety of molecular abnormalities, including NPM, FLT3 ITD, CEBPA, TP53, ASXL 1, BCOR, RUNX1, SF3B1, and others. While a targeted NGS panel may be useful to detect known genetic abnormalities for risk stratification, some important genes such as CEBPA (a GC-rich area which is difficult to amplify by PCR) and FLT3 ITD (variably sized due to internal tandem duplications) may require more specialized NGS-based approaches.[5]
2. *Response assessment by NGS-based minimal residual disease (MRD):* The approaches to MRD measurement in AML are enumerated below. NGS-based MRD holds an advantage especially at the time of subsequent relapse, when small subclones present at diagnosis may be picked up as the dominant clone subsequently at relapse.[6]
3. *Identification of novel fusion partners:* RNA-based NGS targeted at the known clinically relevant genes to identify novel fusion partners, expanding our understanding of the molecular drivers of AML.[6]
4. *Identification of potentially targetable lesions:* Potentially targetable lesions are being increasingly explored in adult as well as pAML, examples of these being FLT3–ITD mutations and IDH1/IDH2 mutations. In fact, the modifying effect of FLT3-ITD inhibitor midostaurin in AML therapy has been a factor in moving FLT3 ITD from adverse risk to intermediate risk (regardless of allelic ratio) in the ELN 2022 risk stratification.[5]

5. What are the implications of risk stratification in AML at therapy onset?

The first important implication is on treatment. While induction courses remain uniform regardless of risk stratification, the choice of method of consolidation may vary. There is consensus that standard risk AMLs will not benefit from hematopoietic stem cell transplantation (HSCT), however, guidelines are less clear in higher-risk cases. Though there has been evidence to suggest that there is a significantly lower relapse risk in patients undergoing allo-HSCT, this may or may not imply an improvement in survival.[4,7-9] Therefore, the International BFM Study Group AML Committee recommends consideration of benefit versus toxicity of allogeneic HSCT at first remission for high-risk and certain intermediate-risk cases who have MRD positive.[3]

The second important implication of risk stratification is on prognostication. Treatment of any pAML is often an arduous journey, and families of children with pAML require careful counseling with due consideration given to treatment-related morbidity and mortality, possibility and costs of an HSCT, and expected survival as well as long-term toxicities. A baseline high-risk stratification [with current event-free survival (EFS) rates of just 28%][10] would require prior preparation of the family with regards to the possibility of relapse and options thereafter.

CASE *(Continued)*

L was started on chemotherapy in February 2018. He received induction containing 3 + 7 regime of daunorubicin and cytarabine. Postinduction marrow was in remission.

6. What is the structure of treatment of a case of AML? When do we assess response?

The current consensus on treatment involves two phases, induction and consolidation. Induction consists of two courses and usually is composed of a backbone of cytarabine with an anthracycline, while consolidation (also called "intensification") consists of two to three courses of high-dose cytarabine with or without mitoxantrone. In higher-risk patients, this consolidation is carried out with HSCT rather than chemotherapy.[11]

The AML committee of the BFM study group recommends response assessment at the end of the first and second course of induction, with complete remission (CR) being defined as <5% blasts in bone marrow, absence of any blasts with Auer rods, and absence of extramedullary disease, having achieved the independence of red cell transfusions, absolute neutrophil counts (ANC) of >1,000/µL and platelet count exceeding 80,000/µL. An additional provision for CR with incomplete recovery (CRi) is allowed in which remaining criteria for remission are met in the absence of ANC or platelet thresholds. CRi is currently a definition used predominantly for trial purposes, however, rather than in routine clinical management.

Apart from molecular genetics and cytogenetics, response to the first course of therapy is the most important indicator of outcome in AML.[3]

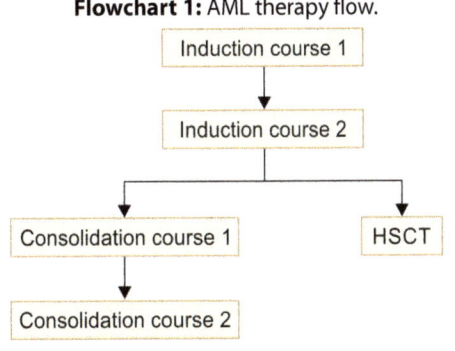

Flowchart 1: AML therapy flow.

(HSCT: stem cell transplantation)

Various studies, including those by the Medical Research Council (MRC) 10 study group and the Nordic group, have found that outcomes varied significantly between those who achieve CR and those who achieve an intermediate response at the end of the first induction, with the British group finding that 5-year survival fell from 53 to 44% and the Nordic group found that EFS fell from 61 to 35%.[9,12] Both these groups, however, used only morphological CR criteria for assessment, which leaves us with the question, what is the role of MRD in AML.

7. What is the role of MRD in AML?

Minimal residual disease, simply put, refers to low levels of residual leukemia that cannot be detected by morphologic assessment alone. The role of MRD has been long well established in the management of pediatric acute lymphoblastic leukemia (ALL), its role in AML is gaining prominence as well. A systematic review and meta-analysis of 81 trials published in 2020 found that the estimated OS and estimated 5-year disease-free survival (DFS) for patients without MRD were 68 and 64%, respectively, which fell to 34 and 25% respectively in those with MRD.[13]

The challenges faced by the widespread adoption of MRD assessment in AML are the lack of standardization and comparability among the various available assays.[8] To address this issue, in 2021, the European Leukemia Net MRD working party published recommendations for technical standards of flow and molecular-based MRD, as well as MRD thresholds and definitions for MRD response. While the full details of this document are beyond the scope of this chapter, briefly; PCR-based MRD monitoring is recommended in patients with mutant NPM1, RUNX1-RUNX1T1, and CBFB–MYH11, and remaining patients should be monitored using multiparametric flow cytometry-based MRD.[8]

Recommended thresholds for MRD negativity are <0.1% of CD45 cells expressing target phenotype in flow-based MRD and a cycling threshold of at least 40 in 2 of 3 replicates (with at least 10,000 copies of the selected housekeeping gene). Optimal thresholds for NGS-based MRD are yet to be defined for various genes and time points.[8]

8. What are the treatment implications if MRD is positive?

Various study groups, including the Nordic group, Children's Oncology Group (COG), and the Italian group, have since explored the implication of MRD on therapy, many finding that a positive MRD (>0.1%) at the end of induction-2 is a poor prognostic feature and has suggested intensification of therapy in such patients including using of HSCT as consolidation therapy. Based on these findings, MRD positivity has been used in addition to molecular genetics to risk stratify AML, especially those patients in intermediate risk categories as per genetics.[14-16] The AML02 multicenter trial used response to treatment as an additional risk stratification factor. Apart from baseline molecular and cytogenetics group, patients with ≥25% blasts post first induction or positive MRD after first-three courses were assigned to the "high risk" strata, in whom HSCT would be done in all cases where feasible. Their findings were that there was no difference in OS between high-risk patients undergoing HSCT ($n = 48$) or receiving chemotherapy; however, when they analyzed only high-risk patients with MRD >1% after induction 1, OS was better among those who underwent HSCT compared with those who did not: 43.5% (12.4) versus 23.1% (10.1; $p = 0.14$), findings that are likely to justify the consideration of HSCT in these patients when logistics and donor availability allow for it.[17]

9. What are the current treatment regimens being used by major study groups?

The most recently concluded AML upfront treatment trial protocols by the MRC and BFM groups, along with the outcomes of both, are given in **Table 2**.

TABLE 2: Summary of recently concluded trials by MRC and BFM groups.

Study	MRC AML 15[18]	BFM AML 2004[19,20]

Stratification	Based on cytogenetics
	Favorable:
	• t(8;21)
	• t(15;17)
	• inv(16)
	(alone or with other abnormalities)
	Intermediate:
	• Abnormalities not classified as favorable or adverse, *or*, lack of identifiable cytogenetic abnormalities
	Adverse:
	• –5
	• –7
	• del(5q) abnormal 3q complex karyotype
		SR:
		• M1/M2 with Auer rods
		• *M4eo or favorable cytogenetics*:
		   – t(8:21)
		   – t(16:16) or inv(16)
		• BM blasts <5% on day 15
		• All FAB M3 patients
		HR:
		• Those not meeting the criteria for SR
		• SR patients found to be positive for FLT3 ITD

Induction	Ara C + DA versus Ara C + DA + Etoposide (ADE) versus Fludarabine + Cytarabine + Idarubicin + G-CSF (FLAG IDA) In induction course 1, all three groups were also randomly assigned to receive/not receive a single dose of GO	Cytarabine + Idarubicin + Etoposide (AIE) versus Cytarabine + L-DNR + Etoposide (ADxE) *Induction 2 for SR patients*: Cytarabine + Idarubicin (AI) *Induction 2 for HR patients*: High-dose cytarabine 3 g/m^2 + High-dose cytarabine and mitoxantrone
Reassessment	18–21 days from the end of course 1 → 15% or more blasts → HR irrespective of the initial risk	• On day 15, patients were stratified into SR or HR • Postinduction 1: Response to induction therapy • Postinduction 2: Decision for HSCT (after 2006)
Consolidation	• Amsacrine + Cytarabine + Etoposide followed by Mitoxantrone + Cytarabine 1 g/m^2 (MACE-MiDAC) versus high-dose ARAC (HiDAC) 3 g/m^2 versus HidAC 1.5 g/m^2 • All three groups were randomly assigned to receive/not receive a single dose of GO in the first course of consolidation • Further all patients were randomized to either receive a third consolidation or stop after two courses (i.e., a total of four vs. five courses)	All SR patients received HAM • *HR patients randomized*: Cytarabine 0.5 g/m^2 + Idarubicin + Cladribine (AI/2-CDA) versus Cytarabine 0.5 g/m^2 + Idarubicin (AI) • *Intensification*: High-dose cytarabine and etoposide in SR, HAM followed by HSCT in HR, 1-year maintenance with IT cytarabine, and randomization between 12 and 18 Gy CRT (stopped in 2009)
HSCT	Permitted for intermediate or HR disease	Pre-2006 HSCT to all HR patients at CR1 when feasible; after 2006 HR patients with BM blasts >5% after second induction

Contd...

Contd...

Study	MRC AML 15[18]	BFM AML 2004[19,20]
Outcomes	*Induction:* • No benefit in rate or durability of response with the addition of Etoposide • FLAG IDA significantly better relapse-free survival but greater hematologic toxicity • The benefit of FLAG IDA in all groups, including poor-risk patients. Idarubicin lower dose of 8 mg/m² also shows benefits • Patients who received only two courses of FLAG IDA (no consolidation) had similar outcomes to DA/ADE with consolidation *Consolidation:* • MACE/MidAC is equivalent to HiDAC in favorable and intermediate risk but superior in adverse risk. (Finding in adult subjects as a proportion of pediatric adverse risk patients was very low) • MACE/MidAC had more hematologic toxicity • No significant difference between HidAC 3 g/m² and 1.5 g/m² • No benefit of a fifth course GO • The benefit of addition of 3 mg/m² single dose in induction in favorable and intermediate groups, not adverse groups • No benefit of the addition of GO in consolidation (*Note:* These conclusions were from a mixed population, not from a pediatric population)	*Induction:* • Benefits seen in patients with t(8:21) with L-DNR • Overall patient population, the initial blast count on day 15 was better with Idarubicin, but two cohorts no longer different on day 28 → reflects prolonged action of L-DNR *Consolidation:* • Similar overall survival with and without the addition of Cladribine • Tolerable toxicity profile of Cladribine
Further studies	*MyeChild 01* is planned to build on findings of previous studies in regard to four main areas: 1. *Randomization 1:* (To find optimum anthracycline to use during induction) Mitoxantrone and Cytarabine versus L-DA and Cytarabine 2. *Randomization 2:* (Dose finding study for GO) single dose 3 mg/m² versus two doses of 3 mg/m² each in induction (further planned to increase to three doses based on safety data) 3. *Randomization 3:* (Addition of Fludarabine to consolidation) Fludarabine and Cytarabine versus high-dose Cytarabine 4. *Randomization 4:* (To check outcomes of reduced intensity conditioning in AML HSCT) RIC versus MAC prior to allogeneic HSCT	*BFM AML 2012* was planned to study the difference in outcomes in pediatric AML patients when cytarabine, liposomal daunorubicin and clofarabine (*ADxC*) were randomized against the standard induction course of cytarabine, etoposide, and L-DNR (*ADxE*). Unfortunately, enrolment was terminated early due to the cessation of availability of L-DNR[21]

(AML: acute myeloid leukemia; ADE: ara-C, daunorubicin, and etoposide; BFM: Berlin-Frankfurt-Munster; BM: bone marrow; CRT: crania radiotherapy; DNR: daunorubicin; FLAG: fludrabine cytarabine G-CSF; GO: gemtuzumab ozogamicin; G-CSF: granulocyte colony-stimulating factor; HiDAC: high dose cytarabine; HSCT: hematopoietic stem cell transplantation; HR: high risk; IDA: idarubicin; L-DA: liposomal daunorubicin; MACE: amsacrine cytarabine etoposide; MRC: Medical Research Council; MiDAC: mitoxantrone and intermediate dose cytarabine; MAC: myeloablative conditioning; RIC: reduced intensity conditioning; SR: standard risk)

10. Apart from chemotherapy, what is the role of targeted therapies in first-time AML?

In 2018, Bolouri et al. published the findings of the COG TARGET initiative, which aimed to describe the molecular landscape of pAML. This data was collected from 1,023 patients who had been enrolled in previous COG AML studies. Some of the key findings were:[22]

- *Most common mutated genes*: RAS, KIT, FLT3
- IDH1 and 2 mutations are exceedingly rare in pAML.
- Epigenetic regulators like KMT2A and WT1 showed a higher mutation rate than in adults.
- Some novel focal deletions (IL9R, MBNL1, ZEB2) and fusion genes (*CBFA2T3-GLIS2, NUP98-NSD1*) seem to be almost exclusively associated with pAML.

Data emerging from this and related studies suggest that there will be an increasing role for targeted therapies in pAML in the years to come. As described in a review by Yu et al. targeted therapies in AML can be broadly classified into three categories:[23]

1. Therapies targeting oncogenic mutations (e.g., FLT3 inhibitors).
2. Therapies targeting metabolic or maintenance pathways (e.g., epigenetic modifiers like hypomethylating agents).
3. Targeted delivery of cytotoxic agents [e.g., antibody drug conjugates (ADC) like gemtuzumab ozogamicin].

Current ongoing studies for some of the important agents in upfront pediatric AML are presented in **Table 3**. The role of targeted therapies in relapsed/refractory pAML will be summarized later in the chapter.

TABLE 3: Studies for targeted therapy in upfront pediatric AML.

Target/Mechanism	Drug	Evidence/Ongoing studies
FLT3 inhibitors	Midostaurin	*NCT03591510:* Ongoing phase II study, in children with FLT ITD allelic ration of 0.5 or greater, previously untreated—phase 1 is a dose-finding study, followed by phase 2 to evaluate efficacy (EFS at 24 months) tolerability and safety[24]
	Gilteritinib	*COG AAML 1831:* Phase III trial ongoing to compare standard chemotherapy with liposomal cytarabine + daunorubicin (CPX 351) with or without Gilteritinib (ongoing)
	Sorafenib	*COG AAML 1031:* Sorafenib + chemotherapy, post-HSCT maintenance sorafenib in high allelic ratio FLT3 ITD + AML improved CR rates and EFS[25]
ADC, CD33 antibody	GO	• *MRC AML 15:* Survival benefit good and intermediate risk cytogenetics[18] • *COG AAML 0531:* One dose each of GO added to ADE induction and MA (MiDAC) consolidation—significant improvement in EFS, no improvement in OS, increased toxicity and neutropenia[26] • *NOPHO AML 2004:* AML patients not undergoing HSCT were randomly assigned to receive two doses of GO postconsolidation, with no improvement in survival compared to no further treatment[27] • *MYECHILD 01:* Ongoing, dose-finding for GO, one dose during induction versus two doses (to increase to three depending on safety data)

(ADC: antibody drug conjugates; AML: acute myelogenous leukemia; CR: complete remission; COG: Children's Oncology Group; EFS: event-free survival; GO: gemtuzumab ozogamicin; HSCT: hematopoietic stem cell transplantation; MRC: Medical Research Council; MA: mitoxantrone and cytarabine; MiDAC: mitoxantrone and intermediate dose cytarabine)

Source: Lonetti A, Pession A, Masetti R. Targeted therapies for pediatric AML: gaps and perspective. Front Pediatr. 2019 Nov 15;7:463.

CASE (Continued)

L received induction-2 (one more cycle of daunorubicin and cytarabine). During the course, he had one episode of invasive aspergillosis, which was successfully treated.

11. Children with AML have a high incidence of infections; what can be done to prevent the same? What is the role of antifungal and antibacterial prophylaxis?

While infectious complications are seen in almost all patients undergoing treatment for cancer, children with leukemia, especially AML, are especially susceptible. Various studies have shown that patients with AML experience, on average, three infectious episodes during therapy, with <3% of all patients remaining free from infections.

Indian studies on AML have shown that infectious complications occur in up to 64% of all patients.[28] One study found that 100% of their AML patients had an episode of febrile neutropenia (FN) during induction chemotherapy, with 65% having positive blood cultures.[29] Patients with AML also have a high incidence of invasive fungal infections with Indian data revealing incidence ranging anywhere between 3 and 55%, with the highest numbers found during induction.[30,31]

The Infectious Diseases Society of America (IDSA) constituted a clinical practice guideline for the use of antibacterial prophylaxis in pediatric cancer and HSCT in which they recommend that one may consider systemic antibacterial prophylaxis administration in children with AML and relapsed ALL receiving intensive chemotherapy expected to result in severe neutropenia (ANC < 500 µL for at least 7 days).[32] The basis of this recommendation is a large study published in 2018 by Alexander et al. that compared levofloxacin versus no prophylaxis in children with acute leukemia and those undergoing HSCT. Of the 200 patients with acute leukemia, they found that the likelihood of bacteremia was significantly lower in the levofloxacin prophylaxis group than in the control group (21.9 vs. 43.4%). FN was also less common in the levofloxacin group (71.2 vs. 82.1%), and there was no significant increase in the risk of invasive fungal disease (IFD), Clostridium difficile-associated diarrhea, or musculoskeletal toxicity in the group receiving levofloxacin.[33] This recommendation has, however, been termed as a weak one by the expert panel due to reservations regarding the emergence of resistant strains as demonstrated in two studies[34,35] also the uncertain implications of widespread use of fluoroquinolones (FQ) prophylaxis over longer treatment periods and the possible emergence of cross-resistant species. At this time, the use of antibacterial prophylaxis in patients with first time AML remains an institutional decision, to be taken after carefully weighing possible risks and benefits.

With regards to antifungal prophylaxis, evidence is clearer, with IDSA making a strong recommendation toward the use of antifungal prophylaxis in children and adolescents with AML receiving treatment expected to cause prolonged or profound neutropenia. The basis for the recommendation is a systematic review that found that compared with no systemic prophylaxis, systemic antifungal prophylaxis significantly reduced proven or probable IFD, proven or probable yeast, and fungal infection-related mortality, with the reduction in probable and proven IFD being the greatest in those at greatest risk for the same. Antifungal prophylaxis is hence widely used in AML. Further, they recommend using a mold-active antifungal, as compared with fluconazole would significantly reduce proven or probable IFD, mold infections, and invasive aspergillosis as well as fungal infection-related mortality.[36]

A systematic review and meta-analysis published in 2020 of five randomized controlled trials (RCTs) with 1,617 participants found that posaconazole prophylaxis significantly reduces the risk of invasive fungal infections as compared to other antifungal agents, however, the fact that the drug is currently only approved in children 13 years of age and above precludes its widespread use in pAML.[37]

12. Is the use of granulocyte colony-stimulating factor (G-CSF) safe in children with AML?

Granulocyte colony-stimulating factor has been used during the therapy of many solid tumors, both as primary prophylaxis to reduce the duration and depth of neutropenia postmyelosuppressive chemotherapy. Its use in AML is less well established. Earlier concerns of G-CSF increasing the risk of relapse have now been largely disproved, with various studies showing no increase in relapse rates and no difference in remission and OS in those patients who receive G-CSF during therapy.[38] The effectiveness of G-CSF in preventing infection in AML is yet to be established. In the AML BFM 98 trial, 538 patients with AML were randomized to receive or not receive prophylactic G-CSF at the end of induction chemotherapy. It was found that there was no significant effect on the incidence of FN, documented infections, infection-associated mortality, or EFS; only the time of neutropenia was significantly reduced.[39]

In contrast, a study from the Korean University AML registry found that prophylactic G-CSF in AML reduced infection-related deaths without affecting remission relapse or OS. The American Society of Clinical Oncology (ASCO), in their clinical practice guidelines on growth factor usage, *do not* recommend the use of prophylactic G-CSF in nonrelapsed AML and recommend its use in the presence of infections only in case of presence of risk factors for poor outcomes, for example, hemodynamic instability. A retrospective study by Relling et al. found an increased risk of therapy-related acute myeloid leukemia (tAML) in patients who received G-CSF along with topoisomerase inhibitors would further caution us in the use of G-CSF in etoposide-containing protocols.[40]

CASE (Continued)

L received two cycles of high-dose ARAC and completed treatment in July of 2018. End of treatment marrow was in remission. Echocardiography done post-treatment revealed diastolic cardiac dysfunction, for which he was started on cardioprotection (enalapril).

13. In addition to infections, drug toxicity contributes to treatment-related mortality. What are the current protocols used, and how effective are they in reducing toxicity?

With gradually improving outcomes in pAML, efforts have been made in recent years to optimize treatment schedules to achieve these outcomes with the least possible toxicity.

As mentioned earlier, the treatment of pAML in most protocols involves a total four or five courses of chemotherapy, of which the latter two or three courses are often consolidation blocks centered around high-dose cytarabine. In an effort to reduce the exposure to cytarabine, the COG group compared the results of the AAML1031 trial using four courses (a cumulative cytarabine dose of 21.6 g/m^2) with those of the AAML0531 trial using five courses (a cumulative cytarabine dose of 45.6 g/m^2), they found that in the subset of low-risk

(LR) patients who had no favorable or unfavorable cytogenetics with the end of induction MRD negative, DFS was significantly less with four courses, OS was also less, but this was not statistically significant. On the other hand, children with favorable risk cytogenetics were not found to have any statistically significant differences in outcomes.[41] The MRC 15 study group, on the other hand, found no benefit in the addition of a fifth course in any of their patients.[18]

The MRC 15 study also had significant findings in the area of cytarabine doses in adults. Compared to 3 g/m^2, 1.5 g/m^2 cytarabine had a trend toward higher relapse risk but no difference in OS. However, it was noted that the 3 g/m^2 arm had a significantly higher requirement of supportive care and hematological toxicity, suggesting that 1.5 g/m^2 may be a sufficient dose in consolidation to achieve remission with reduced toxicity however this remains to be studied in the pediatric age group.[18]

Etoposide, an important drug used as a part of induction in many AML protocols, is known to cause therapy-related leukemia. Various studies have looked into the dose of etoposide at which this risk increases, with one study finding a 3.3% risk of secondary leukemia in 6 years in doses as low as <1.5 g/m^2.[42] Many trials used etoposide as a part of their induction chemotherapy, with some adding etoposide into later courses as well. The COG 0531 used 1.75 g/m^2 of etoposide, the COG 1031 between 1.5 and 2.2 g/m^2 depending on randomization, and the ADE arm of MRC 15 used 1 g/m^2 of etoposide.[26,43] The MRC 15 trial compared the traditional ADE with an etoposide free arm using only 12 hourly cytarabine with three doses of daunorubicin and found that they were equivalent with respect to relapse risk, deaths in remission, relapse-free survival, and OS, opening up the possibility of using etoposide-free protocols in the future with a corresponding decrease in secondary leukemia.[18]

14. Which patients may require dosage modification during treatment?

Though comorbidities at treatment initiation are a concern encountered more frequently in the elderly, it is important to take into account any possible requirements of dosage modification prior to initiation of therapy. As a part of baseline workup, the BFM AML study group recommends the following:[3]

Assessment of WHO performance status:
1. Physical examination for syndromes and comorbidities
2. Biochemistry (liver and renal functions)
3. Coagulation tests
4. Chest X-ray, 12 lead electrocardiogram (ECG), and echocardiography
5. Hepatitis A, B, C, and cytomegalovirus (CMV).

In addition, each individual centers have various protocols for screening for infections at baseline prior to treatment induction; for example, at our center we screen with a tuberculin skin test, computed tomography (CT) of the chest and paranasal sinuses, and a serum galactomannan, while some other centers also include a rectal screening swab for extended-spectrum beta-lactamase resistant organisms.

The following situations may warrant dosage modification:
- *Cardiac dysfunction:* A left ventricular ejection fraction of 45% is the most commonly used threshold while deciding on the use of anthracyclines in therapy. This cutoff is largely based on adult studies, especially in patients with breast cancer. In patients with cardiac dysfunction detected at baseline, an option of HidAC-based therapy instead of

anthracycline-based may be considered; however therapy must be decided based on the risk–benefit of the individual case.

- *Liver dysfunction:*
  - Anthracyclines are metabolized primarily by the liver, and administration of anthracyclines in the context of liver dysfunction may worsen doxorubicin-related toxicity, especially myelosuppression. A study done over 40 years ago by Benjamin et al. exploring bilirubin adjusted dosage of doxorubicin recommended the following modifications **(Table 4)**:[44]

TABLE 4: Anthracycline dose modification in liver dysfunction.[44]

Bilirubin mg/dL	Transaminases	Dose
3.0–5.0	Any	50%
5.0–7.0	Any	25%
>7.0	Any	With hold
<3.0	Any	No adjustment

Adapted from: Benjamin RS, Wiernik PH, Bachur NR. Adriamycin chemotherapy-efficacy, safety and pharmacologic basis of an intermittent single high-dosage schedule, Cancer 1974:33(1)19-27.

The above cutoffs have widely been incorporated into practice. It is important to bear in mind that these cutoffs are based on adult studies, and metabolism in the pediatric age group may vary.

Subsequently Donelli et al. 1998 suggested no dosage adjustment below 3.0 mg/dL and to withhold the drug above that cutoff.[45] Some isolated case reports have described unmodified doses even in bilirubin >5.0 mg/dL.

- Cytarabine is metabolized in the liver, but a part of it is excreted unchanged by the kidney. Following rapid intravenous (IV) infusion of cytarabine, 90% of the dose is excreted as inactive metabolite uridine arabinoside while 10% is excreted unmetabolized. Though uniform recommendations are lacking, Floyd et al. suggest a 50% reduction of cytarabine dose in the presence of elevated transaminases.[46] The Indian Collaborative Childhood Leukemia group (ICiCLe) suggests the following dose adjustments in their ALL protocols **(Table 5)**.

TABLE 5: Cytarabine dose modification in liver dysfunction.

Bilirubin mg/dL	Transaminases	Dose reduction
2.0–3.0	>3 × ULN	50%
3.0–5.0		25%
>5.0		Withhold

(ULN: upper limits of normal)
Adapted from: Indian Collaborative Childhood Leukemia group (ICiCLE) protocol for ALL treatment.

- Etoposide toxicity depends on liver function in two different ways. It is metabolized by the liver and partially cleared in the bile; hence liver dysfunction causes delayed clearance. The other mechanism is due to reduced serum albumin, which results in a greater fraction of unbound etoposide. Studies have shown that mild to moderate liver

dysfunction (1–2 mg/dL) may not effect etoposide metabolism, but higher bilirubin levels may require dose reduction, though specific guidelines are lacking.[47]
- *Renal dysfunction:* Dosages of anthracyclines, etoposide, and cytarabine all require adjustment as per the glomerular filtration rate (GFR) of the patient are given in **Table 6**.[48]

TABLE 6: Anthracycline, etoposide and cytarabine dose modification in renal dysfunction.

Drug	Creatinine/Creatinine clearance	Adjustment
Daunorubicin	>3 mg/dL	50% of the dose
Etoposide	15–50 mL/min	75% of the dose
	<15 mL/min	Withhold
Cytarabine	40–60 mL/min	• If dose >2 g/m^2, decrease to 1 g/m^2 • If dose 0.75–1 g/m^2, decrease to 0.5 g/m^2
	<40 mL/min	If dose >0.75 g/m^2/dose, divide to give 200 mg/m^2/day

Adapted from: McLeod HL, Clinically relevant drug-drug interactions in oncology, Br J Clin Pharm. 1998:45(6) 539-44.

- *Malnutrition:* A study in Brazil on the nutritional status at diagnosis of cancer found that up to 23% of the screened children were undernourished (MUAC for age Z scores).[49] A similar study in Pakistan, specifically on children with AML, found that 22.3% of patients were moderately malnourished and 15.5% were severely malnourished, and this significantly impacted outcome, with worse OS and DFS and higher treatment-related mortality in children with malnutrition.[50] Children who are malnourished at the onset of chemotherapy may require dosage adjustment, but, more importantly require aggressive nutritional rehabilitation. A comparative experimental study in Netherlands on pediatric cancer patients with malnutrition found that while 21% of children on nonstructured nutritional rehabilitation achieved their target weight in 16 weeks, protocolized tube feeding resulted in 100% of the patients achieving target weight,[51] evidence that suggests that a structured tube feeding regimen may be of value in such patients.

REFERENCES

1. Arber DA, Orazi A, Hasserjian RP, Borowitz MJ, Calvo KR, Kvasnicka HM, et al. International consensus classification of myeloid neoplasms and acute leukemia: integrating morphological, clinical, and genomic data. Blood. 2022;140(11):1200-28.
2. Döhner H, Estey E, Grimwade D, Amadori S, Appelbaum FR, Büchner T, et al. Diagnosis and management of AML in adults: 2017 ELN recommendations from an international expert panel. 2017;129(4):424-47.
3. Creutzig U, van den Heuvel-Eibrink MM, Gibson B, Dworzak MN, Adachi S, de Bont E, et al. Diagnosis and management of acute myeloid leukemia in children and adolescents: recommendations from an international expert panel. Blood. 2012;120(16):3187-205.
4. Rasche M, Zimmermann M, Borschel L, Bourquin JP, Dworzak M, Klingebiel T, et al. Successes and challenges in the treatment of pediatric acute myeloid leukemia: a retrospective analysis of the AML-BFM trials from 1987 to 2012. Leukemia. 2018;32(10):2167-77.
5. Döhner H, Ebert B, Godley L, Levine R, Ossenkoppele G. Diagnosis and management of AML in adults: 2022 ELN recommendations from an International Expert Panel. 2022;58.

6. Levine RL, Valk PJM. Next-generation sequencing in the diagnosis and minimal residual disease assessment of acute myeloid leukemia. Haematologica. 2019;104(5):868-71.
7. Gibson BES, Wheatley K, Hann IM, Stevens RF, Webb D, Hills RK, et al. Treatment strategy and long-term results in paediatric patients treated in consecutive UK AML trials. Leukemia. 2005;19(12):2130-8.
8. Heuser M, Freeman SD, Ossenkoppele GJ, Buccisano F, Hourigan CS, Ngai LL, et al. 2021 Update on MRD in acute myeloid leukemia: a consensus document from the European LeukemiaNet MRD Working Party. Blood. 2021;138(26):2753-67.
9. Abrahamsson J, Forestier E, Heldrup J, Jahnukainen K, Jónsson ÓG, Lausen B, et al. Response-guided induction therapy in pediatric acute myeloid leukemia with excellent remission rate. J Clin Oncol. 2011;29(3):310-5.
10. Conneely SE, Stevens AM. Acute myeloid leukemia in children: emerging paradigms in genetics and new approaches to therapy. Curr Oncol Rep. 2021;23(2):16.
11. Rubnitz JE, Kaspers GJL. How I treat pediatric acute myeloid leukemia. Blood. 2021;138(12):1009-18.
12. Wheatley K, Burnett AK, Goldstone AH, Gray RG, Hann IM, Harrison CJ, et al. A simple, robust, validated and highly predictive index for the determination of risk-directed therapy in acute myeloid leukaemia derived from the MRC AML 10 trial: simple highly predictive index for directing therapy in AML. Br J Haematol. 1999;107(1):69-79.
13. Short NJ, Zhou S, Fu C, Berry DA, Walter RB, Freeman SD, et al. Association of measurable residual disease with survival outcomes in patients with acute myeloid leukemia: a systematic review and meta-analysis. JAMA Oncol. 2020;6(12):1890.
14. Buldini B, Rizzati F, Masetti R, Fagioli F, Menna G, Micalizzi C, et al. Prognostic significance of flow-cytometry evaluation of minimal residual disease in children with acute myeloid leukaemia treated according to the AIEOP-AML 2002/01 study protocol. Br J Haematol. 2017;177(1):116-26.
15. Tierens A, Bjørklund E, Siitonen S, Marquart HV, Wulff-Juergensen G, Pelliniemi TT, et al. Residual disease detected by flow cytometry is an independent predictor of survival in childhood acute myeloid leukaemia; results of the NOPHO-AML 2004 study. Br J Haematol. 2016;174(4):600-9.
16. Loken MR, Alonzo TA, Pardo L, Gerbing RB, Raimondi SC, Hirsch BA, et al. Residual disease detected by multidimensional flow cytometry signifies high relapse risk in patients with de novo acute myeloid leukemia: a report from Children's Oncology Group. Blood. 2012;120(8):1581-8.
17. Rubnitz JE, Inaba H, Dahl G, Ribeiro RC, Bowman WP, Taub J, et al. Minimal residual disease-directed therapy for childhood acute myeloid leukaemia: results of the AML02 multicentre trial. Lancet Oncol. 2010;11(6):543-52.
18. Burnett AK, Russell NH, Hills RK, Hunter AE, Kjeldsen L, Yin J, et al. Optimization of chemotherapy for younger patients with acute myeloid leukemia: results of the Medical Research Council AML15 Trial. J Clin Oncol. 2013;31(27):3360-8.
19. Creutzig U, Zimmermann M, Bourquin JP, Dworzak MN, Fleischhack G, Graf N, et al. Randomized trial comparing liposomal daunorubicin with idarubicin as induction for pediatric acute myeloid leukemia: results from study AML-BFM 2004. Blood. 2013;122(1):37-43.
20. Creutzig U, Zimmermann M, Dworzak M, Bourquin JP, Neuhoff C, Sander A, et al. Study AML-BFM 2004: improved survival in childhood acute myeloid leukemia without increased toxicity. Blood. 2010;116(21):181.
21. Waack K, Schneider M, Walter C, Creutzig U, Klusmann JH, Rasche M, et al. Improved outcome in pediatric AML - the AML-BFM 2012 Study. Blood. 2020;136(Supplement 1):12-4.
22. Bolouri H, Farrar JE, Triche T, Ries RE, Lim EL, Alonzo TA, et al. The molecular landscape of pediatric acute myeloid leukemia reveals recurrent structural alterations and age-specific mutational interactions. Nat Med. 2018;24(1):103-12.
23. Yu J, Jiang PYZ, Sun H, Zhang X, Jiang Z, Li Y, et al. Advances in targeted therapy for acute myeloid leukemia. Biomark Res. 2020;8(1):17.

24. Reinhardt D, Zwaan CM, Hoenekopp A, Niolat J, Ifrah S, Noel-Baron F, et al. Phase II Study of Midostaurin + Chemotherapy in Pediatric Patients with Untreated, newly diagnosed, FLT3-mutated acute myeloid leukemia (AML). Blood. 2019;134(Supplement_1):3835.
25. Pollard JA, Alonzo TA, Gerbing R, Brown P, Fox E, Choi J, et al. Sorafenib in combination with standard chemotherapy for children with high allelic ratio FLT3/ITD+ acute myeloid leukemia: a report from the Children's Oncology Group Protocol AAML1031. J Clin Oncol Off J Am Soc Clin Oncol. 2022;40(18):2023-35.
26. Gamis AS, Alonzo TA, Meshinchi S, Sung L, Gerbing RB, Raimondi SC, et al. Gemtuzumab ozogamicin in children and adolescents with de novo acute myeloid leukemia improves event-free survival by reducing relapse risk: results from the randomized phase III Children's Oncology Group Trial AAML0531. J Clin Oncol. 2014;32(27):3021-32.
27. Hasle H, Abrahamsson J, Forestier E, Ha SY, Heldrup J, Jahnukainen K, et al. Gemtuzumab ozogamicin as postconsolidation therapy does not prevent relapse in children with AML: results from NOPHO-AML 2004. Blood. 2012;120(5):978-84.
28. Gupta A, Singh M, Singh H, Kumar L, Sharma A, Bakhshi S, et al. Infections in acute myeloid leukemia: An analysis of 382 febrile episodes. Med Oncol. 2010;27(4):1037-45.
29. Philip C, George B, Ganapule A, Korula A, Jain P, Alex AA, et al. Acute myeloid leukaemia: challenges and real world data from India. Br J Haematol. 2015;170(1):110-7.
30. Bansal S, Advani S. Pattern of bloodstream infections in patients with hematological malignancies in a tertiary care centre. Indian J Cancer. 2014;51(4):447.
31. Jain H, Rengaraj K, Sharma V, Bonda A, Chanana R, Thorat J, et al. Infection prevalence in adolescents and adults with acute myeloid leukemia treated in an Indian Tertiary Care Center. JCO Glob Oncol. 2020;(6):1684-95.
32. Lehrnbecher T, Fisher BT, Phillips B, Alexander S, Ammann RA, Beauchemin M, et al. Guideline for antibacterial prophylaxis administration in pediatric cancer and hematopoietic stem cell transplantation. Clin Infect Dis. 2020;71(1):226-36.
33. Alexander S, Fisher BT, Gaur AH, Dvorak CC, Luna DV, Dang H, et al. Effect of levofloxacin prophylaxis on bacteremia in children with acute leukemia or undergoing hematopoietic stem cell transplantation: a randomized clinical trial. JAMA. 2018;320(10):995-1004.
34. Saini L, Rostein C, Atenafu EG, Brandwein JM. Ambulatory consolidation chemotherapy for acute myeloid leukemia with antibacterial prophylaxis is associated with frequent bacteremia and the emergence of fluoroquinolone resistant E. Coli. BMC Infect Dis. 2013;13(1):284.
35. Michael C, Neil S, Lucinda B, Claire G, Mark H, Peter S, et al. Antibacterial prophylaxis after chemotherapy for solid tumors and lymphomas. N Engl J Med. 2005;353(10):988-98.
36. Lehrnbecher T, Fisher BT, Phillips B, Beauchemin M, Carlesse F, Castagnola E, et al. Clinical practice guideline for systemic antifungal prophylaxis in pediatric patients with cancer and hematopoietic stem-cell transplantation recipients. J Clin Oncol. 2020;38(27):3205-16.
37. Wong TY, Loo YS, Veettil SK, Wong PS, Divya G, Ching SM, et al. Efficacy and safety of posaconazole for the prevention of invasive fungal infections in immunocompromised patients: a systematic review with meta-analysis and trial sequential analysis. Sci Rep. 2020;10(1):14575.
38. Feng X, Lan H, Ruan Y, Li C. Impact on acute myeloid leukemia relapse in granulocyte colony-stimulating factor application: A meta-analysis. Hematology. 2018;23(9):581-9.
39. Lehrnbecher T, Zimmermann M, Reinhardt D, Dworzak M, Stary J, Creutzig U. Prophylactic human granulocyte colony-stimulating factor after induction therapy in pediatric acute myeloid leukemia. Blood. 2007;109(3):936-43.
40. Relling MV, Boyett JM, Blanco JG, Raimondi S, Behm FG, Sandlund JT, et al. Granulocyte colony-stimulating factor and the risk of secondary myeloid malignancy after etoposide treatment. Blood. 2003;101(10):3862-7.

41. Getz KD, Alonzo TA, Sung L, Meshinchi S, Gerbing RB, Raimondi S, et al. Cytarabine dose reduction in patients with low-risk acute myeloid leukemia: A report from the Children's Oncology Group. Pediatr Blood Cancer. 2022;69(1):e29313.
42. Zhang W, Gou P, Dupret JM, Chomienne C, Rodrigues-Lima F. Etoposide, an anticancer drug involved in therapy-related secondary leukemia: Enzymes at play. Transl Oncol. 2021;14(10):101169.
43. Aplenc R, Meshinchi S, Sung L, Alonzo T, Choi J, Fisher B, et al. Bortezomib with standard chemotherapy for children with acute myeloid leukemia does not improve treatment outcomes: a report from the Children's Oncology Group. Haematologica. 2020;105(7):1879-86.
44. Benjamin RS, Wiernik PH, Bachur NR. Adriamycin chemotherapy—efficacy, safety, and pharmacologic basis of an intermittent single high-dosage schedule. Cancer. 1974;33(1):19-27.
45. Donelli MG, Zucchetti M, Munzone E, D'Incalci M, Crosignani A. Pharmacokinetics of anticancer agents in patients with impaired liver function. Eur J Cancer. 1998;34(1):33-46.
46. Floyd J, Mirza I, Sachs B, Perry MC. Hepatotoxicity of chemotherapy. Semin Oncol. 2006;33(1):50-67.
47. Superfin D, Iannucci AA, Davies AM. Commentary: oncologic drugs in patients with organ dysfunction: A summary. Oncologist. 2007;12(9):1070-83.
48. McLeod HL. Clinically relevant drug-drug interactions in oncology. Br J Clin Pharmacol. 1998;45(6):539-44.
49. Viani K, Barr RD, Filho VO, Ladas EJ. Nutritional status at diagnosis among children with cancer referred to a nutritional service in Brazil. Hematol Transfus Cell Ther. 2021;43(4):389-95.
50. Ghafoor T, Ahmed S, Khalil S, Farah T. Impact of malnutrition on treatment outcome of paediatric acute myeloid leukemia. J Coll Physicians Surg Pak. 2020;30(10):1021-5.
51. den Broeder E, Lippens RJ, van't Hof MA, Tolboom JJ, van Staveren WA, Hofman Z, et al. Effects of naso-gastric tube feeding on the nutritional status of children with cancer. Eur J Clin Nutr. 1998;52(7):494-500.

EXPERT OPINION

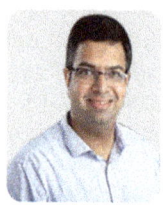

Venkatraman Radhakrishnan MD DM MSc
Professor and Head
Department of Medical Oncology, Cancer Institute (W.I.A)
38, Sardar Patel Road, Chennai, Tamil Nadu, India, Pin: 600036

1. Are all AMLs the same? How do you treat AML according to the risk stratification? What are the implications of risk stratification in AML at therapy onset?

Not all AMLs are the same. There is evidence that adult and pAML are biologically different. Compared to adult AMLs, pAMLs are less likely to be associated with underlying myelodysplastic syndrome (MDS). Inherited causes of AML, like Downs syndrome and bone marrow failure syndromes, are common in children. Adolescents and young adults likely behave more like adult AML than pAML. A normal karyotype is less common in children compared to adults (10 vs. 40%). MLL mutation is more common in children <2 years of age (<5% in adults, up to 60% in infants). Genomic alterations (TET2, DNMT3A, RUNX1) are rare in children. Pediatric patients have higher FLT3 mutations and lesser NPM1 mutations compared to adults. IDH, DNMT3, and TP53 mutations are more common in adults.

Pediatric acute myeloid leukemia can be risk stratified based on:
- Cytogenetic risk stratification at diagnosis.
- MRD at the end of induction chemotherapy.

The choice of chemotherapy is not influenced by the risk stratification. However, patients with intermediate and adverse risks have poor outcomes and should be offered transplants in their first remission.

2. Do you think NGS/chromosomal microarray analysis (CMA)/array comparative genomic hybridization (aCGH) has any role in the management of AML upfront?

Data is evolving. NGS can pick up mutations at a lower level. However, the importance of many mutations detected by NGS in pAML remains unknown. Conventional karyotyping should be done for all patients at diagnosis. If NGS is not available or expensive, then PCR testing for common core binding factor (CBF) translocations (8;21, inv 16) and mutations (NPM, FLT3, CEBPA, and IDH) should be performed.

3. Do you recommend doing pretreatment infections work in AML? What is the role of doing rectal swabs? Is there any role of low-dose chemotherapy upfront when AML patients present with infection?

Patients presenting with fever or features of infection should be evaluated to identify the focus of infection. We get a baseline HRCT chest to rule out fungal infections in asymptomatic patients. We do not do rectal swabs but send stool cultures to identify multidrug resistant (MDR) bacteria colonization. We have published a study to show that stool MDR colonization is associated with increased mortality during leukemia induction. Rectal swabs can cause mucosal damage and, therefore, should be avoided.

4. Which induction regimen do you follow at your center and why? What is your experience of treating AML induction with three drugs regimen [ara-C, daunorubicin, and etoposide (ADE)] versus two drugs (AD)?

We conducted a trial comparing daunorubicin and ARA-C (DA) induction chemotherapy versus ADE in pAML. The study randomized 149 patients. There was no difference in EFS, OS, and toxicities between the DA and ADE arms. However, in subgroup analysis, patients <10 years of age, those with extramedullary disease, and normal nutrition status had better survival with the ADE regimen. We have devised an algorithm based on age, nutritional status, and extramedullary disease to decide if DA or ADE induction should be used.

5. What is the role of MRD in the management of AML? What dose of cytosine arabinoside (ARA-C) do you prefer for the consolidation for a favorable risk AML with the end of induction negative MRD (ARA-C 3 g/m^2 vs. 1.5 g/m^2)?

The role of MRD in AML is evolving. A cut of 0.1% MRD is taken positive. There is no consensus on the timing and level of MRD. Patients with MRD-positive diseases do worse than MRD-negative diseases. Patients with CBF AML can have MRD positivity for longer, which does not seem to affect the prognosis. MRD might be helpful in deciding which patients with intermediate risk should be taken up for transplant.

6. What is the role of maintenance chemotherapy in AML? Share your experience.

We do not practice maintenance chemotherapy. There is no clear evidence that maintenance chemotherapy in AML improves survival.

7. Apart from chemotherapy, what is the role of targeted therapies in upfront AML?

Targeted therapy is well established in adult AML. These include FLT3 inhibitors and BCL2 inhibitors. Trials for these targeted agents are currently ongoing for pAML.

CHAPTER 4

Acute Myeloid Leukemia Relapse

Kritika Setlur, Aditya Kumar Gupta

CASE VIGNETTE

(Case vignette continues from chapter 3)
L was under regular follow-up in our survivor clinic. 15 months after treatment completion, he was noted to have persistent thrombocytopenia, a bone marrow aspirate was done to rule out relapse. Bone marrow aspiration (BMA) showed 17% blasts and flow cytometry confirmed an acute myeloid leukemia (AML) relapse.

1. What is the prognosis for a patient with AML relapse? What are the risk factors to be considered at relapse and what are the investigations that may contribute to our understanding of the risk of relapse?

Studies on adult relapsed AML to identify prognostic factors in patients with AML relapse have yielded two prognostic scores, the GOELAMS score developed and validated on a cohort of patients from France and Israel showed that the three most important prognostic factors were:[1]
1. Time of relapse (>12 months vs. 6–12 months or refractory)
2. Molecular status [FMS-like tyrosine kinase-internal tandem duplication (FLT3-ITD) + or -]
3. Cytogenetics (favorable/intermediate vs. poor)

Based on the presence of none of these poor prognostic factors, versus presence of one factor versus presence of 2/3 factors, the patients could be divided into favorable, intermediate, and poor risk at relapse, with 2-year overall survival (OS) of the favorable group being 58% and that of the poor risk group being just 12%.

Another prognostic score developed for adult patients is the European Prognostic Index, developed on a cohort of 667 adult patients, later validated by a study group of 599 patients from the MD Anderson Cancer Center found the following factors predictive of outcomes:[2]
- Relapse-free interval (<6 months, 7–18 months, >18 months)
- Cytogenetics at diagnosis [t(8;21), inv(16) or others]
- Age at first relapse (<35, 36–45 or >45)
- Stem cell transplantation before first relapse.

Though prognostic scores have not been developed for the pediatric population, tabulated below are some of the prognostic features identified by various large study groups **(Table 1)**.

Identification of molecular defects at relapse is important. In addition to prognostication, the other application of identifying molecular defects at relapse is the use of targeted therapy for certain driving mutations, more about which is covered subsequently.

TABLE 1: Prognostic factors in relapsed AML.

Study group	Prognostic factors

BFM: Relapsed AML 2001/01[3]	• Favorable:
	  – Time to relapse (>1 year)
	  – Age <10 years at relapse
	  – Favorable cytogenetics
	  – No HSCT during initial treatment

Japanese AML 99[4]	• Poor prognosis:
	  – Early relapse (<1 year)
	  – FLT3-ITD positive

Japanese Pediatric Leukemia Lymphoma Study group AML 05R[5]	• Poor prognosis:
	  – FLT3-ITD positive
	• Favorable prognosis:
	  – t(8;21) and inv(16)

NOPHO[6]	• Favorable prognosis:
	  – Time to relapse (>1 year)
	  – t(8;21) and inv(16)
	  – No HSCT during initial treatment

(AML: acute myeloid leukemia; BFM: Berlin-Frankfurt-Münster; HSCT: hematopoietic stem cell transplantation; NOPHO: Nordic Society for Pediatric Hematology and Oncology)

What is important to note is, cytogenetics as well as molecular profile of AML at relapse do not necessarily match that at first diagnosis.[7] Molecular as well as karyotypic evolution and devolution are known. In fact, karyotypic instability (i.e., either the loss or gain of aberrations at relapse) is per se associated with poor outcomes.[8] This highlights the need for a fresh molecular as well as cytogenetic workup at the time of relapse.

2. What are the salvage options in a patient with AML relapse?

Managing a relapsed AML involves selection of a chemotherapy regimen that is intense enough to induce remission and at the same time does not cause undue toxicity. Various treatment regimens have been explored, some of which are summarized below **(Table 2)**.

TABLE 2: Salvage options in relapsed AML.

Study group/Trial	Drugs used	Remission/Survival outcomes	Toxicity
Webb et al. children who relapsed following MRC AML 10, 1999[9]	• ADE • DAT (daunorubicin, cytarabine, thioguanine) • MACE • FLAG (Fludarabine + cytarabine + GCSF) • MidAC	Remission rates ADE—69% DAT—57% MACE—67% FLAG—88% MidAC—33%	

Contd...

Contd...

Study group/Trial	Drugs used	Remission/Survival outcomes	Toxicity
Wells et al. Children's Cancer Group 2851, 2003[10]	Mitoxantrone and cytarabine	Remission rates: 76%	Induction mortality rate: 3%
Kaspers et al. BFM group, 2013[11]	FLAG versus FLAG + liposomal daunorubicin	Remission rates: 69% in FLAG/L-DNR 59% in FLAG OS was similar in both groups	Grade 3 and 4 cardiotoxicity seen in 2.7% in FLAG/L-DNR, 0.6% in FLAG Rest of toxicities similar in both groups, predominant toxicity-hematological
Anders et al. 2017[12]	HIDAC	Remission rates: 62%	Febrile neutropenia: 38%
Mustafa et al. 2018[13]	FLAG ± idarubicin	Remission rate of 68% Survival till HSCT 48%	• Hematological toxicity 96% • Febrile neutropenia 53% • NEC 28% • Toxic deaths 6%
Moritake et al. Japanese pediatric leukemia/Lymphoma Study Group, 2020[5]	FLAG versus Etoposide + cytarabine + mitoxantrone (ECM)	Remission rates: 63% for ECM 65.8% for FLAG	
Ruan et al. 2021[14]	Cladribine + HIDAC + mitoxantrone GCSF till recovery of counts (CLAG-M) versus	Remission rates: 80% in CLAG-M 51% in MEC/IEC	Most common toxicity was hematological occurring in all patients of both groups
	Mitoxantrone/idarubicin + etoposide + LDAC (MEC/IEC)	3-year PFS: 52.6% in CLAG-M 34.9% in MEC/IEC	Febrile neutropenia 55% in CLAG-M and 42.9% in MEC/IEC
Ramaswamy et al. 2022[15]	Clofarabine topotecan, vinorelbine, thiotepa	Remission rate: In first relapse 71.4% OS of responders: 50%	• More than Grade 3 febrile neutropenia in 66.7% • Documented bacteremia 15.1%

(AML: acute myeloid leukemia; BFM: Berlin-Frankfurt-Münster; FLAG: fludarabine cytarabine GCSF; GCSF: granulocyte colony stimulating factor; HSCT: hematopoietic stem cell transplant; HIDAC: high-dose cytarabine; L-DNR: liposomal daunorubicin; MidAC: mitoxantrone + cytarabine; MACE: amsacrine cytarabine etoposide; OS: overall survival; PFS: progression-free survival)

CASE *(Continued)*

L was given two cycles of fludarabine cytarabine granulocyte colony-stimulating factor-idarubicin (FLAG-IDA) after which his BMA showed complete morphological remission and minimal residual disease (MRD) was negative. He was planned for consolidation by hematopoietic stem cell transplantation (HSCT).

3. Who are the preferred donors for HSCT in AML? Is there a role for autologous transplants in AML?

While the role of HSCT in AML at CR1 depends on a combination of molecular and cytogenetic risk as well as response to therapy, in CR2 HSCT represents the best chance of long-term survival. The preferred donor for transplant is a matched sibling or matched unrelated donors (MUDs). Mismatched or haploidentical HSCT may be used in the absence of a matched donor in patients who are early relapses or very high-risk disease (e.g., FLT3 ITD positive at relapse).[16]

With regards to the role of autologous transplant in CR1, Locatelli et al. found no advantage of auto-HSCT over consolidation chemotherapy. With the advent of better immunological control over graft versus host disease (GVHD) and other transplant-related complications, the practice of autologous HSCT in CR1 has gone out of practice.[16]

In relapsed AML, however, Godder et al. found that while outcomes were poor in patients with a short duration of CR1 (<12 months), outcomes in patients with a CR1 of more than a year were much better with a 3-year OS of 60%.[17] This suggests that in patients with late relapse, autologous HSCT may be considered as an option for therapy in the absence of a suitable donor and logistics for an allogeneic HSCT.[3]

4. What are the outcomes when transplant is performed with a positive MRD? Can a transplant be done without achieving morphological remission?

While morphological remission is an important prerequisite for successful HSCT in AML, the role of MRD negativity prior to transplant is less well established. The Berlin-Frankfurt-Münster (BFM) study group analyzed outcomes of 108 pediatric AML patients [all harboring recurrent abnormalities, i.e., 8;21, inv16, t(9;11), KMT2A-MLLT3 or FLT3-ITD]. Patients who underwent HSCT with negative MRD had a 5-year OS of 83%, significantly more than the OS of 57% in those who had a positive MRD.[18]

In the population of AML patients in whom complete remission (CR) is not achieved, either in upfront disease (primary refractory) or during relapse (refractory relapse), data on HSCT outcomes in a nonremission marrow is available. Jabbour et al. compared outcomes in 28 cases of refractory AML who underwent HSCT versus 149 patients who only received chemotherapy. At the end of 3 years, OS was 39% in the HSCT arm and only 2% in those who received chemotherapy. A retrospective study on the European Society for Blood and Marrow Transplantation (EBMT) registry also showed a similar OS of 35.3–39.7% depending on the type of conditioning used. This highlights that though outcomes are worse in the absence of morphological remission, HSCT represents the best survival option in refractory patients. This could in part be attributed to the role of graft versus leukemia effect in AML transplant, as well as improvements in post-transplant supportive care.[18,19]

5. What is the preferred conditioning regimen in AML transplant?

Though there is no "conditioning of choice", total body irradiation (TBI) has not been shown to have any benefit in comparison to chemotherapy only regimens in AML.[16] The BFM group in their recommendations for management of AML also advocates the use of myeloablative chemotherapy over TBI in the pediatric age group due to concerns over the latter causing increased late effects and secondary malignancies. A retrospective study in 204 European Group for Blood and Marrow Transplantation Centers comparing outcomes of HSCT while using TBI versus Busulfan–Cyclophosphamide versus Busulfan–Melphalan–Cyclophosphamide found that the best outcomes were of patients conditioned with Bu–Mel–Cy with OS of 76.6% (vs. 64 and 64.5%) and relapse free survival (RFS) of 74.5% (vs. 58 and 61.9%) with a similar nonrelapse mortality to both other modalities. The only drawback was a slightly increased incidence of acute GVHD III and IV.[20]

In the recent years there has been a growing interest in the usage of "reduced toxicity conditioning". These are regimens that are myeloablative but with minimal nonhematologic toxicity. One of the ways to achieve this in AML has been to replace cyclophosphamide with Fludarabine.[21] A retrospective study comparing the use of Bu–Cy with Flu–Blu (12.8 mg/kg) in 71 pediatric AML in either CR1 or CR2 found that engraftment rate of the two groups were similar (91% Bu–Cy and 87.5% Flu–Blu), with a lower therapy related mortality (TRM) in the Flu–Blu group (4.1 vs. 14.9%). The relapse-free survival of Bu–Cy at 2 years was higher (70.2 vs. 52%) but the incidence of grade III and IV a GVHD as well as chronic graft versus host disease (cGVHD) was slightly higher (57.1 vs. 41% for acute, 46.5 vs. 28.5% for chronic). However, none of these findings reached statistical significance and the study concluded that while FluBlu is a good alternative myeloablative option, neither regimen can be recommended over the other.[22]

By reducing the dose of Bulsufan in Bu–Flu to 8 mg/kg (as opposed to the traditional 12 mg/kg) we may produce a "reduced intensity conditioning" regimen. Defined by Champlin[23] in the first International Workshop of Nonmyeloablative Stem Cell Transplantation, reduced intensity conditioning (RIC) regimen is one that:

- Results in reversible myelosuppression (usually within 28 days) when given without stem cell support.
- Results in mixed chimerism in a proportion of patients at time of first assessment (28–35 days poststem cell transplantation).
- Is associated with low rates of nonhematologic toxicity.

Reduced intensity conditioning has been studied increasingly in adult leukemias as the lower toxicity allows its use in patients who would fail to tolerate traditional myeloablative conditioning (MAC) due to either their age or comorbidities. RIC in the pediatric population in the context of hematological malignancies is less well studied, however a retrospective analysis of 180 cases of pediatric AML in 2014 by Bitan et al. found that the OS in RIC and MAC were comparable (45 and 48%), as were the relapse rates (39 and 39%) and transplant-related mortality (16 and 16%). The number of patients in this analysis having received RIC was small ($n = 39$), but this data suggested that further studies into RIC in pediatric AML would be justified.[24] The Japan Society for Hematopoietic Cell Transplantation registry data suggests that AML with Down's syndrome is a specific population in which RIC has clearly better outcomes than MAC.[25] A phase I study in 2016 explored usage of RIC followed by gemtuzumab ozogamicin immunotherapy consolidation post-transplant and found an OS of 61% at 5 years with an event-free survival (EFS) of 78%, a follow-up Phase II study is underway.[26]

Some other novel drugs that have been used as a part of conditioning in an effort to reduce toxicity are threosulfan and Clofarabine, both of which have shown promising results.[27,28]

6. What are the outcomes in patients with AML relapse who are treated with chemotherapy only?

A 2020 systematic review of studies on relapsed pediatric AML included five studies comparing outcomes of relapsed AML treated on chemotherapy alone with those treated with auto/allo-HSCT, with OS ranging between 18 and 50% in the chemotherapy only arms. Four of those studies found a worse OS in patients treated with chemotherapy only.[29] The fifth by Wells et al. found a better OS in chemotherapy only as compared to allogeneic HSCT however, this study included only 13 patients in the chemotherapy only arm and the follow up period was relatively short (2 years).[10]

7. What are the evolving targeted therapies for relapsed AML?

Some of the new therapeutic targets identified in relapsed AML as well as the drugs under trial in pediatrics for the same are given in **Table 3**.

TABLE 3: Potential targeted therapies in relapsed and refractory pediatric AML.

Target	Drug	Study
CD 33+	Gemtuzumab ozogamicin	Zahler et al.: Phase I study, RIC followed by allo-HSCT followed by GO consolidation—5-year OS 61%[26]
Mesothelin	Anetumab ravtansine	COG AAML 2011, phase I, in development[30]
KMT2A fusion	DOT1L (disruptor of telomeric silencing 1-like) inhibitor—pinometostat	Shukla et al.: Phase I, acceptable safety, transient reduction in bone marrow and peripheral blasts in 40% patients[31]
	Menin inhibitor SNDX 5613	PedAL initiative (COG), underway[30]
MDM2	Aileron (ALRN) 6924	Phase I trial, ongoing[30]
FLT3	Quizartinib	Cooper et al.: Phase I study, determined to be safe, phase I/II study underway[30,32]

(COG: Children's Oncology Group; FLT: FMS-like tyrosine kinase; GO: gemtuzumab ozogamicin; HSCT: hematopoietic stem cell transplantation; OS: overall survival)

CASE *(Continued)*

L underwent a HSCT with the donor being a fully matched sibling, conditioning was done with Busulfan and Fludarabine. During the pretransplant period he was found to have cardiac dysfunction and started on cardio protection. Post-transplant, L remains well and in remission.

8. What are the important considerations during survivorship for a case of AML/AML relapse?

The St Jude lifetime cohort study found that survivors of childhood AML (both those treated with chemotherapy only and those who underwent a hematopoietic stem cell transplant), when followed to the age of 40 years, had a higher cumulative burden of chronic health conditions than healthy controls. Specifically, findings suggested that those patients that underwent an HSCT had a significantly higher incidence of metabolic and endocrine derangements, with a 45% prevalence of hypertriglyceridemia, 47% prevalence of hypercholesterolemia, and 27% prevalence of primary hypothyroidism. Impaired reproductive function was detected specifically in those patients who underwent TBI, and the prevalence of the same is likely to fall with wider adoption of non-TBI based conditioning.

In the category of patients who were treated with only chemotherapy, the most prevalent late effects were cardiovascular, with 11.9% prevalence of cardiomyopathy and 53.7% prevalence of hypertension. Neurocognitive dysfunction across all domains were higher in survivors regardless of treatment modality.[33] Further when comparing the two treatment groups, the Nordic Society for Pediatric Hematology and Oncology (NOPHO) AML group found that those patients who underwent an HSCT had significantly more physical health limitations as compared to those who received chemotherapy alone, and up to 16% of the HSCT survivors reported that their health problems prevented them from either attending school or retaining employment.[34]

Another important domain explored by the Children's Oncology Group (COG) study group was the risk taking behaviors and the psychological late effects of AML treatment. They found that while the prevalence of smoking, alcohol, and other substance abuse were no higher than that of the normal population, AML adolescent and adult survivors are likely to suffer from significant psychosocial sequelae, with 8% of the young adult survivors and 15% of the adolescent survivors reporting a feeling of sadness/hopelessness which limited their activities. This was especially prevalent in survivors with cancer-related anxiety or other chronic health conditions.[35]

It is important to follow up survivors closely for potential late effects, the COG has suggested guidelines for long-term follow up for childhood, adolescent, and young adult survivors, of which those relevant to most commonly used modalities in AML are summarized below.[36]

TABLE 4: Late effects in survivors of AML.

Exposure	Potential late effects	Recommendation
Any cancer experience	Psychosocial, mental health disorders, risky behaviors, chronic pain and disability, fatigue	• Yearly psychosocial assessment: 　– Education/vocation 　– Depression 　– Anxiety 　– Post-traumatic stress 　– Social withdrawal
High-dose cytarabine	Neurocognitive deficits	Baseline neuropsychological evaluation for all, and periodic follow-up based on any evidence of impaired educational/vocational progress
	Leukoencephalopathy	Yearly history and physical examination for motor/sensory deficits, seizures, spasticity, ataxia, dysarthria, hemiparesis
Anthracycline antibiotics	Cardiomyopathy, left ventricular dysfunction, arrhythmias	• Yearly history and physical examination • Echo at baseline, and periodically based on cumulative dose (elaborated later)

Contd...

Contd...

Exposure	Potential late effects	Recommendation
Hematopoietic stem cell transplant	• Hepatic toxicity	• Baseline liver functions, ferritin, and subsequently as clinically indicated
	• Osteonecrosis	• Especially in those on chronic corticosteroids for cGVHD, yearly history of joint pain, immobility, limitation of motion, and musculoskeletal examination
	• Osteopenia, osteoporosis	• DEXA scan at baseline and repeat as clinically indicated
	• *Disability secondary to cGVHD*:	
	– Nails, skin	• Yearly physical examination for alopecia, skin dyspigmentation, scleroderma, nail hypoplasia
	– Xerostomia and dental health	• Yearly history and examination of oral cavity, 6 monthly dental examination and cleaning
	– Xerophthalmia	• Yearly history for dry eyes, and ophthalmological examination
	– Esophageal strictures	• Yearly history of dysphagia or heartburn
	– Joint contractures	• Yearly musculoskeletal examination
	– Immunological deficiencies	• Generally IgA deficiency or hypogammaglobulinemia, yearly history and examination for chronic conjunctivitis, chronic sinusitis, chronic bronchitis
	– Pulmonary toxicity	• Prone for bronchiolitis obliterans, chronic bronchitis, bronchiectasis, especially in the presence of TBI, busulfan, carmustine, lomustine
		• Yearly history and respiratory examination, with a baseline PFT (DLCO and spirometry) and Chest X-ray, repeat as indicated (abnormal results or progressing symptoms)

(cGVHD: chronic graft versus host disease; DEXA: dual energy X-ray absorptiometry; DLCO: diffusion capacity of the lung for carbon monoxide; Ig: immunoglobulin; PFT: pulmonary function tests; TBI: total body irradiation)

Adapted from: Hudson MM, Landier W, Eshelman D, Forte K, Darling J, Hester A, et al. Long-term follow-up guidelines for survivors of childhood, adolescent and young adult cancers, version 2.0. Children's Oncology Group. 2006.

9. How do we prevent, manage, and follow-up on cardiotoxicity?

In addition to cardiotoxicity caused by anthracyclines, patients with AML also experience frequent infections which may trigger sepsis-induced cardiac dysfunction. Patients treated under the AAML 0531 clinical trial had a 12% prevalence of cardiotoxicity when followed up for a period of 5 years with 70% of incidents occurring during therapy. EFS and OS were both significantly worse in these patients, in part because this protocol required discontinuation of anthracycline after the development of left ventricular systolic dysfunction (LVSD), highlighting the need for strategies to limit cardiotoxicity.[37]

Prevention of cardiotoxicity may be carried out at two main levels:[38-40]

1. *Primary prevention:* Concentrating on the reduction of anthracycline exposure and chest RT exposure (sometimes known as "primordial prevention"), cardioprotective measures and reducing coexisting risk factors for cardiac morbidity.

2. *Secondary prevention:* Early detection and intervention of evolving left ventricular (LV) dysfunction, guided by laboratory findings such as echocardiographic abnormalities, biomarkers like troponin or natriuretic peptides.

Primary prevention strategies may be broadly divided into nonpharmacological and pharmacological.

Nonpharmacological:
- *Genetic testing:* Certain genetic polymorphisms have been implicated in an increased susceptibility to cardiotoxicity secondary to anthracycline use. Some of these include topoisomerase 2B [mediates reactive oxygen species (ROS) generation], carbonyl reductase (CBR, conversion of anthracycline to alcohol metabolites), and C282Y allele of the *HFE* gene (mediates iron accumulation) as well as various prooxidant enzymes like nicotinamide adenine dinucleotide phosphate (NADPH) oxidase. Though guidelines for testing these mutations have not been developed; this is a future area of interest.[39-41]
- Reduction of other cardiovascular disease (CVD) risk factors, as per American Heart Association (AHA) scientific statement, cardiovascular risk reduction in high-risk pediatric patients, interventions on weight management, heart-healthy diet, exercise, and avoidance of tobacco exposure.

Pharmacological:
- *Delivery time:* It has been found that while the anticancer activity of anthracyclines is dependent on the total plasma exposure, i.e., the area under the curve, the cardiotoxicity relates directly to the peak plasma level (which drives entry of the drug into cardiac tissue). This concept gave rise to the practice of slow infusions for anthracyclines in AML. Evidence, however, suggests that longer infusion times exacerbate side effects such as myelotoxicity, alopecia, and mucositis. It was also found that there was increased accumulation of the drug in blood cells, increasing DNA oxidative damage, and in turn possibly predisposing further to secondary AML.[39] A randomized controlled trial comparing bolus and infusion doses of doxorubicin found that there was no statistically significant difference in cardiac function even at 8 years post therapy.[42]
- *Liposomal formulations:* The molecules of liposomal anthracycline formulations exceed the size of endothelial gap junctions in cardiac tissue, hence it is hypothesized that these formulations may minimize cardiotoxicity. A liposomal formulation of daunorubicin and cytarabine (1:5 molar ratio) has been tried in therapy of adult as well as pediatric AML. This formulation has been found to accumulate selectively in AML blasts as compared to normal peripheral mononuclear cells. Another available formulation is DaunoXome [liposomal daunorubicin (L-DNR)].

Adult studies have shown that usage of liposomal doxorubicin (as compared to free doxorubicin) resulted in a 50% reduction in cardiac dysfunction (both clinical and nonclinical).[43] In the pediatric setting, the BFM group has studied L-DNR and found that its efficacy is similar to that of IDA in de novo pediatric AML, but there was no increase in cardiotoxicity despite using a higher equivalent dose (80 mg/m^2 of L-DNR compared to IDA equivalent to 60 mg/m^2 of daunorubicin).[44] In the setting of relapsed pediatric AML, the BFM group compared FLAG alone versus FLAG with L-DNR, the rationale being to intensify therapy without too much increase in morbidity in this group of heavily pretreated patients. This combination resulted in better early response and the OS of both arms was similar as was then the incidence of grade 3 and 4 toxicity. These findings suggest that liposomal formulations would be useful to mitigate cardiotoxicity without compromising on leukemia-free survival.[11] Unfortunately DaunoXome is no longer being produced as a commercial formulation. Studies are underway by the COG group for the use of CPX 351 (L-DNR with cytarabine) in pediatric AML. The cost and availability of these formulations would remain a limiting factor in our setting.

- *Dexrazoxane:* The cardiotoxicity of anthracyclines is largely mediated by ROS that are formed as a byproduct of anthracycline reduction. The ROS in combination with iron available in the cardiac tissue mediates oxidative stress, DNA damage, and death of cardiomyocytes. Dexrazoxane acts by binding to iron preventing it from forming iron-oxygen complexes.[39] It is currently the only Food and Drug Administration (FDA)-approved drug for the prevention of anthracycline-induced cardiotoxicity and was approved in 2014 for children 0–16 years of age. Used as an infusion before anthracycline administration, the dosage depends on the equivalent cardiotoxicity of each anthracycline agent. With daunorubicin, dexrazoxane is used in a 5–10:1 ratio. The AAML 1031 trial for de novo pediatric AML used dexrazoxane in 9% of their patients and found that while LVSD was not entirely prevented, the rate of decrease in LV ejection fraction was slower in patients receiving dexrazoxane.[45] Concerns over the increase in the risk of secondary malignancy have precluded its widespread use in pediatrics, and availability in our country remains a limiting factor.[46]

Secondary prevention involves two main components, which are, monitoring for early signs of cardiotoxicity and early corrective measures (modification of chemotherapy and cardiac remodeling drugs).

- *Monitoring:* Serial precycle 2D echocardiograms to detect early signs of LVSD. Parameters used for this include left ventricular fractional shortening (LVFS), global longitudinal strain (GLS), and left ventricular ejection fraction (LVEF). While LVFS is easy to measure, it has poor reliability and high inter acquisition variability. LVEF (by Simpson's method) while more challenging to measure, has better reproducibility and is recommended as the primary screening modality. GLS is yet to be validated in the podiatric population and may be used as an adjunct. Close monitoring for fall in these parameters heralds onset of LVSD and would provide a point for early intervention.[44]
- *Corrective measures:* Considering the efficacy of anthracyclines in disease control, interruptions or delay of chemotherapy should be minimized. However, delay may be considered in case transient worsening of cardiac dysfunction secondary to sepsis is suspected. Drugs that reduce cardiac remodeling, like angiotensin converting enzyme (ACE) inhibitors and beta blockers have been used in multiple adult studies and may be considered in cases of early cardiac dysfunction in pediatrics as well.

Monitoring of cardiac function after treatment completion **(Flowcharts 1, 2 and 3)**:

Flowchart 1: Cardiac function monitoring: <1 year.

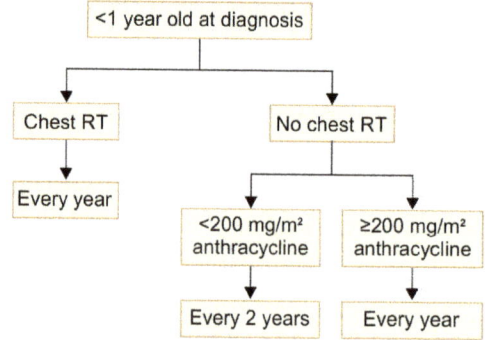

Flowchart 2: Cardiac function monitoring: 1–4 years.

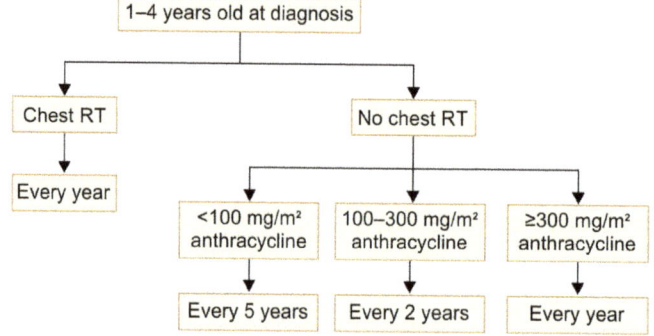

Flowchart 3: Cardiac function monitoring: ≥5 years.

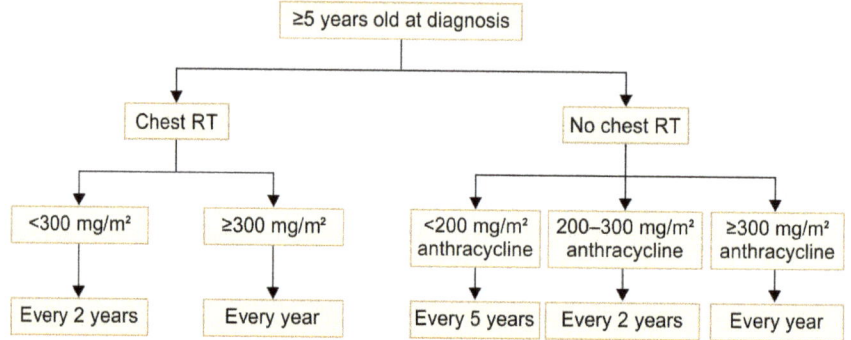

Source: (Flowcharts 1-3) Hudson MM, Landier W, Eshelman D, Forte K, Darling J, Hester A, et al. Long-term follow-up guidelines for survivors of childhood, adolescent and young adult cancers, version 2.0. Children's Oncology Group. 2006.

10. What is the incidence of secondary malignancies in AML, and how do we follow-up for the same?

On analysis of a cohort of 501 AML patients in St Jude Children's Hospital, it was found that at 15 years post-treatment, there was a 1.34% incidence of second malignancy (i.e., five patients). Of these, two patients developed malignancies in the head and neck area after having received craniospinal irradiation. Of the remaining three, two patients who had developed mucoepidermoid carcinoma of the parotid gland had received high-dose chemotherapy followed by HSCT. The fifth developed acute lymphoblastic leukemia (ALL). Drugs given during AML therapy that predispose to secondary malignancies include etoposide, anthracyclines, and alkylating agents. Follow-up for secondary malignancies after therapy of AML involves a yearly history and examination as well as yearly complete blood count (CBC) and differential count, for up to 10 years after exposure.[47]

■ REFERENCES

1. Chevallier P, Labopin M, Turlure P, Prebet T, Pigneux A, Hunault M, et al. A new Leukemia Prognostic Scoring System for refractory/relapsed adult acute myelogeneous leukaemia patients: A GOELAMS study. Leukemia. 2011;25(6):939-44.
2. Giles F, Verstovsek S, Garcia-Manero G, Thomas D, Ravandi F, Wierda W, et al. Validation of the European prognostic index for younger adult patients with acute myeloid leukaemia in first relapse. Br J Haematol. 2006;134(1):58-60.
3. Sander A, Zimmermann M, Dworzak M, Fleischhack G, von Neuhoff C, Reinhardt D, et al. Consequent and intensified relapse therapy improved survival in pediatric AML: results of relapse treatment in 379 patients of three consecutive AML-BFM trials. Leukemia. 2010;24(8):1422-8.
4. Nakayama H, Tabuchi K, Tawa A, Tsukimoto I, Tsuchida M, Morimoto A, et al. Outcome of children with relapsed acute myeloid leukemia following initial therapy under the AML99 protocol. Int J Hematol. 2014;100(2):171-9.
5. Moritake H, Tanaka S, Miyamura T, Nakayama H, Shiba N, Shimada A, et al. The outcomes of relapsed acute myeloid leukemia in children: results from the Japanese Pediatric Leukemia/Lymphoma Study Group AML-05R study. Pediatr Blood Cancer. 2021;68(1):e28736.
6. Karlsson L, Forestier E, Hasle H, Jahnukainen K, Jónsson ÓG, Lausen B, et al. Outcome after intensive reinduction therapy and allogeneic stem cell transplant in paediatric relapsed acute myeloid leukaemia. Br J Haematol. 2017;178(4):592-602.
7. Flach J, Shumilov E, Porret N, Shakhanova I, Legros M, Kronig MN, et al. Experiences with next-generation sequencing in relapsed acute myeloid leukemia: a patient case series. Mediterr J Hematol Infect Dis. 2020;12(1):e2020068.
8. Klein K, Beverloo HB, Zimmermann M, Raimondi SC, von Neuhoff C, de Haas V, et al. (2021). Prognostic significance of chromosomal abnormalities at relapse in children with relapsed acute myeloid leukemia: a retrospective cohort study of the Relapsed AML 2001/01 Study. [online] available from https://onlinelibrary.wiley.com/doi/10.1002/pbc.29341 {Last accessed October, 2022].
9. Webb DK, Wheatley K, Harrison G, Stevens RF, Hann IM. Outcome for children with relapsed acute myeloid leukaemia following initial therapy in the Medical Research Council (MRC) AML 10 trial. MRC Childhood Leukaemia Working Party. Leukemia. 1999;13(1):25-31.
10. Wells RJ, Adams MT, Alonzo TA, Arceci RJ, Buckley J, Buxton AB, et al. Mitoxantrone and cytarabine induction, high-dose cytarabine, and etoposide intensification for pediatric patients with relapsed or refractory acute myeloid leukemia: Children's Cancer Group Study 2951. J Clin Oncol Off J Am Soc Clin Oncol. 2003;21(15):2940-7.
11. Kaspers GJL, Zimmermann M, Reinhardt D, Gibson BES, Tamminga RYJ, Aleinikova O, et al. Improved outcome in pediatric relapsed acute myeloid leukemia: results of a randomized trial on liposomal daunorubicin by the International BFM Study Group. J Clin Oncol. 2013;31(5):599-607.
12. Anders B, Veltri L, Kanate AS, Shillingburg A, Shah N, Craig M, et al. Outcomes of six-dose high-dose cytarabine as a salvage regimen for patients with relapsed/refractory acute myeloid leukemia. Adv Hematol. 2017;2017:6464972.
13. Mustafa O, Abdalla K, AlAzmi AA, Elimam N, Abrar MB, Jastaniah W. FLAG/FLAG-IDA regimen for children with relapsed/refractory acute leukemia in the era of targeted novel therapies. J Oncol Pharm Pract. 2019;25(8):1831-8.

14. Ruan M, Liu L, Zhang A, Quan Qi B, Liu F, Liu T, et al. Improved outcome of children with relapsed/refractory acute myeloid leukemia by addition of cladribine to re-induction chemotherapy. Cancer Med. 2021;10(3):956-64.
15. Ramaswamy K, Steinherz PG, Agrawal AK, Forlenza CJ, Mauguen A, Roshal M, et al. Clofarabine with topotecan, vinorelbine, and thiotepa reinduction regimen for children and young adults with relapsed AML. Blood Adv. 2022;6(8):2688-94.
16. Gibson BES, Sauer MG, Amrolia P. Acute myeloid leukemia in children. In: Carreras E, Dufour C, Mohty M (Eds). The EBMT Handbook: Hematopoietic Stem Cell Transplantation and Cellular Therapies [Internet], 7th edition. Berlin: Springer; 2019.
17. Godder K, Eapen M, Laver JH, Zhang MJ, Camitta BM, Wayne AS, et al. Autologous hematopoietic stem-cell transplantation for children with acute myeloid leukemia in first or second complete remission: A prognostic factor analysis. J Clin Oncol. 2004;22(18):3798-804.
18. Pigazzi M, Benetton M, Walter C, Hansen M, Skou AS, Da Ros A, et al. Impact of minimal residual disease (MRD) assessed before transplantation on the outcome of children with acute myeloid leukemia given an allograft: a retrospective study by the I-BFM Study Group. Blood. 2020;136(Supplement 1):38-9.
19. Gyurkocza B, Lazarus HM, Giralt S. Allogeneic hematopoietic cell transplantation in patients with AML not achieving remission: Potentially curative therapy. Bone Marrow Transplant. 2017;52(8):1083-90.
20. Lucchini G, Labopin M, Beohou E, Dalissier A, Dalle JH, Cornish J, et al. Impact of conditioning regimen on outcomes for children with acute myeloid leukemia undergoing transplantation in first complete remission. An analysis on behalf of the pediatric disease working party of the European Group for blood and marrow transplantation. Biol Blood Marrow Transplant. 2017;23(3):467-74.
21. Visani G, Malagola M, Guiducci B, Lucesole M, Loscocco F, Gabucci E, et al. Conditioning regimens in acute myeloid leukemia. Expert Rev Hematol. 2014;7(4):465-79.
22. Paina OV, Rakhmanova ZZ, Kozhokar PV, Frolova AS, Tsvetkova LA, Ekushov KA, et al. Comparison of FLU-BU12 conditioning with the standard BU-CY myeloablative regimen in high-risk pediatric ACUTE myeloid leukemia patients undergoing allogeneic stem cell transplantation. Blood. 2020;136:30-1.
23. Champlin R, Khouri I, Komblau S, Molidrem J, Giralt S. Reinventing bone marrow transplantation. Nonmyeloablative preparative regimens and induction of graft-vs-malignancy effect. Oncology (Williston Park). 1999;13(5):621-8; discussion 631, 635-8, 641.
24. Bitan M, He W, Zhang MJ, Abdel-Azim H, Ayas MF, Bielorai B, et al. Transplantation for children with acute myeloid leukemia: a comparison of outcomes with reduced intensity and myeloablative regimens. Blood. 2014;123(10):1615-20.
25. Muramatsu H, Sakaguchi H, Taga T, Tabuchi K, Adachi S, Inoue M, et al. Reduced intensity conditioning in allogeneic stem cell transplantation for AML with Down syndrome: RIC for AML With DS. Pediatr Blood Cancer. 2014;61(5):925-7.
26. Zahler S, Bhatia M, Ricci A, Roy S, Morris E, Harrison L, et al. A phase I study of reduced-intensity conditioning and allogeneic stem cell transplantation followed by dose escalation of targeted consolidation immunotherapy with gemtuzumab ozogamicin in children and adolescents with CD33+ acute myeloid leukemia. Biol Blood Marrow Transplant. 2016;22(4):698-704.
27. Kussman A, Shyr D, Hale G, Oshrine B, Petrovic A. Allogeneic hematopoietic cell transplantation in chemotherapy-induced aplasia in children with high-risk acute myeloid leukemia or myelodysplasia. Pediatr Blood Cancer. 2019;66(1):e27481.
28. Versluys AB, Boelens JJ, Pronk C, Lankester A, Bordon V, Buechner J, et al. Hematopoietic cell transplant in pediatric acute myeloid leukemia after similar upfront therapy; a comparison of conditioning regimens. Bone Marrow Transplant. 2021;56(6):1426-32.
29. Hoffman AE, Schoonmade LJ, Kaspers GJ. Pediatric relapsed acute myeloid leukemia: a systematic review. Expert Rev Anticancer Ther. 2021;21(1):45-52.

30. Chen J, Glasser C. New and emerging targeted therapies for pediatric acute myeloid leukemia (AML). Children. 2020;7(2):12.
31. Shukla N, Wetmore C, O'Brien MM, Silverman LB, Brown P, Cooper TM, et al. Final report of phase 1 study of the DOT1L inhibitor, pinometostat (EPZ-5676), in children with relapsed or refractory MLL-r acute leukemia. Blood. 2016;128(22):2780.
32. Cooper TM, Cassar J, Eckroth E, Malvar J, Sposto R, Gaynon P, et al. A phase I study of quizartinib combined with chemotherapy in relapsed childhood leukemia: A Therapeutic Advances in Childhood Leukemia & Lymphoma (TACL) Study. Clin Cancer Res Off J Am Assoc Cancer Res. 2016;22(16):4014-22.
33. Bhatt NS, Baassiri MJ, Liu W, Bhakta N, Chemaitilly W, Ehrhardt MJ, et al. Late outcomes in survivors of childhood acute myeloid leukemia: a report from the St. Jude Lifetime Cohort Study. Leukemia. 2021;35(8):2258-73.
34. Wilhelmsson M, Glosli H, Ifversen M, Abrahamsson J, Winiarski J, Jahnukainen K, et al. Long-term health outcomes in survivors of childhood AML treated with allogeneic HSCT: A NOPHO-AML Study. Bone Marrow Transplant. 2019;54(5):726-36.
35. Schultz KAP, Chen L, Chen Z, Zeltzer LK, Nicholson HS, Neglia JP. Health and risk behaviors in survivors of childhood acute myeloid leukemia: A report from the Children's Oncology Group. Pediatr Blood Cancer. 2010;55(1):157-64.
36. Hudson MM, Landier W, Eshelman D, Forte K, Darling J, Hester A, et al. Long-term follow-up guidelines for survivors of childhood, adolescent and young adult cancers, version 2.0. Children's Oncology Group. 2006.
37. Getz KD, Sung L, Ky B, Gerbing RB, Leger KJ, Leahy AB, et al. Occurrence of treatment-related cardiotoxicity and its impact on outcomes among children treated in the AAML0531 clinical trial: A report from the Children's Oncology Group. J Clin Oncol. 2019;37(1):12-21.
38. Dixon SB, Howell CR, Lu L, Plana JC, Joshi VM, Luepker RV, et al. Cardiac biomarkers and association with subsequent cardiomyopathy and mortality among adult survivors of childhood cancer: A report from the St. Jude Lifetime Cohort. Cancer. 2021;127(3):458-66.
39. Menna P, Salvatorelli E. Primary prevention strategies for anthracycline cardiotoxicity: a brief overview. Chemotherapy. 2017;62(3):159-68.
40. Bansal N, Adams MJ, Ganatra S, Colan SD, Aggarwal S, Steiner R, et al. Strategies to prevent anthracycline-induced cardiotoxicity in cancer survivors. Cardio-Oncol. 2019;5(1):1-22.
41. Witteles RM, Bosch X. Myocardial protection during cardiotoxic chemotherapy. Circulation. 2015;132(19):1835-45.
42. Lipshultz SE, Miller TL, Lipsitz SR, Neuberg DS, Dahlberg SE, Colan SD, et al. Continuous versus bolus infusion of doxorubicin in children with ALL: long-term cardiac outcomes. Pediatrics. 2012;130(6):1003-11.
43. Blair HA. Daunorubicin/cytarabine liposome: A review in acute myeloid leukaemia. Drugs. 2018;78(18):1903-10.
44. Creutzig U, Zimmermann M, Bourquin JP, Dworzak MN, Fleischhack G, Graf N, et al. Randomized trial comparing liposomal daunorubicin with idarubicin as induction for pediatric acute myeloid leukemia: Results from Study AML-BFM 2004. Blood. 2013;122(1):37-43.
45. Getz KD, Sung L, Alonzo TA, Leger KJ, Gerbing RB, Pollard JA, et al. Effect of dexrazoxane on left ventricular systolic function and treatment outcomes in patients with acute myeloid leukemia: a report from the Children's Oncology Group. J Clin Oncol Off J Am Soc Clin Oncol. 2020;38(21):2398-406.
46. Narayan HK, Getz KD, Leger KJ. Minimizing cardiac toxicity in children with acute myeloid leukemia. Hematology. 2021;2021(1):368-75.
47. Leung W, Ribeiro R, Hudson M, Tong X, Srivastava D, Rubnitz J, et al. Second malignancy after treatment of childhood acute myeloid leukemia. Leukemia. 2001;15(1):41-5.

EXPERT OPINION

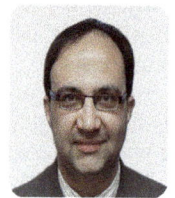

Sameer Bakhshi
Professor
Department of Medical Oncology
Dr BRA Institute Rotary Cancer Hospital
All India Institute of Medical Sciences
New Delhi, India

1. Do you think next-generation sequencing (NGS) has any role in the management of AML upfront or at relapse?

Based on the present evidence of targeted therapy in pediatric AML, I feel that doing NGS will not add any advantage beyond routine cytogenetics and the known available molecular markers as needed for risk stratification. Likewise, even at relapse, NGS is unlikely to add any benefit. However, if a patient with AML is refractory, I would suggest getting NGS for evaluating any available targets and possible any experimental modes of therapy. Notably, the data does not support any benefit of exploring such targets by NGS in a refractory setting in general because quite often even if a target is detected, the same may not be the driver for that malignancy. It is also to be noted that in Indian setting even if this was detected, the drug for that target may be far too expensive for routine clinical use in families for the masses.

2. What salvage do you use in a relapsed AML and why? What have been your centers experience with it?

I generally prefer to use ADE regimen and our own experience suggests that the same may be offered even in an outpatient setting with manageable toxicity provided a daily follow-up can be ensured, and that the CR rate in a relapse setting is close to 70%. I would however add that there is no BEST regimen in a relapse setting and would suggest that any regimen with an anthracycline and cytosine arabinoside as may be a reasonable option. While I would prefer to have an anthracycline in the reinduction regimen at relapse, the setting of the patient as above in the index case with cardiomyopathy would not permit the use of anthracyclines. In that situation, I would use high-dose cytosine arabinoside as the induction regimen.

3. Do you think metronomic chemotherapy has a role in AML-upfront or at relapse?

Acute myeloid leukemia is not exquisitely chemosensitive like ALL, and therefore I believe that intensive regimen is still the best option. However, in those with refractory disease and perhaps in a very poor performance status, a combination of cyclophosphamide and VP-16 is attempted, although there is no proven benefit. Personal experiences suggest that occasionally in refractory setting, the benefit may be observed although in the absence of a proper control population, it is difficult to state whether that benefit is driven by the metronomic therapy or due to the disease biology itself.

4. Is there any situation when a relapsed AML becomes MRD negative after salvage chemotherapy, that you would avoid HSCT in?

It is desirable that at relapse the patient is MRD negative prior to transplant and the fact that the patient is MRD negative would not take me away from the decision to transplant. Irrespective of MRD, I would take the patient for transplant. If patient is not in morphological CR, in my personal experience whosoever I have transplanted has relapsed.

5. Hematopoietic stem cell transplantation for AML. Please comment briefly regarding the choice of donor, conditioning regimen, and GVHD prophylaxis.

First choice would be a matched sibling donor followed by haploidentical or MUD. If the registry for MUD is not robust or if the center is not very well equipped with haploidentical transplant or cost is a major obstacle for the family, the option to go with an autologous transplant in the absence of a matched sibling donor for those with late relapses of AML is an acceptable option.

The conditioning regimen preferred is myeloablative with cyclophosphamide and busulfan.

The GVHD prophylaxis is cyclosporine with methotrexate, cyclosporine is continued till around 4 months with tapering thereafter and stoppage before 6 months from the day of transplant.

CHAPTER 5

Difficult Situations in Leukemia

5.1 INFANTILE LEUKEMIA

Gargi Das, Jagdish P Meena

CASE VIGNETTE

Master K is a 6.5-month-old infant, who presented with fever and excessive irritability for 3 months, with progressive pallor and abdominal distension for 2 months. He is the second born child of a nonconsanguineous couple with a smooth perinatal transition. On examination he had a liver and spleen, palpable 5 and 6 cm from the costal margins.

Complete blood count (CBC) revealed a hemoglobin (Hb) of 4.2 g/dL, total leukocyte count (TLC) of 43,600/μL, and platelet count of 39,000/μL. Peripheral smear revealed few myelocytes and metamyelocytes along with 18% blasts. A bone marrow (BM) aspirate revealed 85% blasts which were negative for myeloperoxidase (MPO). Flow cytometry revealed 84% CD45 dim positive blasts which were positive for CD19, cCD79a, CD81, CD58, NG2, and HLA-DR. They were negative for CD38, CD123, CD20, CD10, cMPO, CD13, CD33, CD7, cCD3, and sCD3. Hence a diagnosis of a B-cell lineage lymphoblastic leukemia was made with a suspicion of an underlying KMT2a rearrangement. Cerebrospinal fluid (CSF) done with BM revealed 10 blasts/μL.

1. What is the most likely leukemia in infants?

Acute lymphoblastic leukemia (ALL) accounts for around 20% of cancers in patients younger than 20 years of age.[1] According to the population-based cancer registry (PBCR 2012–14 report), childhood cancer accounts for 0.7–4.4% of total cancer diagnoses.[2] A recent review summarizing the outcome of ALL in various hospital-based studies, showed overall survival (OS) between 45 and 81% and event-free survival (EFS) between 41 and 70%.[3] Infantile leukemia does not have similar outcomes, and is of special interest in various cooperative group trials.[4] There is a slight predominance of lymphoid over myeloid cases within infant leukemia. It is also noteworthy that in infants, the incidence of ALL is lower than in children aged 1–14 years old and approximately the same as adolescents.[5] In contrast, the incidence of acute myeloid leukemia (AML) in infants is approximately twice that of older children and adolescents. Interestingly, females have a higher risk of developing infant leukemia than males.[5]

2. Is there a difference in presentation of infants and older children with ALL?

The differences in presentation of leukemia between infants and children are given in **Table 1**.[5-8]

TABLE 1: Presentation differences in infants and older children with ALL.

Characteristics	Infants	Older children
Hyperleukocytosis	More	Less
Hepatosplenomegaly	Bulkier	Less bulky
CNS positivity	More common	Less common
Leukemia cutis	More common	Less common
Outcome of infant ALL	EFS around 50%	EFS in western cooperative groups around 85%

(ALL: acute lymphoblastic leukemia; CNS: central nervous system; EFS: event-free survival)

3. What is the expected flow cytometry?

Infant ALL is mostly a B-lineage ALL (96% B-ALL vs. 4% T-ALL). It is mostly CD10 negative and shows more myeloid antigen coexpression than children or adolescents with ALL, indicating origin from very immature lymphoid progenitors.[6] NG2 may also be expressed and point toward an underlying *mixed lineage leukemia* (*MLL*) mutation.[9]

In AML, KMT2A-r is associated with monocytic differentiation. Infant leukemia cases can be of ambiguous lineage, either due to a mixed phenotype [mixed phenotype acute leukemia (MPAL)], or lack of differentiation markers (acute undifferentiated leukemia).[10]

CASE *(Continued)*

In the above case, CD10 negativity and NG2 positivity pointed toward a *MLL* diagnosis.

4. What are the gene rearrangements seen in Infant ALL?

Infant leukemias are characterized cytogenetically by balanced chromosomal translocations involving the histone lysine methyltransferase 2A gene (KMT2A), (formerly known as *MLL* gene) at chromosome 11q23.[10] KMT2A rearrangement is seen in 5–8% of childhood ALL in western cohorts[11] and somewhere between 1 and 3% in children with ALL from India.[12] In infants however, KMT2A rearrangements are much more prevalent, seen in approximately 70–80% of infants.[10] Interestingly, in childhood AML, KMT2A-r is more common overall (15–20%), but is also particularly common in the infant age group (around 50%).[13] KMT2A-r results in the fusion of the N terminus of the wild-type (WT) *KMT2A* gene with the C terminus of a partner gene. The translocator partner genes (TPGs) involved in the rearrangement with KMT2A in infants with ALL, as seen in the data obtained from 2,345 acute leukemia patients, were AF4 (40%), AF9 (18%), ENL (18%), AF10 (9%), ELL (3%), AF6 (1%), EPS15 (1%), and other genes (9%).[14] Infantile AML had predominantly AF10 (27%), AF9 (25%), and ELL (15%) as partner genes, while pediatric ALL includes AF9 (29%), AF4 (22%), ENL (12%), and AF10 (12%) as most common TPGs.[14] Infant ALL with KMT2A rearrangements have worse prognosis than children with ALL and KMT2A rearrangements. In a retrospective review of 497 children with

MLL translocation treated by 11 different cooperative groups in the United States, Canada, and Europe; MLL-rearranged ALL in children of all ages had a relatively poor outcome, but infants fared worst of all.[6]

5. What is the difference between WT-MLL and fusion MLL protein?

Mixed lineage leukemia is an enzyme that changes the methylation of histones (protein components of chromatin around which DNA is wound) and thus changes gene transcription (expression). Leukemic cells with *MLL* translocations express both WT-MLL and MLL fusion protein. The fusion protein binds to a subset of the target genes to which WT-MLL normally binds, and it alters the level of their transcription to favor oncogenesis. WT-MLL are generally more stable and are required for maintenance of normal hematopoiesis.[15] Hence in any child, a MLL break-apart FISH (fluorescence in situ hybridization), would suggest involvement with a pathogenic partner gene. If the break-apart FISH is negative, we would consider it as WT-MLL (or germline MLL). Risk stratification of infantile ALL are also dependent on this factor.

6. What are the cytogenetics and outcomes of patients without KMT2A rearrangement in infantile ALL?

Data on infants with ALL, without *KMT2A* gene rearrangements (KMT2A-g or MLL-G), is typically small. MLL-R infants are younger than their MLL-G counterparts. MLL-G cases share same genetic abnormality and risk stratification as older children with ALL. The frequency of good-risk cytogenetic abnormalities [hyperdiploidy and t(12;21)] among MLL-G infants was significantly lower, whereas the frequency of poor risk abnormalities [t(9;22) and t(1;19)] was similar. Low FLT3 expression was found to be associated with an excellent outcome in infants with ALL.[16] Hence, MLL-G infants behave similarly to older children, when classified into the same good risk, intermediate risk (IR), and poor risk cytogenetic subgroups as childhood ALL. This suggested that some MLL-G infants, especially those with good-risk cytogenetics, may benefit from treatment on childhood protocols, which are generally less intensive and less toxic than infant ALL regimens.[16]

7. What were the major prognostic factors of infantile ALL, as determined by studies of childhood ALL?

In the past, all leukemias were treated uniformly. Combined analysis of various childhood ALL protocols identified key biological and clinical prognostic features of infants with ALL. Presence of *MLL-r* gene, hyperleukocytosis, absence of CD10 antigen, age <6 months at diagnosis, and poor prednisolone response were independently associated with an inferior outcome.[4] This leads to various cooperative groups treating infantile ALL separately with its own risk stratification.

CASE *(Continued)*

Karyotype sent for this child was normal and break-apart FISH revealed a break in the *MLL* gene. Subsequently a fusion FISH was performed, which revealed a KMT2A-AF4 rearrangement [t(4;11)].

8. How would you risk stratify this child of infantile ALL?

The current risk stratification uses the stratification before starting management of ALL (Table 2).[10]

TABLE 2: Risk stratification of infant ALL.

Risk	Interfant	COG	JPSLG	Approximate EFS (%)
High	KMT2A-r and age <6 months and WBCs ≥300,000/μL and/or poor prednisolone response	KMT2A-r and age <3 months	KMT2A-r and (age <6 months or CNS involvement)	20
Intermediate	KMT2A-r and not high risk	KMT2A-r and not high risk	KMT2A-r and not high risk	50
Low	WT-KMT2A	WT-KMT2A	WT-KMT2A	75

(ALL: acute lymphoblastic leukemia; CNS: central nervous system; COG: Children's Oncology Group; EFS: event-free survival; JPSLG: Japanese Pediatric Leukemia/Lymphoma Study Group; WT: wild-type; WBCs: white blood cells)

The above child had a TLC of 43,600/μL at presentation, was >6 months of age and had a central nervous system (CNS)-3 disease (CNS leukemia). He had a rearranged MLL gene. He would be classified as IR as per the Interfant group and high risk (HR) as per the Japanese study group. Main difference would be that he would be an upfront hematopoietic stem cell transplantation (HSCT) candidate as per the Japanese trials, but as per Interfant, minimal residual disease (MRD) would guide decision to transplant.

9. Is there any difference in the outcomes of the patients categorized into the three risk groups in MLL-10 (Japanese group) and Interfant-06?

TABLE 3: Comparison of risk groups as per MLL-10 and Interfant-06.

	LR, KMT2A-g	MR, KMT2A-r without HR features	HR, KMT2A-r, <6 months and WBC ≥300,000/μL	3- and 5-year EFS (%)
LR, KMT2A-g	15	–	–	93.3
IR, KMT2A-r and age ≥180 days and no CNS leukemia	–	19	0	94.4
HR, MT2A-r and either age <180 days or CNS leukemia	–	23	33	56.6
3- and 5-year EFS (%)	93.3	82.4	45.2	

(CNS: central nervous system; EFS: event-free survival; HR: high risk; LR: low risk; MR: medium risk; MLL: mixed lineage leukemia; WBC: white blood cell)

The comparison is provided in **Table 3**. It is noteworthy that all patients who were HR in the Interfant-06 trial were HR in the MLL-10 trial. The difference is in the medium risk (MR)/IR group. There was a group in the IR category of Interfant-06, who were categorized as HR in the MLL-10 trial, owing to better survival in this group.

10. **The above child had CSF positive for blasts. Would he require cranial radiotherapy (CRT)? Describe the early efforts in improving survival and assessing efficacy of various modes of CNS prophylaxis.**

The initial evidence for development of infant-specific protocols for treatment of ALL, came from a retrospective review of 115 infants with ALL. 4-year EFS was 23%, with early recurrence, rather than excessive toxicity contributing to the poor EFS.[17] This preempted a pilot trial from the Children's Cancer Group (CCG), the *CCG-192P* trial, which included intensive, high-dose chemotherapy (standard childhood ALL induction and consolidation), and CRT for infants. CNS relapse rates reduced and EFS improved significantly (36% at 4 years), but remained less than in older patients treated with this protocol.[18] Nonetheless this proved that intensive therapy was well tolerated in infants and can be a viable option in this cohort of patients. The subsequent *CCG-107* and *CCG-1883* trials *omitted CRT as CNS prophylaxis and gave high-dose methotrexate and intrathecal (IT) therapy instead.* Both studies intensified systemic chemotherapy, administered in five phases with dosages calculated on body surface area. CCG-1883 was further intensified postinduction, primarily with the addition of high-dose cytarabine. Complete remission (CR) rate was around 90% for both trials and there was an improvement in 5-year EFS (37.6 vs. 32.6%) and OS (50.2 vs. 42.8%) when comparing CCG-1883 with CCG-107, with tolerable toxicities and low incidence of CNS relapse (5 vs. 20% in historical controls). However, EFS was still low as compared to older children and marrow relapses remained the primary mode of treatment failure.[19] Simultaneously, the Pediatric Oncology Group (POG), introduced a new therapy designed specifically for infant ALL, *POG-8493*. Treatment was based upon body weight rather than surface area. Induction included, cyclophosphamide, vincristine (VCR), Ara-C, and prednisone (COAP); consolidation therapy with teniposide (VM-26) and Ara-C; and continuation therapy with alternating pulses of COAP with VM-26/Ara-C separated by a methotrexate and 6-MP backbone plus CNS therapy consisting of standard triple intrathecal therapy (TIT), and avoided the use of radiotherapy in this population. CR rate was 89.3% and EFS was around 30%, and marrow relapses remained high.[20] There was a *general consensus that inducing CR was easy, but preventing early marrow relapses still remained a challenge.*

Based on the above evidence, CRT is not used prophylactically in management of infants with ALL. As child is <3 years of age, the benefit of using CRT to treat CNS leukemia maybe outweighed by its severe late effects on a developing brain. On the MLL 10 protocol, this child would have automatically qualified for a HSCT, but in the Interfant 06 protocol, MRD at beginning of OCTADAD guides if transplant is to be done.

11. **What is the ideal protocol for this child with infant ALL?**

a. **Describe the first trials in infant All, where *MLL* was used to risk stratify patients.**

By the early 1990s, the *MLL* gene was identified as a poor prognostic factor in infantile ALL and the subsequent trials *CCG-1953 and POG-9407*, considered early intensification of chemotherapy based on body surface area and used HSCT for infants with MLL rearranged ALL. These trials reported high incidence of toxic deaths during therapy. Moreover when comparing infants with MLL-rearranged ALL receiving HSCT with those who did not, the EFS and OS were comparable, suggesting no benefit in the routine use of HSCT for infant

ALL.[8,21,22] Across the pacific, the JPLSG was founded in 2003, and was the first group to include MLL rearrangement in risk stratification and subsequent management.[4] In the *MLL-96* trial, MLL-rearranged ALL received HSCT, while the MLL WT/germline patients were treated like older children and received continuous chemotherapy for 83–85 weeks. CR was induced in 90.5% with MLL-r ALL and in 100% with MLL-g. In the MLL-r subgroup, the estimated 3-year EFS 34% compared with 92.3% in the MLL-g subgroup.[23] The *MLL-98* trial was also similar, however instituted more intense chemotherapy and early HSCT (within 3–5 months of therapy initiation). The CR rate was 91.0%, and the 3-year OS and EFS were 58.2 and 43.6%, respectively. Post-transplant EFS was 64.4% with only the timing of HSCT (first remission versus others) proving to be a significant risk factor by multivariate analysis ($p < 0.0001$).[24] These results were unlike the results by the early CCG/POG trials and suggest that *early introduction of HSCT, possibly with a less toxic conditioning regimen, may improve the prognosis for infants with MLL-r ALL*. Another important conclusion is that *infants with germline MLL had a better prognosis and could be treated with protocols meant for older children with ALL*. Other relevant conclusion was the *need for more effective postremission therapy*, as a high proportion of relapse (61.7%) occurred before HSCT. Age <6 months was the only independent prognostic factor associated with inferior outcome for MLL-rearranged infants (5-year EFS 27.8% <6 months vs. 52.9% >6 months) with CNS disease at diagnosis identified on univariate analysis.[25]

b. Is there a role of AML like in induction in treatment of infantile ALL?
Yes, based on in vitro drug sensitivity experiments of *infant ALL cells, blasts were shown to have high sensitivity to cytarabine and high resistance against major key ALL drugs, prednisolone and asparaginase*.[26] A "hybrid chemotherapy" incorporating AML-oriented drugs (e.g., cytarabine, anthracyclines, and etoposide) to ALL chemotherapy backbone was proposed by the Interfant ALL study group (consists of 17 European pediatric hematology oncology treatment groups). It is the largest consortium with multicenter participants, tasked to study and improve survival in infants with ALL.[4] The first and largest collaborative trial the *Interfant 99*, was conducted to treat both acute lymphoblastic and myeloid leukemia but with no irradiation and only small amounts of anthracyclines and alkylating agents and also to assess the efficacy of a late intensification course with high doses of both cytarabine and methotrexate between reinduction and maintenance phases.[4,10] The induction phase consisted of a standard four-drug induction for patients with acute lymphoblastic leukemia, with the addition of low-dose cytarabine. Those with good prednisolone response were labeled as standard risk (SR), while those with poor prednisolone response (absolute blast count >1,000), were included in HR. The MARAM phase was a slightly modified consolidation course that included high-dose cytarabine and high-dose methotrexate. OCTADAD was a reinduction block derived from the consolidation phase of the Berlin-Frankfurt-Münster (BFM) trials for treatment of acute leukemia, except that prednisone was replaced by dexamethasone. HR patients could receive HSCT, if 5/6 or 6/6 HLA matched donor was available.[26] After 20 weeks, a late intensification randomization was done. SR patients, who were randomly assigned to the intervention group were treated with the intensification (VIMARAM) phase (similar to the MARAM maintenance block but with the addition of VCR), followed by a standard maintenance phase after 2 weeks of recovery (maintenance 1B; which includes 6MP, methotrexate and pulses of prednisolone

and VCR). HR patients, randomly assigned to receive VIMARAM, were given the intensified maintenance treatment after 2 weeks of recovery (maintenance 1A; which includes 6MP, methotrexate, etoposide and Ara-C pulses). At 4 years, EFS was 47% and OS was 55.3%. Of 445 patients in CR after 5 weeks of induction treatment, 191 were randomized: 95 patients to receive a late intensification course, and 96 to a control group. Disease-free survival (DFS) at 4 years did not differ between the two groups, signifying *no benefit from late intensification course with high-dose methotrexate and cytarabine.*[27] The *Interfant-06* trial studied the role of early intensification of two AML induction blocks versus BFM style 1b postinduction in MR and HR patients (refer to **Table 2**). Patients in the MR and HR groups were randomly assigned to receive the lymphoid course low-dose cytosine arabinoside, 6-mercaptopurine, cyclophosphamide (Ib) or experimental myeloid courses, namely Ara-C, daunorubicin, etoposide (ADE), and mitoxantrone, Ara-C, etoposide (MAE). 6-year EFS and OS was 46.1 and 58.2%, respectively. The 6-year probability of DFS was comparable for the randomized arms (ADE + MAE 39.3 vs. IB 36.8% $p = 0.47$). The 6-year EFS rate of patients in the HR group was 20.9% with around 50% receiving HSCT (due to early events). Hence, *outcome with myeloid-type chemotherapy course did not significantly improve outcome for infant ALL.*[28]

CASE *(Continued)*

At our center, we follow the Interfant 06 protocol. This child was an IR/MR as per stratification and was swiftly started on the induction protocol. Child had a good prednisolone response on day 8. Plan was to do weekly TITs till CSF cleared with two addition TITs after clearance. CSF cleared by week 2 and he went on to receive 2 more TITs in induction. MRD at end of induction was not detectable (<0.01% by flow cytometry).

12. Is there a role of MRD assessment in infantile ALL?

The prognostic significance of MRD, was analyzed for the first time in Interfant-99, with high MRD ($>10^{-4}$) significantly associated with lower DFS.[29] All subsequent trials use MRD to guide therapy.

CASE *(Continued)*

After induction of Interfant 06, child received consolidation protocol 1b followed by MARMA (including high-dose Ara-C and high-dose methotrexate) block of chemotherapy only protocol. This child remained MRD negative (<0.01% by flow cytometry) after MARMA and hence we decided to forgo transplant and continue the child on a chemotherapy only protocol.

13. When would you have considered HSCT in this child?

When compared with MLL-rearranged infants who received chemotherapy alone after first CR, infants who received HSCT had significantly improved DFS and OS. This difference is particularly for a subgroup of HR MLL-rearranged infants with unfavorable prognostic features, including age <6 months and either poor day 8 prednisone response or white blood cell (WBC) >300,000 cells/μL at diagnosis, although this subgroup also had a high early failure rate, with a third having an event before the median time to transplantation.[4] The early use of HSCT was studied in the Japanese *MLL-03 study*. Short-course intensive chemotherapy was followed by early HSCT within 4 months for all KMT2A rearranged leukemias. The 4-year EFS and OS rates were 43.2 and 67.2%, respectively. A univariate analysis showed younger age (<90 days at diagnosis), CNS disease, and prednisone poor-response (PPR) was significantly associated with poor prognosis ($p < 0.05$). In a multivariate analysis, younger age at diagnosis tended to be associated with poor outcome (hazard ratio = 1.969, 95% CI = 0.903–4.291, $p = 0.088$). Considering the risk of severe late effects and balancing risk with benefit, it was suggested to *restrict HSCT to specific subgroups with poor risk factors*.[30] The *MLL-10* trial of the JPLSG stratified patients and transplanted patients only those with KMT2A rearrangement and age <6 months and with CNS leukemia (HR group). IR (KMT2A rearranged without HR features) and low risk (LR) group received chemotherapy only. The 3-year EFS for LR and IR was 93.3 and 94.4%, respectively, while 3-year EFS rate for HR was 56.6%. This way they restricted using HSCT for all KMT2A rearranged leukemias.[31] Hence, to summarize, *data is not so conclusive, but a small subset of HR infant ALL (age <6 months, TLC >300 × 10^9/L, and persistence of MRD) benefit from HSCT in CR1.*

CASE (Continued)

This patient was characterized as MR group as per the Interfant group risk stratification. In our institute we go ahead with HSCT only if the patient was in the HR group to begin with or IR and MRD positive (>0.01% by flow cytometry) at the beginning of OCTADAD. We prefer an early transplant (<4 months from diagnosis), if logistics permits. We prefer a matched sibling donor (MSD) transplant. If MSD not available, we hunt for a matched unrelated donor (MUD) transplant, but go ahead with a haploidentical transplant if funds do not permit a donor search or if donor is unavailable.

14. Which conditioning regimen is used in infantile ALL, if at all transplantation is considered?

Most cooperative group trials use cyclophosphamide (or fludarabine) and busulfan (±melphalan) with standard infection and graft versus host disease (GVHD) prophylaxis. Total body irradiation (TBI)-based conditioning is not used owing to the severe late effects observed.

15. What are the prognostic factors in this child with infantile ALL?

Prognostic factors as per the latest trials of infant ALL are given in **Table 4**.

TABLE 4: Prognostic factors for infants with ALL.

Trial	Poor prognostic factor
Interfant 06	• t(4;11) and t(11;19) have worse prognosis than t(9;11) >All three do worse than germline KMT2A ALL infants • Age <6 months • WBC ≥300 × 10^9/L • Poor prednisolone response
MLL-10	• Female gender • Age <180 days • MRD positive at end of consolidation

(ALL: acute lymphoblastic leukemia; MLL: mixed lineage leukemia; MRD: minimal residual disease; WBC: white blood cell)

CASE (Continued)

So in our case, apart from the t(4;11) rearrangement, all other factors were favorable (age was >6 months, WBC was <300,000/µL, good prednisolone response, male gender, and most importantly MRD negativity at end of consolidation). However, it may be argued, that this child, like many other children in low–middle income countries, presented very late (a history of 3 months) and may have had some form of alternate therapy before reaching the healthcare facility. Nonetheless he had a good prednisolone response and MRD negativity, which have been seen to override all other factors.

16. What is the likelihood that this child will relapse and what are the risk factors at the time of relapse?

As per Interfant 99, probability of relapse is high (around 45%), occurring mostly within the first year of diagnosis (median time 10 months). Most relapses were seen to occur in the BM (71.8%), whereas others were isolated extramedullary ($n = 23$) or combined relapses ($n = 32$). Patients in the HR group relapsed earlier than patients in the SR group (median: 9 vs. 12 months, $p = 0.042$) and germline MLL patients relapsed later and less frequently. Patients were mainly (75%) treated with salvage chemotherapy followed by HSCT. Salvage chemotherapy can be in the form of any protocol used for relapsed ALL (UK-ALL R3 protocol or BFM-REZ 2002 protocol). OS following HSCT was around 20% and this was significantly better than chemotherapy only protocols. Higher WBC count, relapse within 1 year and BM only relapse had poorer prognosis in the multivariable model.[32] The role of immunotherapy [blinatumomab or chimeric antigen receptor (CAR) T cells] on relapsed infants with ALL is evolving, with current evidence limited to pilot trials.

CASE (Continued)

Child completed maintenance therapy in August 2021 and remains alive and well.

17. What are the novel therapies being studied for infantile ALL?

High FLT3 protein levels are expressed in the leukemic blasts of infants with MLL-rearranged ALL, even in the absence of FLT3 activating mutations, which occur in <20% of infants with MLL-rearranged ALL.[33] *FLT3 inhibitor, lestaurtinib* potentiates chemotherapy-induced cytotoxicity in preclinical models. In the *COG AALL0631*, after chemotherapy induction, KMT2A-r infants received either chemotherapy only or chemotherapy plus lestaurtinib. There was no difference in 3-year EFS between patients treated with chemotherapy plus lestaurtinib ($n = 67$, 36%) versus chemotherapy only ($n = 54$, 39%, $p = 0.67$).[34] Safety and efficacy of *clofarabine* is being tested in the MLL-17 trial. Hypomethylating agents like azacytidine and decitabine, *histone deacetylase inhibitors like vorinostat and panabinostat and BCL-2 inhibitors like venetoclax* are being tested.[10] Mutations in NRAS and KRAS are seen in 14% of KMT2A-r infant ALL. Hence, preclinical studies for *MEK inhibitors* are underway.[10] Blinatumomab has been tested in 11 infants treated on the Interfant chemotherapy backbone. An EFS of 50% has been reported, which is superior to historical controls. *CAR T cells* are also in preclinical studies.[10]

18. What are the expected late effects in this child?

Not much has been reported on late effects in infant ALL. A review of survivors treated on the MLL-03 protocol revealed serious growth failure, especially in children who received TBI. This was followed closely by dental late effects and thyroid dysfunction.[35]

REFERENCES

1. Noone AM, Cronin KA, Altekruse SF, Howlader N, Lewis DR, Petkov VI, et al. Cancer incidence and survival trends by subtype using data from the surveillance epidemiology and end results program, 1992-2013. Cancer Epidemiol Biomarkers Prev. 2017;26(4):632-41.
2. https://ncdirindia.org/NCRP/ALL_NCRP_REPORTS/PBCR_REPORT_2012_2014/ALL_CONTENT/Printed_Version.htm.
3. Arora R, Arora B. Acute leukemia in children: a review of the current Indian data. South Asian J Cancer. 2016;5(3):155-60.
4. Kotecha RS, Gottardo NG, Kees UR, Cole CH. The evolution of clinical trials for infant acute lymphoblastic leukemia. Blood Cancer J. 2014;4(4):e200.
5. Brown P. Treatment of infant leukemias: challenge and promise. Hematol Am Soc Hematol Educ Program. 2013;2013:596-600.
6. Silverman LB. Acute lymphoblastic leukemia in infancy. Pediatr Blood Cancer. 2007;49(Suppl 7):1070-3.
7. Creutzig U, Zimmermann M, Bourquin JP, Dworzak MN, Kremens B, Lehrnbecher T, et al. Favorable outcome in infants with AML after intensive first- and second-line treatment: an AML-BFM study group report. Leukemia. 2012;26(4):654-61.
8. Hilden JM, Dinndorf PA, Meerbaum SO, Sather H, Villaluna D, Heerema NA, et al. Analysis of prognostic factors of acute lymphoblastic leukemia in infants: report on CCG 1953 from the Children's Oncology Group. Blood. 2006;108(2):441-51.
9. Swerdlow SH (Ed). WHO Classification of Tumours of Haematopoietic and Lymphoid Tissues, 4th edition. International Agency for Research on Cancer; 2008.
10. Brown P, Pieters R, Biondi A. How I treat infant leukemia. Blood. 2019;133(3):205-14.
11. Behm FG, Raimondi SC, Frestedt JL, Liu Q, Crist WM, Downing JR, et al. Rearrangement of the MLL gene confers a poor prognosis in childhood acute lymphoblastic leukemia, regardless of presenting age. Blood. 1996;87(7):2870-7.
12. Agarwal M, Seth R, Lall M. Study of cytogenetic alterations and association with prognostic factors in Indian children with B-lineage acute lymphoblastic leukemia. Clin Lymphoma Myeloma Leuk. 2020;20(7):e346-e351.
13. Harrison CJ, Hills RK, Moorman AV, Grimwade DJ, Hann I, Webb DKH, et al. Cytogenetics of childhood acute myeloid leukemia: United Kingdom Medical Research Council Treatment Trials AML 10 and 12. J Clin Oncol. 2010;28(16):2674-81.
14. Meyer C, Burmeister T, Gröger D, Tsaur G, Fechina L, Renneville A, et al. The MLL recombinome of acute leukemias in 2017. Leukemia. 2018;32(2):273-84.
15. Grembecka J, Cierpicki T. Stabilizing the mixed lineage leukemia protein. N Engl J Med. 2017;376(17):1688-9.
16. De Lorenzo P, Moorman AV, Pieters R, Dreyer ZE, Heerema NA, Carroll AJ, et al. Cytogenetics and outcome of infants with acute lymphoblastic leukemia and absence of MLL rearrangements. Leukemia. 2014;28(2):428-30.
17. Reaman G, Zeltzer P, Bleyer WA, Amendola B, Level C, Sather H, et al. Acute lymphoblastic leukemia in infants less than one year of age: a cumulative experience of the Children's Cancer Study Group. J Clin Oncol. 1985;3(11):1513-21.
18. Reaman GH, Steinherz PG, Gaynon PS, Bleyer WA, Finklestein JZ, Evans R, et al. Improved survival of infants less than 1 year of age with acute lymphoblastic leukemia treated with intensive multiagent chemotherapy. Cancer Treat Rep. 1987;71(11):1033-8.

19. Reaman GH, Sposto R, Sensel MG, Lange BJ, Feusner JH, Heerema NA, et al. Treatment outcome and prognostic factors for infants with acute lymphoblastic leukemia treated on two consecutive trials of the Children's Cancer Group. J Clin Oncol. 1999;17(2):445-55.
20. Frankel LS, Ochs J, Shuster JJ, Dubowy R, Bowman WP, Hockenberry-Eaton M, et al. Therapeutic trial for infant acute lymphoblastic leukemia: The Pediatric Oncology Group experience (POG 8493). J Pediatr Hematol Oncol. 1997;19(1):35-42.
21. Salzer WL, Devidas M, Carroll WL, Winick N, Pullen J, Hunger SP, et al. Long-term results of the pediatric oncology group studies for childhood acute lymphoblastic leukemia 1984-2001: A report from the Children's Oncology Group. Leukemia. 2010;24(2):355-70.
22. Salzer WL, Jones TL, Devidas M, Hilden JM, Winick N, Hunger S, et al. Modifications to induction therapy decrease risk of early death in infants with acute lymphoblastic leukemia treated on Children's Oncology Group P9407. Pediatr Blood Cancer. 2012;59(5):834-9.
23. Isoyama K, Eguchi M, Hibi S, Kinukawa N, Ohkawa H, Kawasaki H, et al. Risk-directed treatment of infant acute lymphoblastic leukaemia based on early assessment of MLL gene status: results of the Japan Infant Leukaemia Study (MLL96). Br J Haematol. 2002;118(4):999-1010.
24. Kosaka Y, Koh K, Kinukawa N, Wakazono Y, Isoyama K, Oda T, et al. Infant acute lymphoblastic leukemia with MLL gene rearrangements: outcome following intensive chemotherapy and hematopoietic stem cell transplantation. Blood. 2004;104(12):3527-34.
25. Tomizawa D, Koh K, Sato T, Kinukawa N, Morimoto A, Isoyama K, et al. Outcome of risk-based therapy for infant acute lymphoblastic leukemia with or without an MLL gene rearrangement, with emphasis on late effects: a final report of two consecutive studies, MLL96 and MLL98, of the Japan Infant Leukemia Study Group. Leukemia. 2007;21(11):2258-63.
26. Pieters R, den Boer ML, Durian M, Janka G, Schmiegelow K, Kaspers GJ, et al. Relation between age, immunophenotype and in vitro drug resistance in 395 children with acute lymphoblastic leukemia-implications for treatment of infants. Leukemia. 1998;12(9):1344-8.
27. Pieters R, Schrappe M, De Lorenzo P, Hann I, De Rossi G, Felice M, et al. A treatment protocol for infants younger than 1 year with acute lymphoblastic leukaemia (Interfant-99): an observational study and a multicentre randomised trial. Lancet. 2007;370(9583):240-50.
28. Pieters R, De Lorenzo P, Ancliffe P, Aversa LA, Brethon B, Biondi A, et al. Outcome of infants younger than 1 year with acute lymphoblastic leukemia treated with the Interfant-06 protocol: results from an International Phase III Randomized Study. J Clin Oncol. 2019;37(25):2246-56.
29. Van der Velden VHJ, Corral L, Valsecchi MG, De Lorenzo P, Cazzaniga G, Panzer-Grümayer ER, et al. Prognostic significance of minimal residual disease in infants with acute lymphoblastic leukemia treated within the Interfant-99 protocol. Leukemia. 2009;23(6):1073-9.
30. Koh K, Tomizawa D, Saito AM, Watanabe T, Miyamura T, Hirayama M, et al. Early use of allogeneic hematopoietic stem cell transplantation for infants with MLL gene-rearrangement-positive acute lymphoblastic leukemia. Leukemia. 2015;29(2):290-6.
31. Tomizawa D, Miyamura T, Imamura T, Watanabe T, Saito AM, Ogawa A, et al. A risk-stratified therapy for infants with acute lymphoblastic leukemia: a report from the JPLSG MLL-10 trial. Blood. 2020;136(16):1813-23.
32. Driessen EMC, de Lorenzo P, Campbell M, Felice M, Ferster A, Hann I, et al. Outcome of relapsed infant acute lymphoblastic leukemia treated on the Interfant-99 protocol. Leukemia. 2016;30(5):1184-7.
33. Stam RW, den Boer ML, Schneider P, Nollau P, Horstmann M, Beverloo HB, et al. Targeting FLT3 in primary MLL-gene-rearranged infant acute lymphoblastic leukemia. Blood. 2005;106(7):2484-90.
34. Brown PA, Kairalla JA, Hilden JM, Dreyer ZE, Carroll AJ, Heerema NA, et al. FLT3 inhibitor lestaurtinib plus chemotherapy for newly diagnosed KMT2A-rearranged infant acute lymphoblastic leukemia: Children's Oncology Group trial AALL0631. Leukemia. 2021;35(5):1279-90.
35. Aoki Y, Hayakawa A, Koike K, Tauchi H. Late effects in survivors of infant acute lymphoblastic leukemia from the 3 consecutive Japanese nationwide clinical trials. Blood. 2019;134(Supplement 1):4559.

EXPERT OPINION

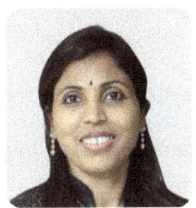

Sirisha Rani S
Senior Consultant in Pediatric Hematology Oncology and BMT
Rainbow Children's Hospital, Hyderabad, India

1. What is the ideal protocol for a child with infant ALL? Which protocol do you choose at your center?

As infant ALL is more aggressive in presentation as being more immature precursor B-cell type, high count, and HR genetics association, it requires a more intense protocol than pediatric ALL protocol. We use Interfant 06 protocol in our center.

2. Is there a role of AML like in induction in the treatment of infantile ALL?

These leukemias are derived from early hematopoietic precursors with myeloid differentiation, and they are more immature with aggressive biology. Infantile ALL response to regular ALL protocol. The inadequate and high association with HR genetics like KMT2A clearly makes it different from pediatric ALL. Hence, there is a role of AML-like induction, like in Interfant protocol that includes cytarabine in the induction.

3. Is there a role of MRD assessment in infantile ALL upfront?

Minimal residual disease's role in assessing treatment response in acute leukemias is well established. Its role in infantile ALL gives a good idea about disease control. The early assessment identifies HR cases early. In HR MRD positivity, early assessment gives adequate time to work up for HSCT and intensity treatment to achieve remission before HSCT.

4. When and how to consider HSCT? Which conditioning regimen is used in infantile ALL if transplantation is considered?

It is indicated to do HSCT after disease remission with induction and then consolidating remission with consolidation. TBI-based conditioning must be avoided in <3 years of age. Using treosulfan, fludarabine, and thiotepa is ideal for conditioning in infantile ALL.

5. Is there any role of the novel therapies in infantile ALL upfront?

Its high association with KMT2A opened a lot of clinical trials to try agents targeting its variants. Various agents described to be effective are FLT3 inhibitors, epigenetic modifiers, RAS pathway inhibitors, immunotherapy agents like blinatumomab, histone deacetylase inhibitors, etc. Among them, FLT3 inhibitor Lestaurtinib is more practical to use in the postinduction phase to enhance the efficacy of consolidation medications.

5.2 ACUTE LEUKEMIA IN DOWN SYNDROME

Gargi Das, Jagdish P Meena

CASE VIGNETTE

Master L is a third born child of a nonconsanguineous couple. He was born by normal vaginal delivery, at term, and had a smooth perinatal transition. At birth, physicians noticed a typical phenotype of upslanting palpebral fissures, flat nasal bridge, flat face, prominent epicanthal folds, simian crease on palms, sandal gap, generalized hypotonia, and a reducible umbilical hernia. A provisional diagnosis of Down syndrome (DS) was made, and a karyotype was sent for analysis. ECHO at birth and at 72 hours of life was essentially normal for age. On day 4 of life, child had a complete blood count (CBC) revealing a hemoglobin (Hb) of 14, total leukocyte count (TLC) of 25,000/µL (neutrophilic predominance), and platelet count of 56,000/µL. Simultaneously physicians noticed increase in size of liver and spleen. On day 6 of life, TLC increased to 45,000/µL. Karyotype on day 14 revealed a trisomy 21.

1. What are the hematological abnormalities seen in DS?

In 95% of DS patients, there is presence of trisomy of the 21st chromosome, while 1% are mosaics and 4% have translocation involving chromosome 21. The constellation of clinical features allows for early detection of DS in infancy.[1] Up to 80, 66, and 34% of newborns with DS have neutrophilia, thrombocytopenia, and polycythemia, respectively.[2] Transient leukemia of DS [TL-DS, previously known as transient abnormal myelopoiesis disorder (TMD)], occurs in 10% of all DS patients and about 20% progress to DS-associated acute leukemia [acute megakaryoblastic leukemia (AMKL)].[3]

2. In the above case, is it suggestive of a TL in DS? What investigations are required to establish this diagnosis?

Progression of trisomy 21 to TL-DS to AMKL is an incremental process of leukemogenesis. TL-DS is a critical model to understand the natural history of AMKL. 20% of TL-DS cases evolve into AMKL either overtly, or following an apparent remission. DS-AMKL leukemogenesis can be explained by three genetic hits. The first hit (first genetic event) is trisomy of chromosome 21, which is inherent to the development of DS. The second hit is a mutation of the X-linked gene *GATA1*, encoding a transcription factor essential for development of the erythroid and megakaryocytic lineages.[4] *GATA1* mutation occurs most likely in utero.[5] A *GATA1* mutant TL-DS clone acquires additional mutations (*CTCF, EZH2, KANSL1, JAK3, MPL, SH2B3,* and *RAS* pathway genes) and progress to myeloid leukemia (ML)-DS (third hit). Moreover, *GATA1* is not seen in remission samples after treatment of ML-DS nor are they commonly present in other DS and non-DS leukemias.[6] As suggested by the British Society of Hematology, TL-DS should be defined as *"the presence of a GATA1 mutation together with a peripheral blood blast percentage >10% and or clinical features suggestive of TL-DS in a child with DS or mosaic trisomy 21."*[7]

CASE (Continued)

In the above case, there is a progressive increase in TLC with decrease in platelet count and newly detected hepatosplenomegaly within first week of life. Another soft pointer is that child has a normal to high Hb. Hence, we should consider a TL-DS in this child. Peripheral smear done in this child revealed 12% blasts and subsequent next-generation sequencing (NGS) revealed a GATA1 mutation, hence the child had TL-DS.

3. What are the clinical features and what do we expect in peripheral smear and flow cytometry in this child?

A good peripheral smear examination, ideally in the first 3 days of life, is done to assess the blast count. Clinical features occur due to spill of megakaryoblastic cells into peripheral blood and spread to distant tissues. Enlargement of the liver, malignant pleural, and pericardial effusions and/or papular or vesiculopustular rash due to deposits containing TL-DS blast cells in the skin occur as part of the TL-DS spectrum. Splenomegaly is found in 30% of cases, although this is often due to portal venous obstruction. Raised transaminases with conjugated hyperbilirubinemia, extreme leukocytosis (with neutrophilia), and coagulopathy are laboratory findings in TL-DS.[7]

Circulating blast cells are megakaryoblastic-pleomorphic, often having prominent nucleoli and basophilic and blebbed cytoplasm. Immunophenotypically they have a phenotype distinct from other leukemias, showing variable coexpression of stem cell markers (CD34 and CD117), myeloid markers CD13/CD33 and platelet glycoproteins (CD36, CD42, and CD61), as well as aberrant expression of CD56 and CD7 and low expression of CD11a.[8] As blast cells in TL-DS are believed to originate in the liver, bone marrow examination is generally not useful.[7]

CASE (Continued)

Flow cytometry of peripheral blasts revealed 37% blasts, positive for CD45 (dim), CD34, CD117, CD13, 33 (dim), CD41, CD61, CD16, and CD56, further cementing the diagnosis of TL-DS.

4. Should all children of DS be tested for GATA1 mutation?

The answer is No. The combination of a GATA1 mutation with no increased blast cell percentage (i.e., <10%) in a neonate with DS has been termed silent TL-DS (rate of transformation to acute leukemia is <3% compared to 20% in clinical TL-DS).[6] Only neonates in whom blast percentage was not assessed or deemed unreliable, we may conduct a GATA1 mutation analysis and follow children accordingly. GATA1 mutation analysis should be performed in an accredited laboratory using a properly standardized, high-sensitivity assay-like NGS.[7]

5. What are the life-threatening symptoms/signs (LTS) of TL-DS?

Early death in TL-DS is seen in 15–23% of patients.[9] The Children's Oncology Group (COG) defined what they believed were "LTS" or to our understanding symptoms which are associated with an increased risk of early death and hence may warrant treatment. The following are the LTS:[7]
- Multiorgan dysfunction
- White blood cell (WBC) count > 100×10^9/L or clinical features of leukostasis

- Hepatic dysfunction (conjugated bilirubin, ascites or massive hepatomegaly)
- Hepatosplenomegaly (beyond umbilicus or causing respiratory or feeding compromise)
- Hydrops fetalis
- Pleural or pericardial effusions
- Renal failure
- Disseminated intravascular coagulation (DIC)/coagulopathy with bleeding.

CASE *(Continued)*

On day 10 of life, it was noticed that this child had increasing liver and spleen. TLC increased to 112,000/µL with 57% blasts in peripheral smear. He was found to be icteric with a total bilirubin of 6 mg/dL with increased conjugate fraction.

6. When do we consider treating a child with TL-DS? Can we observe this child alone, or does he warrant therapy?

In the COG A2971 study, it was found that majority of children had a spontaneous disappearance of the peripheral blast cells at a median of 36 days. Blasts usually disappear by 4–10 weeks and no study has shown any spontaneous resolution after 6 months of age.[10] Cases of TL-DS lacking LTS should be monitored with a CBC and liver function tests including conjugated bilirubin until there is spontaneous remission. All children with previous TL-DS or silent TL-DS should be monitored for progression to ML-DS with 3 monthly clinical review and CBCs with peripheral smear until the age of 2 years. If the CBC and film are normal and there are no clinical features of ML-DS, monitoring should continue 6 monthly until the age of 4 years. Abnormal blood counts should prompt early bone marrow evaluation along with a *GATA1* mutation analysis (if not done previously).[7] In case of LTS, we should consider early treatment. TL-DS blasts are highly sensitive to cytarabine (Ara-C). Hence, cytarabine should be given without delay at a dose of 1–1.5 mg/kg/day for 5–7 days either intravenously or subcutaneously. Repeated courses of cytarabine can be considered to achieve control where severe liver dysfunction persists. Hepatomegaly may take weeks/months to resolve. Exchange transfusion or leukapheresis can be considered to lower counts, but are not definitive means of treatment. Treatment with Ara-C, does not reduce future risk of ML with DS (ML-DS).[7]

CASE *(Continued)*

The above child had features of LTS (increasing counts, increasing organomegaly, and rising bilirubin), and hence would benefit from low-dose Ara-C, which he was given for 7 days, following which his TLC decreased to 57,000/µL by day 20 and 23,000/µL by day 31. Blasts also reduced to <10% gradually over next 3 weeks and bilirubin improved to normal for age by day 21. His hepatosplenomegaly resolved by 9 months of age. He was followed up clinically and by TLC and remained well till 2 years of age.

At 27 months of life he presented to our outpatient department with fever, progressive pallor, and petechiae for 1 month. On examination, child was found to have liver and spleen palpable 5 and 7 cm below costal margins. CBC revealed Hb of 8.6 g/dL, TLC of 65,140/µL and platelet count of 32,000/µL. Peripheral smear revealed 80% blasts, probably myeloid in morphology with salmon colored granules and prominent hofs. Peripheral blood flow cytometry revealed 82% CD45 dim+ blasts which were heterogeneously positive for CD34, dim positive for CD13, and moderate to strong positive for CD33, CD117, CD11b, CD7, CD38, CD41, and CD61. Blasts were negative for cMPO, cCD79a, cCD3, sCD3, CD4, CD16, CD123, HLA DR, CD64, CD56, CD14, and CD235a. Findings were suggestive of an AMKL.

7. What are the characteristics of leukemia in DS?

Children with DS have a 20-fold increased risk of developing leukemia. 1–2% of DS patients develop ML-DS by 4 years of age. 20% of them have a history of TL-DS. Older children with DS have increased frequency of acute lymphoblastic leukemia (ALL). DS account for around 4% of acute myeloid leukemia (AML).[11] ML-DS has a superior prognosis compared to childhood AML, with an event-free survival (EFS) close to 80% in part due to exquisite sensitivity to cytarabine and also due to clinical features like low initial WBC count, no central nervous system (CNS) involvement, and fewer cytogenetic abnormalities.[12]

8. What are the peripheral smear, bone marrow, and flow cytometric abnormalities in Down with AML?

There is a high prevalence of AMKL in DS patients.[11] Peripheral smear usually shows blasts and erythroid precursors. Platelet counts are decreased with occasional giant platelets. The bone marrow aspirate reveals unique looking blasts with round to irregular nuclei and moderate amount of basophilic cytoplasm and cytoplasmic blebs. Cytoplasm may have coarse basophilic granules. Dysgranulopoiesis and dysplastic erythroid precursors maybe seen. Bone marrow may have increased fibrosis and hence sometimes it is a dry tap necessitation a bone marrow biopsy. Immunophenotyping reveals, negative myeloperoxidase (MPO), positive prematurity markers (CD117), and myeloid marker (CD13, 33, and 11b) along with positivity for megakaryoblast markers (CD41, 42b, and 61).[8]

CASE (Continued)

Molecular analysis was negative for *NPM1, CEBPa,* and *FLT3-ITD* and *TKD* mutation but positive for a *GATA1* mutation. **Figure 1** shows the karyotype of the child.

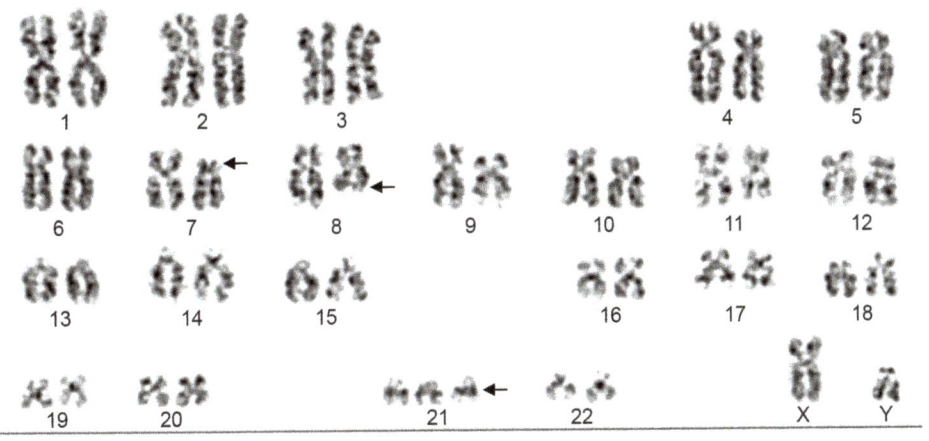

47, XY, del(7)(p11), del(8)(q22), +21

Fig. 1: Karyotype of index child.

9. What is the interpretation of the karyotype?

The child has a 47XY karyotype with trisomy 21 (the first hit, along with GATA1, the second hit) and has additional mutations including deletion of chromosome 7 [del(7)(p11)] and deletion 8 [del(8)(q22)]. These two mutations are probably the third hit which triggered the ML in this child with DS.

10. What are the precautions we need to keep in mind when treating this child with DS?

It is important to note that though the survival in ML-DS is more, these patients have poor tolerance to chemotherapy and the philosophy of management of DS includes a good balance between efficacy and tolerability. ML-DS blasts are exquisitely sensitive to cytarabine (Ara-C) as they generate increased intracellular concentrated of Ara-C triphosphate. Hence, cytarabine can be intensified to improve outcome in ML-DS. These blasts are also sensitive to anthracyclines. Overexpression of the chromosome 21 localized gene, carbonyl reductase, catalyzes the reduction of anthracyclines to cardiotoxic alcohol metabolites, increasing cardiotoxicity. Hence, anthracyclines can be reduced to maintain equal efficacy at reduced cost of cardiotoxicity.[13] Good supportive care is central to management of ML-DS.

11. Briefly discuss the evolution of clinical trials including DS patients with AML.

The progress in ML-DS chemotherapy regimens can be understood by tracking its historical evolution. We have tried to discuss the trials of ML-DS via the following questions.

a. What were the outcomes of ML-DS patients treated on non-DS AML protocols?

Before 1990, ML-DS were treated on individualized protocols, receiving minimal chemotherapy due to the impression that DS patients could not tolerate chemotherapy. This approach was largely ineffective.[14] Subsequently, they started treatment of ML-DS on protocols used for non-DS AML patients. This improved their outcomes dramatically. **Table 1** highlights the complete remission (CR) rates and survival [overall survival (OS) and EFS] of DS patients in non-DS AML trials.[11]

b. Do ML-DS patients require separate trials?

Table 2 highlights key characteristics of trials treating AML separately. ML-DS 2006 is the European trial while COG are North American cooperative group trials.

c. What is the role of etoposide?

Etoposide has been used variably in previous trials. Etoposide was associated with increased myelosuppression and toxicity and hence eliminated in the COG A2971 trial, maintaining good survival as compared to legacy trials.[16] The COG AAML-0431 trial, reintroduced etoposide, probably because daunorubicin doses were decreased to reduce cardiotoxicity.[13]

d. What is maintenance therapy?

Maintenance chemotherapy was eliminated in the early 1990s.[11] COG A2971 had maintenance IT Ara-C,[16] but subsequently was removed in the COG AAML-0431[13] trial as there was no increased risk of CNS disease or relapse.

TABLE 1: Non-DS AML trials on which DS patients were included.

Study (year)	N	CR (%)	OS (%)	EFS (%)	Special note
POG 8498	12	100	100	100	ML-DS patients were younger (<2 years of age) and more likely to have AMKL. HiDAC in induction and consolidation improved survival
CCG 2861/ CCG2891	110	88	88	68	• Intensive chemotherapy increases TRM and hence marrow recovery necessary before start of next cycle • Also studied role of transplant in CR1, but concluded high TRM
MRC 10/ MRC 12	46	89	74	74	• 11% died during induction. High TRM. High anthracycline dose led to increased TRM • Most TRMs were infections or cardiac complications
NOPHO-84/ NOPHO-88	23	74	79	–	• All four trials concluded importance of HiDAC in chemotherapy regimen of ML-DS and importance of allowing full bone marrow recovery before starting second cycle • DS patients in BFM 98 were treated with reduced anthracycline and HiDAC and had better survival than non-DS patients
AML BFM 93	44	82	79	68	
AML BFM 98	66	100	98	89	

(AML: acute myeloid leukemia; AMKL: acute megakaryoblastic leukemia; BFM: Berlin-Frankfurt-Münster; CR: complete remission; DS: Down syndrome; EFS: event-free survival; HiDAC: high-dose cytarabine; ML: myeloid leukemia; OS: overall survival; TRM: treatment-related mortality)

e. What is CNS therapy?

As per COG A2971 protocol, incidence of CNS disease in ML-DS was low, hence subsequent COG AAML-0431 reduced IT Ara-C doses from seven to two. Moreover, CNS relapse is an extremely low occurrence in the contemporary COG protocols for ML-DS.[13]

f. Can high-dose Ara-C not be used in trials?

According to a trial by the Japanese childhood AML study group. Remission induction chemotherapy consisted of pirarubicin, etoposide, and Ara-C (low dose 100 mg/m^2/day for 7 days). Patients who achieved CR received four courses of intensification therapy of the same regimen. 97.2% achieved a CR and 4-year EFS and OS was 83.3 and 83.7%, respectively.[18] Based on the above trial and results of the COG A2971 where it was reported that there was increased toxicity in cycle 2 [high-dose cytarabine (HiDAC)] in previous trials and good survival of minimal residual disease (MRD) negative patients, it was decided to deintensify therapy [remove high-dose Ara-C in patients who were MRD negative (SR ML-DS)] in the subsequent COG AAML 1531 trial. The survival of SR ML-DS was EFS 85.6% (inferior to 92.7% of 0431, p value = 0.0002). Moreover, survival following relapse was poor, hence subsequent COG trials will use COG AAML 0431 as the backbone.[17]

TABLE 2: Exclusive ML-DS trials.

Study	N	Induction	Intensification	Cumulative dose (mg/m²)	CR/EFS/OS (%)	TRM
ML-DS 2006[15] (Based on older BFM studies)	170	Cycle 1: AIE [Ara-C (A) Idarubicin (I) Etoposide (E)] Cycle 2: AI	Cycle 1: hAM (HiDAC and mitoxantrone) Cycle 2: HA (HiDAC) No maintenance therapy Four doses intrathecal therapy	Ara-C: 27,400 Etoposide: 450 Idarubicin: 34 Mitoxantrone: 14 DNR equivalent: 260	85/87/89	2.9% Mostly infectious complications. Reduced from previous ALL-BFM 98 trial
COG A2971[16]	132	Four cycles of CI-TAD (continuous infusion of 6 thioguanine + Ara-C + DNR) Cumulative in first two cycles Ara-C: 1,600 mg/m² DNR: 160 mg/m²	HiDAC + L-asparaginase Maintenance with three doses of CNS consolidation with IT cytarabine (total seven doses)	Ara-C: 27,200 DNR: 320 Etoposide: 0	84/79/84	3%
COG AAML-0431[13]	205	Cycle 1, 3, 4: CI-TAD Cycle 2: HiDAC + L-asparaginase HiDAC introduced early in induction Cumulative in first two cycles Ara-C: 24,800 mg/m² DNR: 80 mg/m²	Cycle 1, 2: Intermediate dose CI Ara-C + etoposide IT Ara-C doses: Two	Ara-C: 27,800 DNR: 240 Etoposide: 750 Reduced DNR dose Increased etoposide	87/90/93 MRD < 0.01%: 95.6% Incidence of relapse was similar, but EFS and OS were better as compared to the A2971 trial DFS MRD− versus MRD+: 92.7 versus 76.2%	1% Mostly in cycle 1 and 2 of induction Similar rates of bacterial infections in non-DS ML No cardiac deaths Comparable TRM to A2971

Contd...

Contd...

Study	N	Induction	Intensification	Cumulative dose (mg/m²)	CR/EFS/OS (%)	TRM
COG AAML-1531[17]	SR: 114 HR: 26	Cycle 1: CI-TAD Followed by MRD analysis If MRD < 0.05%: Standard risk Received cycle 2 and 3: CI TAD Removed HiDAC in cycle 2 as Increased toxicity in cycle 2 in previous trials MRD– patients did very well Japanese trials for SR ML-DS patients without HiDAC did well If MRD > 0.05%: High risk Cycle 1, 3, 4: CI-TAD Cycle 2: HiDAC + L-asparaginase	SR/HR: Cycle 1, 2—intermediate dose CI Ara-C + etoposide IT Ara-C doses: Two		Interim results as a communication in blood journal: Survival of SR ML-DS EFS 85.6% (inferior to 92.7% of 0431) Survival following relapse was poor	

(ALL: acute lymphoblastic leukemia; BFM: Berlin-Frankfurt-Münster; CNS: central nervous system; COG: Children's Oncology Group; CI-TAD: continuous infusion of 6 thioguanine + AraC + daunorubicin; CR: complete remission; DNR: daunorubicin; DS: Down syndrome; EFS: event-free survival; HR: high risk; HiDAC: high-dose cytarabine; MRD: minimal residual disease; ML: myeloid leukemia; OS: overall survival; SR: standard; TRM: treatment-related mortality)

CASE (Continued)

This child was started on the COG A2971 protocol. Child was admitted for all induction cycles. He had severe FN episodes during cycle 1, 2, and 3 of induction. His MRD was <0.01% after one cycle of induction. Echocardiogram was done prior to each cycle and was normal. He received consolidation and intrathecal therapy subsequently on daycare basis. He is currently 4 years post-treatment completion and is alive and well.

12. What are the relevant prognostic features in a child with DS?

Myeloid leukemia Down syndrome following TL-DS had similar outcomes to de novo ML-DS. Older age portends poorer survival. Better outcome is seen if there is early bone marrow response (<5% blasts by day 14).[16] MRD > 0.01% was associated with significantly inferior survival in the COG AAML 0431 trial and stood out as the single most factor affecting inferior survival in the multivariate analysis.[13]

13. How would you treat an ML-DS in low- and middle-income country (LMIC) setting? Is it reasonable to treat them on historical non-DS AML trials?

The most important factor for treating ML-DS in LMICs is access to good supportive care. In our experience at AIIMS, majority of ML-DS patients die due to treatment-related mortalities (TRMs) during induction. Hence, we must counsel our patients to stay near the hospital following chemotherapy initiation or keep them admitted for the whole duration of induction, ensure blood donations, and counsel parents regarding basic hygiene and importance of reporting to hospital within 1 hour of fever. We must keep them under strict follow-up in case they are discharged after chemotherapy. As for the choice of protocol, this issue can be controversial. Some centers in India use ML-DS based protocols, while some centers use non-DS AML protocols (MRC 12 or 15) with reduced doses (50–75%). For example, the MRC 15 protocol at 75% dose gives a cumulative of 29,700 mg/m^2 of Ara-C, 225 mg/m^2 of daunorubicin (DNR), and 750 mg/m^2 of etoposide. Cumulative doses are like the COG AAML 0431 trial, but the difference is that the benefit of high-dose Ara-C in induction is lost.

14. Differences between AMKL in DS and non-DS patients.

Acute megakaryoblastic leukemia accounts for 4–15% of newly diagnosed childhood AML. AMKL in patients without DS (non-DS AMKL) is frequently associated with poor outcomes. In a study performed to understand the genomic landscape of non-DS AMKL, RNA and exome sequencing on specimens from 99 patients (75 pediatric and 24 adults) were performed identifying seven subgroups. They included patients with CBFA2T3-*GLIS2* rearrangements (18.6%), *KMT2A* rearrangements (17.4%), HOX rearrangements (14.9%), *NUP98-KDM5A* fusions (11.6%), and *RBM15-MKL1* fusions (10.2%). *GATA1* mutation was seen 9.2% of patients and no mutation or translocation was seen in 18.4% of patients. Specifically, *CBFA2T3-GLIS2* and *KMT2A*r were found to have significantly inferior EFS and OS and may benefit from allogeneic stem cell transplant (SCT) in first CR. *NUP98-KDM5A* cases also demonstrated a trend toward poor outcomes and warrant close monitoring and consideration of allogeneic SCT as well. Conversely, *GATA1* and *HOX*r subgroups carried significantly superior outcomes[19] and may be treated with chemotherapy alone.

REFERENCES

1. Kliegman R, Stanton B, St Geme JW, Schor NF, Behrman RE, Nelson WE (Eds). Nelson Textbook of Pediatrics. Netherlands: Elsevier; 2020.
2. Choi JK. Hematopoietic disorders in Down syndrome. Int J Clin Exp Pathol. 2008;1(5):387-95.
3. Blaney SM, Adamson PC, Helman L (Eds). Pizzo and Poplack's Pediatric Oncology, 8th edition. Philadelphia: Wolters Kluwer Health; 2021.
4. Khan I, Malinge S, Crispino J. Myeloid leukemia in Down syndrome. Crit Rev Oncog. 2011;16(1-2):25-36.
5. Shimada A, Xu G, Toki T, Kimura H, Hayashi Y, Ito E. Fetal origin of the GATA1 mutation in identical twins with transient myeloproliferative disorder and acute megakaryoblastic leukemia accompanying Down syndrome. Blood. 2004;103(1):366.
6. Bhatnagar N, Nizery L, Tunstall O, Vyas P, Roberts I. Transient abnormal myelopoiesis and AML in Down syndrome: an update. Curr Hematol Malig Rep. 2016;11(5):333-41.
7. Tunstall O, Bhatnagar N, James B, Norton A, O'Marcaigh AS, Watts T, et al.; British Society for Haematology. Guidelines for the investigation and management of transient leukaemia of Down syndrome. Br J Haematol. 2018;182(2):200-11.
8. Swerdlow SH, Campo E, Harris NL (Eds). WHO Classification of Tumours of Haematopoietic and Lymphoid Tissues, 4th edition. France: International Agency for Research on Cancer; 2017.
9. Massey GV, Zipursky A, Chang MN, Doyle JJ, Nasim S, Taub JW, et al.; Children's Oncology Group (COG). A prospective study of the natural history of transient leukemia (TL) in neonates with Down syndrome (DS): Children's Oncology Group (COG) study POG-9481. Blood. 2006;107(12):4606-13.
10. Gamis AS, Alonzo TA, Gerbing RB, Hilden JM, Sorrell AD, Sharma M, et al. Natural history of transient myeloproliferative disorder clinically diagnosed in Down syndrome neonates: a report from the Children's Oncology Group Study A2971. Blood. 2011;118(26):6752-9.
11. Caldwell JT, Ge Y, Taub JW. Prognosis and management of acute myeloid leukemia in patients with Down syndrome. Expert Rev Hematol. 2014;7(6):831-40.
12. Lanzkowsky P, Lipton JM, Fish JD (Eds). Lanzkowsky's Manual of Pediatric Hematology and Oncology, 7th edition. Netherlands: Elsevier; 2021.
13. Taub JW, Berman JN, Hitzler JK, Sorrell AD, Lacayo NJ, Mast K, et al. Improved outcomes for myeloid leukemia of Down syndrome: A report from the Children's Oncology Group AAML0431 trial. Blood. 2017;129(25):3304-13.
14. Gamis AS. Acute myeloid leukemia and Down syndrome evolution of modern therapy—state of the art review. Pediatr Blood Cancer. 2005;44(1):13-20.
15. Uffmann M, Rasche M, Zimmermann M, von Neuhoff C, Creutzig U, Dworzak M, et al. Therapy reduction in patients with Down syndrome and myeloid leukemia: The international ML-DS 2006 trial. Blood. 2017;129(25):3314-21.
16. Sorrell AD, Alonzo TA, Hilden JM, Gerbing RB, Loew TW, Hathaway L, et al. Favorable survival maintained in children who have myeloid leukemia associated with Down syndrome using reduced-dose chemotherapy on Children's Oncology Group trial A2971: A report from the Children's Oncology Group. Cancer. 2012;118(19):4806-14.
17. O'Dwyer KM. Back to HiDAC: Administering the optimal treatment for children with Down syndrome and acute myeloid leukemia. The Hematologist. 2022;19(2).
18. Kudo K, Kojima S, Tabuchi K, Yabe H, Tawa A, Imaizumi M, et al.; Japanese Childhood AML Cooperative Study Group. Prospective study of a pirarubicin, intermediate-dose cytarabine, and etoposide regimen in children with Down syndrome and acute myeloid leukemia: The Japanese Childhood AML Cooperative Study Group. J Clin Oncol. 2007;25(34):5442-7.
19. de Rooij JDE, Branstetter C, Ma J, Li Y, Walsh MP, Cheng J, et al. Pediatric non-Down syndrome acute megakaryoblastic leukemia is characterized by distinct genomic subsets with varying outcomes. Nat Genet. 2017;49(3):451-6.

EXPERT OPINION

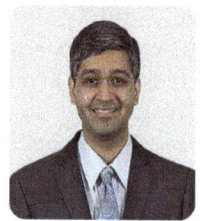

Chetan Anil Dhamne
Associate Professor, Pediatric Oncology
Tata Memorial Hospital, Dr. E Borges Road, Parel, Mumbai 400012

Epidemiology of ML-DS—statistical jugglery!

Children with DS are at an increased risk of both AML and ALL, with a 10–20-fold associated risk of leukemia as compared to those without DS. The risk increases 50-fold for children under 5 years. Within the 5-year age range, the risk is 150-fold for AML and 40-fold for ALL. Overall, 2% of DS children will develop leukemia by 5 years of age.

About 10% of DS children develop the transient myeloproliferative disorder (TMD) or transient abnormal myelopoiesis (TAM). Of these, 15% succumb to the disease. Of the ones who recover, 20–30% develop AMKL by 4 years of age, and 70–80% undergo spontaneous remission without further recurrence.

1. How do you treat TAM?

Transient abnormal myelopoiesis generally presents between 3 and 7 days of life and is generally self-limited. Occasionally children with DS present with hyperleukocytosis, hepatosplenomegaly, hydrops fetalis, pleural effusion, ascites, or DIC. In cases of hyperleukocytosis (WBC > 100,000/cumm) or hydrops fetalis, exchange transfusion is effective, followed by low-dose cytarabine. Cytarabine at 20 mg/m^2/day is generally initiated for children with high or rising WBC count and may be given up to 7 days. Other hematological abnormalities like polycythemia and thrombocytosis can be present in children with DS that are self-limited. TAM is generally resolved within 3-4 months of life. About 20% of these children develop AMKL between 1 and 4 years of life, and caregivers should be made aware of early signs of leukemia like easy bruising, petechiae, recurring fevers, bone pain, the onset of lethargy, or change in feeding patterns.

2. What are the clinical and laboratory characteristics of AML in DS?

In a child with DS, a diagnostic marrow will often yield a dry tap with <20% blast due to underlying myelofibrosis (nonrepresentative sample). Therefore, a diagnosis of AML in DS is not dependent on blast count (20% cutoff). More than 80% of AML in DS presents with megakaryocytic differentiation (AMKL). On flow cytometry, blasts are classically positive for CD41 and CD61. If negative, check for CD42b as a marker for megakaryocytic differentiation. CD36 is bright with an aberrant expression of CD7. Most cases present before 4 years of age and have *GATA1* mutations. Monosomy 7 does not confer an adverse prognosis. Having said that, additional cytogenetic abnormalities with complex cytogenetics may be present and represent a more unfavorable risk group, especially those who do not achieve MRD negativity after first cycle of induction (AAML1331 protocol). DS can also present with nonmegakaryocytic leukemia, predominantly M0 [Berlin-Frankfurt-Münster (BFM)] M1/M2 (COG), and have a prognosis similar to the M7 subgroup if <4 years of age. DS AML presenting after 4 years of age do poorly.

Acute megakaryoblastic leukemia may be preceded by MDS presenting with anemia and thrombocytopenia. These patients respond well to chemotherapy, but there is no urgency to start treatment in a clinically stable child. Delay in treatment does not compromise efficacy and outcomes. CNS involvement in ML-DS is rare at diagnosis and even at relapse.

3. Challenges in treating AML with DS.

Acute myeloid leukemia blasts are highly sensitive to chemotherapy, especially cytarabine. The incidence of resistant AML (5%) and risk of relapse (10%) are low. The greatest challenge is mucositis and infection-related mortality. Therefore, most protocols have evolved around reduction in doses of chemotherapy, especially anthracyclines (cardiotoxicity). In addition to dose reduction, contemporary protocols also reduce dose intensity allowing for complete count recovery prior to initiating the next cycle of chemotherapy.

In addition to hematological complications, children with DS also have problems with vision, hearing, congenital heart disease, thyroid-related disorders, obstructive sleep apnea, and atlantoaxial instability that the pediatric oncologist should be aware of. Identifying these problems and managing the child in collaboration with a multidisciplinary team will improve the quality of life for these children.

4. What are the outcomes of AML with DS?

Outcomes of ML-DS on COG, BFM, and Japanese protocols exceed 85% with reduced anthracycline dose and minimal intrathecal chemotherapy. Outcomes of relapsed AML with DS are exceedingly poor (<20%). But there is no indication for HSCT in the first remission. Thus, ML-DS should be treated on a reduced dose with reduced intensity protocols to achieve good outcomes.

5.3 PHILADELPHIA-POSITIVE ACUTE LYMPHOBLASTIC LEUKEMIA

Himani Bhasin, Rachna Seth

CASE VIGNETTE

I, a 3-year-old female presented with complaints of fever, weight loss, bilateral neck swelling, and epistaxis. On examination, she had significant bilateral cervical lymphadenopathy, ecchymotic patches over both arms and hepatosplenomegaly (liver 5 cm, spleen 4 cm below the right and left costal margin, respectively). Her complete blood count reported hyperleukocytosis, anemia, and thrombocytopenia. Peripheral smear showed 35% blast. On investigating further, her bone marrow aspiration reported 80% blast, which on flow cytometry was positive for CD45, CD10, CD34, CCD79a, CD38, CD304, CD73, CD123, HLA-DR, and negative for MPO, CD13, CD33, CD3, CD7, CD117, and CD56, suggestive of B acute lymphoblastic leukemia (B-ALL). Her cytogenetics was normal (46, XX). Her bone marrow FISH (fluorescence in situ hybridization) was positive for translocation (9:22) (q34;q11.2) (BCR/ABL) in 34% cells. She was diagnosed as a case of Philadelphia-positive (Ph+) precursor B-ALL or Ph+ B-ALL and was started on high-risk (HR) arm of Indian Collaborative Childhood Leukaemia group (ICiCLe) protocol along with imatinib mesylate.

1. What is Ph+ B-ALL or Ph+ ALL?

Acute lymphoblastic leukemia is the most common childhood malignancy, accounting for approximately 75% of childhood leukemias.[1] Ph+ ALL is a separate subtype of B-precursor ALL, resulting from a reciprocal translocation between chromosomes 9 and 22 t(9;22)(q34;q11.2). This subgroup is more common in adults, approximately 25% of adults with ALL are Ph+. Pediatric Ph+ ALL is less frequent occurring in 3–5% of cases.[2]

The diagnosis is established by identifying BCR-ABL1 translocation and/or fusion transcript. The outcome and prognosis of Ph+ ALL is dismal when treated with standard ALL chemotherapy alone due to lower complete remission (CR) rate, increased risk of induction failure, central nervous system (CNS) leukemia, and early relapse as compared to Ph– ALL. Historically hematopoietic stem-cell transplantation (HSCT) in CR1 was considered as gold standard therapy for maintaining CR.

Lately, with advent of tyrosine kinase inhibitors (TKIs) such as imatinib mesylate, the treatment of Ph+ ALL has changed to incorporate the combination of chemotherapy with TKI as the first line of management of Ph+ ALL. The use of TKIs has radically improved the disease-free survival (DFS) from 25–30% to 50–60%, and overall survival (OS) from 30–40% to 80%, respectively.[3] It has been possible to achieve CR1 in >90% of such patients.[4]

2. What is the epidemiology of Ph+ ALL?

The incidence of Ph ALL increases with age, from <5% in younger children to 20–25% in older adults. The population-based studies indicate that the incidence does not continue to increase beyond the fourth decade.[5] However, more studies are warranted specially in pediatric population to precisely define its ethnic, geographical, and epidemiological spectrum.

3. Briefly explain the molecular biology of Philadelphia chromosome.

In 1960, Nowell and Hungerford first described Ph chromosome in the leukemia cells of a chronic myeloid leukemia (CML) patient and from there the name Ph+ ALL was derived after the name of city. In 1973, Janet Rowley reported Ph chromosome as a der (22) product of the reciprocal t(9;22)(q34;q11.2) translocation. The wild *breakpoint cluster region (BCR)* gene on chromosome 22 encodes a 160-kD phosphoprotein associated with serine/threonine kinase activity. The proto-oncogene Abelson murine leukemia virus homolog (ABL1) on chromosome 9, normally encodes a cytoplasmic and nuclear protein tyrosine kinase (TK), which plays a vital role in variety of cellular processes such as cell division, cell differentiation, cell adhesion, and the stress response through RAS and other signaling pathways.

The resultant *BCR-ABL1 fusion* gene engendered by in frame fusion of 3' portion of the ABL1 *tyrosine kinase* gene (exons 2–11, chromosome 9) to the 5' portion of *BCR* gene on chromosome 22 (Philadelphia chromosome). On chromosome 22 there are three main regions where breakpoints cluster within the *BCR* gene. Depending upon the position of the breakpoint, the expression of the *fusion* gene in ALL varies and three types of chimeric messenger ribonucleic acids (mRNAs) are formed as described below.[2,6,7]

1. *Major "CML" BCR (M-BCR):* Breakpoint occurs within a 5.8 kb region spanning BCR exons 12–16 (exons b1–b5, M-BCR) and produces larger 210 kDa protein known as p210 BCR-ABL1 protein, which is found in CML, 25% adult Ph+ ALL, and 10% pediatric Ph+ ALL patients.
2. *Minor "ALL" BCR (m-BCR):* If breakpoint occurs further upstream, between exons e20 and e2 (minor BCR, m-BCR) a smaller p190 (185–190 kDa) gene product is formed. It retains only the first exon of BCR. This is found in 90% of pediatric and adult Ph+ ALL patients. This patient group has exhibited more favorable prognosis than the p210 group as they tend to show an early response and postinduction CR.
3. *"Micro" BCR (μ-BCR):* Rarely translocations occurs involving "μ"-BCR breakpoint between exons 19 and 20 resulting in p230 fusion protein. It is seen in CML variant with neutrophilia and occasionally in classic CML.

4. Are p210 and p190 fusion proteins different?

Both p210 and p190 proteins qualitatively have analogous activities, and both can transform human and murine bone marrow cells. Of the two, the "ALL-type" p190 has higher TK activity and is the stronger transforming agent, thereby resulting in more aggressive phenotype. In contrast p210 results in more indolent chronic leukemia phenotype. In animal models, p190BCR–ABL1-induced exclusively B-lymphoid leukemia with a short latency, while p210BCR–ABL1 led to development of both lymphoid and myeloid leukemias with a longer latency. The suggested mechanism is the greater specific kinase activity and wider substrate array of the p190BCR–ABL1 fusion protein. In addition, p190BCR–ABL1 produces robust STAT1, STAT5, and STAT6 phosphorylation in Baf3 cells than p210BCR–ABL1.[2,8-11]

5. How does the Philadelphia chromosome affects the downstream molecular pathway?

The nuclear ABL1 protein TK is associated with cell cycle control. Under physiological conditions the N-terminus of ABL1 negatively regulates ABL1 kinase activity. The BCR-ABL1 fusion results in loss of this physiological N-terminal inhibitory domain of ABL1 leading to constitutive upregulation of BCR/ABL1 TK activity. These activated kinases disturb downstream signaling pathways, causing enhanced proliferation, differentiation arrest, and resistance to cell apoptosis. The loss of this crucial regulatory domain is a key event leading to ABL1-facilitated leukemogenesis. The only exon of BCR that is constantly retained in all fusions is exon 1. It encodes a coiled-coil domain facilitating dimerization and autophosphorylation (amino acids 1–63), a docking site for the adaptor protein GRB-2 (phosphorylated tyrosine 177), and a tyrosine kinase domain (TKD) (amino acids 298–413). The exact role of the BCR-TKD is unclear.[2,11]

6. What are the other concurrent genetic abnormalities associated with Ph+ ALL?

In Ph+ ALL, in addition to classical BCR-ABL1 fusions several other recurrent mutations, deletions of the lymphoid-specific transcriptional regulators are often identified. The common co-occurring genetic abnormalities are described below.

- *IKZF1 deletions and point mutations:* It is the most frequent genetic abnormality identified in Ph+ ALL. Approximately 70–80% of Ph+ ALLs have somatic mutations in IKZF1 (90% deletions and 10% point mutations) and these are associated with unfavorable outcome. Ikaros plays a role in propelling B-lymphoid development and suppress hematopoietic stem cell (HSC)-specific gene expression programs during initial lineage specification. Few studies suggest that during leukemogenesis first hit is BCR-ABL1 fusion, and second hit IKZF1 mutations occur later. The concept of "convergent" evolution of IKZF1 mutations, i.e., identifying different subclones carrying different IKZF1 mutations within the same patient, was also proposed in some models. Wild type IKZF1 shows remarkable favorable response with TKI and as per EsPhALL and AALL 0622, these patients must be spared from HSCT in CR1.[12-14]

  IKZF1 mutations are of three types.
  1. *Haploinsufficiency or near haploinsufficiency (55%):* Results from monoallelic null mutations.
  2. *Absent Ikaros (12%):* Complete absence of Ikaros due to biallelic deletions.
  3. *Dominant-negative (DN) form of Ikaros (33%), IK6:* Occurs secondary to in-frame deletion of exons 4–7, which deletes the DNA-binding domain and leads to cytosolic accumulation of the mutant protein. This form is more severe than monoallelic null mutations as Ik6 associates with the wild type Ikaros and probably traps it in the cytoplasm.

  Of these, haploinsufficiency and DN form (associated with profound reduction in Ikaros function) are common in Ph+ ALL, on contrary in non-BCR-ABL1 ALL or "Ph-like"

ALL subset IKZF1 mutations resulting in less severe reduction in Ikaros function, i.e., haploinsufficiency is more common (55–70%).[2]

- *PAX5 mutations:* Occur in about one-third of B-ALL, and approximately 50% of Ph+ ALL patients.[2] PAX5 is a transcription factor expressed during B-cell development, and controls lineage identity and commitment. Loss of PAX5 leads to a differentiation block at the pro- to pre-B-cell stage and allows transdifferentiation of committed pro-B cells into other lineages. It also confers survival advantage by allowing certain degree of self-renewal onto this population, and can cause B-cell lymphomas (BCLs). Unlike Ikaros, PAX5 lacks any effect on HSC transcriptional programs and thus its loss is not associated with unfavorable outcome.[14-19]
- *EBF1 mutations:* Occur in about 14% of Ph+ ALL. Early B-cell factor 1 is a transcription factor mediating B-cell lineage commitment and it coregulate target genes with PAX5. Animal models have reported that loss of Ebf1 leads to a differentiation block at the pre- to pro-B-cell stage. Unlike Ikzf1 and Pax5 it does not cause spontaneous hematologic malignancies.[2]
- *CDKN2A/B deletions:* Found in approximately 50% of Ph+ ALL as compared to 30% in non-Ph+ B-ALL. The products of the *CDKN2A* and *CDKN2B* genes, p16INK4A and p15INK4B, inhibits cyclin-dependent kinases. Loss of CDKN2A/B locus in HSC has been linked to HSC self-renewal. CDKN2A/B deletion or hypermethylation does not alter the outcome for pediatric ALL, whereas inactivation of the locus predicts a worse outcome in adults. Deletions as well as epigenetic silencing (promoter hypermethylation) are increasingly being identified at relapse as opposed to the time of initial diagnosis, suggesting their role in facilitating relapse, and resistance to therapy.[2]
- Additional genetic abnormalities:
  - *Epigenetic abnormalities:* Ph+ ALL has a characteristic DNA methylation profile harboring approximately 350 differentially methylated regions (DMRs). Whether differential methylation is a consequence of the BCR-ABL1 fusions or co-occurring genetic abnormalities, and whether it plays a role in malignant transformation, resistance or relapse is unknown. Reactivation of silenced CDKN2A/B by demethylating agents may have therapeutic benefit and demethylating agents are currently in clinical trials for relapsed and refractory ALL. Literature is scant regarding the involvement of other epigenetic mechanisms Ph+ ALL, such as covalent modifications of histones or nucleosome positioning.[2]
  - *Copy number abnormalities and mutations downstream of BCR/ABL1:* Have negative prognostic impact.
  - *Cytogenetic aberrations:* +der (22), $\geq$ 50 chromosomes, 7/del(7p), abnormal (9p), and +8. These have negative prognostic impact (AALL 0031).

7. What are the clinical features of Ph+ ALL?

The clinical presentation of Ph+ ALL are similar to other forms of ALL with other recurrent cytogenetic abnormalities. However, studies have shown some clinical, epidemiological, and molecular characteristics that are associated with Ph+ ALL **(Box 1)**.[2,20]

> **BOX 1:** Salient clinical features of Ph+ ALL.

Clinical presentations:
- 3% pediatric ALL (western data), 15% (India)
- 5–15% adolescent ALL
- 25% adult ALL (most common)
- Most cases CD10+ B-ALL
- Rare T-ALL
- Coexpression of myeloid markers common
- Older age
- CNS involvement
- Higher TLC and peripheral blast count
- Biologically heterogeneous disease with large individual differences in response to chemotherapy

(CNS: central nervous system; Ph+ ALL: Philadelphia-positive acute lymphoblastic leukemia; TLC: total leukocyte count).

8. How to differentiate Ph+ ALL from CML blast crisis?

Occasionally, a child with underlying CML may present with lymphoid blast crisis masquerading Ph+ ALL and it becomes a challenging to differentiate between the two entities. Certain soft pointers which may guide in differentiating both conditions are given in **Box 2**.[2,21]

> **BOX 2:** Salient differentiating features between Ph+ ALL and CML blast crisis.

- *Basophilia:* >20% of basophils are sufficient to classify the CML in accelerate phase. Conversely, basophilia is a very rare condition in de novo *BCR-ABL1* leukemias.
- *Marked splenomegaly*
- *p210 BCR-ABL1 protein:* About 90% of pediatric Ph+ ALL patients harbor classic ALL-type p190 translocation. However, 10–15% of pediatric Ph+ ALL may have p210 BCR-ABL1 protein (not enough to support diagnosis of CML).
- *Presence of concurrent genetic abnormalities such as IKZF1 or CDKN2A/2B genes deletions.* These aberrations are absent in CML-BC.
- *FISH positivity for BCR-ABL1 in nonleukemic cells at end of induction/peripheral neutrophils:* Strongest evidence of underlying diagnosis of CML.

(BC: blast crisis; CML: chronic myeloid leukemia; FISH: fluorescence in situ hybridization; Ph+ ALL: Philadelphia-positive acute lymphoblastic leukemia)

9. How to manage a case of Ph+ ALL and explain how the advent of TKIs has become the major game changer in the management of Ph+ ALL?

The underlying key mechanism involved in leukemogenesis is the constitutive phosphorylation of protein TK as a consequence of *BCR-ABL1* gene fusion. Inhibition of this TK activity appears to be the most acceptable treatment possibility. In the present era, TKIs have become an integral component of treatment backbone of Ph+ ALL. Unfortunately, due to the small number of pediatric Ph+ ALL patients, randomized trials focusing on treatment are still lacking. The evolution of management of Ph+ ALL can be broadly discussed under the two headings of pre-TKI era and TKI era.

Pretyrosine Kinase Inhibitor Era

Historically, prior to the discovery of TKIs, the outcome of the children with Ph+ ALL treated with standard chemotherapy alone was exceptionally poor.

The International Ponte di Legno Childhood ALL consortium reported 7-year event-free survival (EFS) and OS rates of 25 and 36% for patients diagnosed between 1985 and 1996, and 32 and 45% for patients diagnosed between 1995 and 2005 and treated without TKI in CR1. Historically, HSCT in CR1 was considered as the standard therapy. Past studies have reported DFS ranging between 40 and 60% in post-HSCT children after CR1 due to significant lower relapse rate. In 1995–2005, the 5-year EFS and OS rates for patients who achieved CR1 (89%) and went on to HSCT were only 34.2 and 48.3%, respectively.[2,22,23]

Post-tyrosine Kinase Inhibitor Era

Discovery of TKIs has revolutionized the treatment of Ph+ ALL with a dramatical improvement in survival rates and overall prognosis. Combination of intensive chemotherapy along with TKIs has become the standard of care for this subpopulation of ALL. Imatinib mesylate was the first TKI discovered. It binds to the inactive moiety of BCR-ABL kinase, which completely blocks its ATP binding site, leading to the inhibition of tyrosine phosphorylation of proteins that are involved in the signal transduction. Past studies conducted by Children Oncology Group (COG) and the European EsPhALL consortium have provided evidence that pediatric Ph+ ALL patients can be effectively treated with a combination of chemotherapy and TKIs, without HSCT, in the first remission (CR1). With TKI monotherapy CR rates of 90–100% can be achieved for CR1, but combination with standard chemotherapy has improved higher long-term DFS and decreased disease recurrence.

The first landmark trial from COG AALL0031 reported improved outcome in Ph+ ALL children, irrespective of HSCT, with continuous imatinib exposure (280 continuous days) with a 3-year EFS of 80 versus 35% and 7-year EFS of 71 versus 21.4% in the historic controls, without any significant increase in toxicity. Post the results of this trial TKIs became an integral part of treatment for Ph+ ALL and HSCT in CR1 was no longer routinely recommended.[20]

The three large European trials, EsPhALL2004, EsPhALL2010, and EsPhALL2017, have further forted the results of the above American trial. The EsPhALL2004 was the largest and the only randomized trial to assess the efficacy of postinduction, short, discontinuous use of imatinib mesylate combined with Berlin-Frankfurt-Münster (BFM) HR backbone based intensive chemotherapy. Postinduction, patients were classified as good risk or poor risk as per EsPhALL risk stratification criteria. The good risk group was randomized to receive chemotherapy with or without imatinib (300 mg/m^2/day). The poor risk group received postinduction imatinib plus chemotherapy.

It reported 10% increase in 4-year DFS with imatinib (72.9%) after induction compared with no use of imatinib (61.7%) in patients with Ph+ ALL receiving BFM chemotherapy and HSCT. The 4-year EFS for poor-risk patients was 53.5%. The limitation was shorter intermittent imatinib exposure of 126 versus 616 days in COG AALL0031 cohort 5. Also, the role of HSCT in CR1 remained unclear for those receiving imatinib, since most patients (77%) of this study underwent transplant.[24]

The EsPhALL2010 further investigated whether earlier and continuous administration of imatinib from day 15 of induction chemotherapy could give better results. The decision for HSCT was based on early morphological response and minimal residual disease (MRD). Imatinib was given till 1 year post-transplant. The CR1 rate was higher 97 versus 78% than in EsPhALL2004. In poor-risk group, CR rate was 92 versus 50% in EsPhALL2004. The 5-year EFS was 57% (vs. 60.3% EsPhALL 2004) and 5-year OS was 71.8% (vs. 71.6% in EsPhALL 2004). Total imatinib exposure was 24 months (not transplanted) and 15 months (transplanted) whereas in EsPhALL2004 it was 5 months (not transplanted) and 3 months (transplanted).[25]

A higher proportion of patients were MRD negative and less percentage of patients underwent HSCT in EsPhALL2010 (38%) than in EsPhALL2004 (81%) but the outcome was similar. They concluded that earlier introduction and continuous use of imatinib along with intensive chemotherapy resulted in comparable EFS and OS, reducing the use of HSCT but might increase the toxicity.

The treatment-related mortality was 16% in EsPhALL and 5% in COG AALL 0622 (described below). The recent EsPhALL 2017/COGAALL1631 (EudraCT 2017-000705-20) is an ongoing trial comparing imatinib (340 mg/m^2) in combination with two different cytotoxic chemotherapy backbones (EsPhALL and COG AALL 0622). The intensive HR blocks are replaced by four cycles of high-dose methotrexate (5 g/m^2) given as CNS-directed therapy and with less intensive delayed intensification (DI) than in EsPhALL2010 and restricting transplant indications to patients with poor MRD response. The results are awaited.

Spanish trial SHOP-2005 concluded intermediate dose of imatinib (260 mg/m^2) given concurrently (day 15 of induction) with chemotherapy and followed by HSCT in pediatric Ph+ ALL significantly improve 3 years EFS (29.6%, nonimatinib vs. 78.7%, in imatinib arm, $p = 0.01$).[26] Another contemporary Japanese leukemia/lymphoma study group JPLSG Ph(+) ALL 04 study conducted from 2004–2008, investigated role of 2-week-imatinib monotherapy immediately before HSCT and reported that imatinib therapy appeared to have antileukemic effects as 47% of patients with detectable MRD before imatinib monotherapy course transitioned to MRD negative status. However, all children underwent HSCT in CR1. The 4-year EFS rates and OS rates were 54 and 78%, respectively. They concluded that a longer use of imatinib concurrently with chemotherapy may eliminate HSCT in a subset of patients with a rapid clearance of the disease.[27]

Total studies from St. Jude's Children Research Hospital evaluated early response to TKIs starting D22 of induction (continuous imatinib 340 mg/m^2 daily—total 15 study, dasatinib 40 mg/m^2 twice daily—total 16 study) in the post-TKI era. MRD was measured on days 15 and 42 of induction. The reported significantly higher postinduction MRD negative rates in TKI arm (81 vs. 19%, $p < 0.001$) as compared to chemotherapy alone arm. The 5-year EFS was higher, (68.6 vs. 31.6%, $p = 0.22$) in TKI era patients. More patients were transplanted in non-TKI arm (79 vs. 19%, $p = 0.002$).[28]

Based on the results of above-mentioned trials, it can be concurred that patients with Ph+ ALL should receive earlier and continuous TKIs in combination with chemotherapy. Early introduction of TKI helps reducing initial leukemic burden significantly and thus less induction failures and reduce the need for HSCT. End induction MRD status should be used for early response assessment and guiding HSCT decisions. Given the results of EsPhALL

2004 and COG AALL0031, it is highly unlikely that another trial will ever be conducted for chemotherapy with/without TKI in pediatric Ph+ ALL. Imatinib was approved by the US Food and Drug Administration (FDA) for treatment of pediatric Ph+ ALL in 2013.

10. Is there a role of other TKIs in the management of Ph+ ALL?

It was established that imatinib improved survival in Ph+ ALL but the outcomes were still inferior as compared to Ph– ALL. Imatinib mesylate significantly improved the CR1 rates in Ph+ ALL but it was noted that approximately 15–20% of patients develop CNS relapse during on-going imatinib therapy. The most plausible explanation given was the poor CNS penetration of imatinib and increased cellular resistance mechanisms like p-glycoprotein mediated efflux precipitating imatinib resistance.[2,29] These concerns lead to the invention of improved TKIs agents targeting additional downstream pathways in addition to the primary ATP binding site of BCR ABL TK, so as to inhibit TK more potently and attempt to overcome the drug resistance. These agents are classified as second and third generation TKIs as described below.

Second-generation Tyrosine Kinase Inhibitor

Dasatinib

Dasatinib has more than 300-fold in vitro potency as compared to imatinib. It binds to both activated and nonactivated conformation of the BCL-ABL kinase, as a type II competitive inhibitor, whereas imatinib, targets only inactivated isoform, thus leads to more stringent inhibition. In addition it harbors different activity profile as described below.

- Inhibits non-BCR/ABL kinases [like steroid receptor coactivator (Src) family]
- Has other specific antileukemic properties involving MAPK or BCL2 pathways
- Blocks Stat-5 downstream pathway of BCR-ABL
- Has higher CNS penetration
- Effective against most imatinib-resistant ALL mutants except Thr315Ile.[29,30]

In a phase I, CA180-018, dose-escalation trial, the dose of dasatinib was increased from 60 to 120 mg/m² in pretreated CML and Ph+ ALL children. The high dose was found to be safe, efficacious, and tolerable in children without any increased toxicity.[31] The results of the above trial along with observation that every patient in ALL0031 COG trial received cranial radiotherapy, which can later cause neurocognitive deficits and risk of brain tumors, formed the basis of COG AALL0622 trial.

In COG AALL0622 trial dasatinib (60 mg/m²) substituted imatinib and was started earlier (on day 15 vs. day 35 in AALL0031) with chemotherapy. Allogenic HSCT was performed for HR (based on MRD) and all patients with a matched sibling donor irrespective of MRD after at least 11 weeks of therapy. Children with overt CNS leukemia received cranial radiation therapy (CRT). The outcomes were comparable to those in COG AALL0031: 5-year OS of 81 versus 86% and 5-year DFS of 68 versus 60% for AALL0031 versus AALL0622, respectively. The cumulative incidence of isolated and combined CNS relapse was 15% (AALL0622—no CRT) versus 6% (AALL0031—all received 12 Gy RT and imatinib). All CNS relapses occurred in SR patients (no CRT) and none occurred in those who underwent HSCT [most received CNS radiation therapy (RT) as part of conditioning]. Based on the above findings we cannot conclude that dasatinib is better than imatinib.[32]

Another COG AALL1122 (CA180-372) trial on dasatinib (60 mg/m², starting day 15) and EsPhALL backbone-based chemotherapy reported this approach as safe and effective in pediatric Ph+ ALL. They observed decreased HSCT in CR1 (14%) (vs. 81% in EsPhALL 2004 and 38% in EsPhALL2010 imatinib trials) with similar 5-year EFS and OS of 54.6 and 81.7% as compared to 60.3 and 71.5% in EsPhALL 2004 and 57 and 71.8% in EsPhALL 2010 trial.[33]

The Chinese CCCG-ALL-2015 open-label phase-3 trial compared the efficacy between dasatinib (80 mg/m²) and imatinib (300 mg/m²) combined with intensive chemotherapy without prophylactic CRT. Both drugs were administered daily, from starting of induction (median—day 8) till end of therapy. The 4-year EFS and OS was 71 and 88.4% in dasatinib arm as compared to 48.9 and 69.2% in imatinib arm, respectively. The 4-year cumulative risk of any relapse, isolated CNS relapse and any CNS relapse was-19.8, 2.7, and 10% in dasatinib arm as compared to 34.4, 2.7, and 9.4% in imatinib arm, respectively. They concluded that dasatinib has superior survival compared with imatinib and it provides excellent control of CNS leukemia without prophylactic CRT. The higher dose of dasatinib (80 vs. 60 mg/m²) was associated with high treatment abandonment rate (4.2%).[34]

The FDA approved dasatinib for use in pediatric Ph+ ALL in November 2017.

Nilotinib

Nilotinib is another second-generation TKI with following characteristics:[2,29,30,35]
- Highly specific BCR-ABL inhibitor
- 30-fold more potent than imatinib
- Active in vitro against majority of BCR-ABL mutants
- Does not inhibit the Src-family kinases.
- CNS penetration of nilotinib is debatable.
- Shown encouraging activity in adult relapsed/refractory Ph+ ALL.
- Not effective against T315I mutation.

Ponatinib

Ponatinib is a third-generation TKI. It is the only TKI available till date which is effective against T315I mutation. It has not been tested in combination with chemotherapy in children with Ph+ ALL. In adults also, the experience with ponatinib is limited.[2,29,30]

11. What is the role of HSCT in Ph+ ALL?

Historically, HSCT was considered as the gold standard therapy for pediatric Ph+ ALL. Past studies have shown that HSCT from matched related donors significantly decreases the relapse rate and improved DFS varying between 40 and 60%. However, the continuing relapse rate and nonrelapse mortality are still considered limiting factors for HSCT.[29]

In COG AALL0031, HSCT did not improve outcomes for patients treated with imatinib in the final cohort. In contrast, outcomes for patients who did not undergo HSCT on EsPhALL appeared inferior to the transplanted cohort (relapse was reported in three of nine good-risk patients and five of seven poor-risk patients). This disparity can be explicated by the longer duration of imatinib administration in AALL0031, i.e., 616 versus 126 days in EsPhALL. However, in both trials, the numbers were extremely small, and more data will be required to define the role of HSCT in Ph+ ALL.

The combined follow-up trials AALL0031/AALL0622 and EsPhALL, AALL1122 (NCT01460160), assessed the effect of earlier, continuous, and longer exposure to dasatinib and imatinib. Only the patients who were MRD positive and have matched related donor underwent HSCT in CR1. In TKI era, robust remissions have been observed with the combination of TKI and intensive chemotherapy regimens in CR1, so the role of HSCT in CR1 remains debatable. HSCT in CR1 is no longer recommended as standard of care therapy. It may be considered if donor is available and clinical status of the recipient is acceptable. Despite disagreement over the role of HSCT in first remission in pediatric Ph+ ALL, HSCT in CR2 is recommended universally. Owing to the small pediatric Ph+ ALL cohort, more studies are warranted to clarify the role of HSCT in this subgroup.

12. Is there any concurrence on the duration TKIs along with chemotherapy in Ph+ ALL?

The optimal duration of TKIs with chemotherapy is still controversial, there are no consensus guidelines till date. Adults studies propose to extend TKI beyond chemotherapy completion, some propose indefinitely. In children, concerns about growth and bone mineral density combined with concomitant use of intensive chemotherapy and radiation along with uncertainty regarding benefit of additional TKI therapy, the current pediatric trials stop TKI therapy when chemotherapy stops at 2–2.5 years postdiagnosis.[36] This approach seems feasible and is not associated with increased risk of relapse. The question is still unanswered whether it is beneficial to extend TKI therapy beyond 2–2.5 years.[2]

13. For how long TKIs should be administered post-HSCT in Ph+ ALL?

Past studies have reported superior outcomes with post-HSCT TKI administration in terms of relapse prevention and incidence of graft versus host disease (GVHD).[37-39] The European Group for Blood and Marrow Transplantation (EBMT) recommends post-HSCT TKI use commencing from day 30 to 50 after HSCT and continuing for at least 1 year. A recent GMALL study randomized Ph+ ALL patient to receive imatinib post-HSCT either prophylactically, or post rise in MRD. In the prophylactic group the molecular recurrence after HSCT was significantly lower (40 vs. 69%; $p = 0.046$). However, there was no difference in the survival rates.[40]

A recent nonrandomized trial in pediatric Ph+ ALL patients reported that the ability to tolerate post-HSCT imatinib was an independent predictor of DFS and OS.[41] In pediatric COG AALL1122, NCT01460160 post-HSCT use of imatinib for up to 12 additional months is optional and at the discretion of the treating investigator. Robust safety data regarding post-HSCT use of TKIs (imatinib, dasatinib, and nilotinib) is available but no comparative data is there. Benefit of post-HSCT TKI needs to be prospectively validated, especially in patients who develop significant GVHD after HSCT.

14. Are we sure of optimal chemotherapy backbone to choose in Ph+ ALL?

The present concerns include the optimal chemotherapy backbone to be combined with TKIs to achieve maximal CR rates balanced against the treatment-related mortality and potential late effects of drugs such as infertility and second malignancies. In addition, intensive chemotherapy compromises the ability to deliver optimal TKI therapy or to combine TKIs with other new targeted therapies.

The COG AALL1122, NCT01460160 trials are investigating dasatinib on AEIOP-BFM ALL 2000 chemotherapy backbone regimen, which had shown promising results in the EsPhALL trial. As compared to AALL0031 backbone, it has significantly reduced cumulative doses of cyclophosphamide, ifosfamide, etoposide, and methotrexate. Despite the changes, the morbidity and mortality associated with this regimen is still substantial. More trials are warranted to identify the optimal chemotherapy regimen in this ALL subset.

15. What all factors lead to TKI resistance?

Despite the advances in treatment strategy, the prognosis of pediatric Ph+ ALL still remains dismal and these children relapse frequently even post-HSCT. The resistance to TKIs is considered as one of the most common cause of treatment failure and disease recurrence. The acquisition of resistance renders the fusion protein completely or relatively unresponsive to TKIs. Resistance to TKIs can be broadly studied under two categories: BCR-ABL dependent and BCR-ABL independent as described in detail below.[2,42]

BCR-ABL Dependent

- *BCR-ABL1 mutations*: Several mutations in TKD make BCR-ABL1 fusion protein entirely or comparatively impassive to imatinib. It is still contentious whether these mutations are acquired during treatment, or whether these are present at the time of initial diagnosis in minor subclones in Ph+ ALL patients.
  - Common mutations are T315I, Y253H, and E255K/V.
  - Occur frequently in Ph+ ALL patients treated with TKI monotherapy.
  - Few studies suggest that BCR-ABL1 mutations known to cause resistance have been identified in minor subclones in 40% of Ph+ ALL patients at initial diagnosis.
  - Seen in 80% of adults with Ph+ ALL relapse.
  - Most resistant clones are sensitive to second-generation TKI—dasatinib and nilotinib.
  - Ponatinib (third-generation TKI) is active against the most common mutation "gatekeeper" T315I mutation, that cause resistance to both first- and second-generation TKIs.
  - Less common in those treated upfront with combination of intensive chemotherapy and TKI as it may help to reduce selective pressure on TKI-resistant subclones.
- *Increased intracellular BCR-ABL1*: Secondary to amplification of *BCR-ABL1* fusion gene or the entire Ph chromosome (10%).

BCR-ABL1 Independent

- *Overexpression of drug exporters:* The role of efflux pumps such as ABCB1/MDR1/PGP and ABCG2/BCRP is well established in the development of TKI resistance in CML. Data is scant regarding their role in Ph+ ALL but results of preliminary studies highlight that overexpression of these drug exporters leads to TKI resistance in Ph+ ALL as well.

- *Upregulation of parallel pathways:* Activation of pathways downstream of BCR-ABL1 such as Ras-Raf, MEK-MAPK, and Src-family kinase pathways, mediates resistance to TKIs, e.g., upregulation of Src-family kinases (have a crucial role in lymphoid blast crisis and Ph+ ALL) mediates resistance to imatinib and nilotinib. Other pathways involved are Janus kinase enzyme (JAK)-STAT pathway, AKT, STAT5, and the BCL6 transcriptional repressor pathways.
- *Additional genetic abnormalities:* Possession of additional genetic abnormalities such as IKZF1 mutations, etc. may interfere with transcriptional regulation and B-cell development. IKZF1 mutations are commonly identified at diagnosis as well as at relapse. It includes both de novo IKZF1 mutation and a subclone with a more severe mutation at relapse that was initially present at a low percentage. The exact mechanism, how Ikaros would specifically cause drug resistance is unclear.
- *Inhibition of apoptosis:* Increased promoter methylation has been described in relapsed ALL specimens. Function of CDKN2A/B is affected by epigenetic silencing or deletion, which results in inability to upregulate p14Arf, thereby causing loss of functional p53. Second postulated mechanism of inactivating p53 in Ph+ ALL involves the overexpression of BCL6. In a murine model of Ph+ ALL, imatinib treatment resulted in BCL6 upregulation and downregulation of p53. Acquisition of p53 mutations at relapse are described in literature, but are rare as compared to the commonly affected IKZF1, PAX5, and CDKN2A/B loci.
- *Resistance to chemotherapeutic agents:* Concomitant resistance to chemotherapy agents can also develop during combined treatment secondary to mutation, amplification, or upregulation of the molecular target, drug exporters, survival pathways, and inhibition of apoptosis. Furthermore, other genetic alterations (such as MSH6, decreased MSH2 protein levels, NR3C1 and CREBBP mutations) are identified in ALL at relapse triggering resistance to specific cytotoxic agents. However, these mechanisms are not specific to Ph+ ALL.

16. How to manage a relapse case of Ph+ ALL and what all factors to be taken into consideration before framing a treatment plan for a relapse Ph+ ALL case?

Despite of using combined TKI and intensive chemotherapy, relapse is seen in approximately 30% of the Ph+ ALL patients. In EsPhALL 2004 trial, nearly 31% of patients relapsed. The proportion of relapse was lower in HSCT arm (26 vs. 53%) as compared to nontransplanted arm. The underlying mechanism could be drug resistance (discussed previously), acquisition of other clonal recurrent genetic abnormalities, etc. owing to the heterogenous biology of the primary disease. The outcome of relapsed Ph+ ALL is poor. Management of relapsed/refractory Ph+ ALL is challenging and till date HSCT post-CR2 is the standard therapy accepted globally. The following factors described below play a role in deciding the further management plan.

Choice of Tyrosine Kinase Inhibitor

It is very crucial to decide which TKI to use at the time of relapse or progression based on the type of mutation identified. It is recommended that all patients should undergo repeat cytogenetics and resistance testing at the time of relapse/progression. To bridge the time gap we can start on same TKI till the reports are available. If BCR-ABL1 amplification is identified we can use higher doses of imatinib or dasatinib. The specific point mutations in BCR-ABL1 can lead to absolute or relative resistance to imatinib and/or dasatinib. In relapsed Ph+ ALL, 70% adults harbor kinase domain point mutation (T315I, E255K, and Y253H—75%). These are less common in children as pediatric protocols use more intensive chemotherapy backbones and no imatinib monotherapy is used unlike adults.[42]

Nontransplanted Relapse

The allogenic HSCT is preferred therapy in CR2. The ALL 0622 trial reported 5-year OS of 87% in SR arm where majority did not undergo transplantation, suggesting that if relapse occurred, salvage by HSCT in CR2 might be helpful. Despite of being heavily pretreated (those not transplanted in CR1), majority are effectively salvaged through reinduction and consolidation followed by HSCT in CR2. Total body irradiation (TBI)-based regimens are preferred. In adults role of TKI combined with blinatumomab is being explored currently.

Previously Transplanted Relapse

It becomes even more challenging to manage when a patient relapses/progresses post-HSCT in CR1. The following options can be considered:
- *Second HSCT:* If previously TBI-based transplant was done, second HSCT with an alternative donor or chimeric antigen receptor T-cell (CAR-T) therapy can be considered.
- *Dasatinib or ponatinib monotherapy:* Past case reports have highlighted the role of dasatinib or ponatinib (in a child with T315I mutation at relapse) monotherapy in post-HSCT relapse as a bridge to second HSCT following CR. The side effects include opportunistic infections and gastrointestinal bleeding.

17. What are the additional adjunctive therapeutic options available in relapsed Ph+ ALL?

The undermentioned are the new agents proposed for the management of Ph+ ALL cases upfront and in relapsed/refractory cases. Currently these are in preliminary stage and more pediatric trials are warranted to establish their role in management of pediatric Ph+ ALL.[11] These are:
- *Blinatumomab (CD19 monoclonal antibody):* In few studies it has been shown to be highly effective in inducing remission in refractory/resistant Ph+ ALL in both adults and children.[43]
- *Ruxolitinib (JAK inhibitor):* When used in combination with dasatinib or nilotinib, it prevents the development of resistance and induces remissions by targeting this parallel downstream signaling pathway.[44]
- *Bosutinib, vandetanib (Src-family kinase inhibitors):* These drugs are alternative which addresses this respective mechanism of resistance and may help to achieve CR.[45]
- *Dasatinib and venetoclax (BCL2 inhibitor, multikinase inhibition):* Their combination has been shown to exhibit in vitro high synergism. More studies are required currently to recommend their routine use in relapse cases.

18. Is MRD assessment mandated in pediatric Ph+ ALL and if yes, what are the methods available?

The prognostic and predictive impact of MRD detection in pediatric Ph+ ALL is yet not well established. However, pre-HSCT MRD is the most important determinant of success after HSCT. Various MRD detection methods used are flow cytometry, reverse transcriptase-polymerase chain reaction (RT-PCR) immunoglobulin (Ig)/T-cell receptor (TCR), quantitative-reverse transcriptase polymerase chain reaction (qRT-PCR) BCR/ABL. In Ph+ ALL children, the universal, faster, and easier approach is qRT-PCR BCR-ABL.

In COG AALL 0031, MRD was assessed by flow cytometry at end of induction (EOI), before administration of imatinib. MRD was important but lost its prognostic significance for EFS if imatinib had been given continuously. In JPLSG Ph+ ALL 04, BCR/ABL1 transcript levels were monitored prospectively. Total of 26 patients underwent HSCT in CR1. Out of these, 17 patients who were MRD negative at HSCT 5 patients relapsed whereas none of the 5 patients with detectable MRD at HSCT relapsed. They concluded that MRD level at EOI (at HSCT) did not correlate with relapse after HSCT.[46]

Zaliova et al. compared MRD detection by BCR/ABL versus Ig/TCR-based method in children and reported limited overall correlation by two methods (correlation coefficient R2.0.64). Though both had similar sensitivity, still 20% of samples negative by Ig/TCR approach were positive by the BCR/ABL method. This was attributed to multilineage involvement. They concluded BCR/ABL-based MRD is a clinically relevant tool and its monitoring enables better and earlier prediction of relapse compared to the standard Ig/TCR methodology.[47]

The EsPhALL study assessed the predictive value of MRD detected by RQ-PCR based on Ig/TCR and BCR/ABL1 methodology. They observed that MRD negativity progressively increased over time by both methods, however, BCR/ABL1 MRD levels were higher than IG/TR MRD at any time point. Thus, the proportion of patients achieving MRD negativity by BCR/ABL1 was always lower than IG/TR. They reported predictive association between early MRD negativity and favorable outcome. Postinduction BCR/ABL1 MRD negative patients had a comparable relapse risk as those who were IG/TR MRD negative. Overall concordance between the two methods was 69%, with significantly higher positivity by BCR/ABL1 and Ig/TR MRD monitoring appears to be more reliable.

Few adult studies have proposed that MRD kinetics is useful in predicting relapse and is the most powerful factor affecting long-term post-HSCT outcome. Attaining deeper molecular responses is associated with improved outcomes especially, deeper molecular responses prior to HSCT is associated with favorable long-term outcomes. Patients who achieved complete molecular remission (CMR) performed well even without HSCT. Thus, MRD monitoring (RT-PCR BCR-ABL1) is useful for management decisions in adult Ph+ ALL. Its prognostic and predictive role in pediatric counterpart is still debatable.

19. Philadelphia chromosome-like ALL—what is it and when to look for it?

Philadelphia chromosome-like acute lymphoblastic leukemia (Ph-like ALL or BCR-ABL1 like ALL) is a lately designated B-cell precursor ALL subtype that display a gene expression profile similar to BCR/ABL1-positive ALL (Ph+ ALL) but lacks the BCR/ABL1 fusion protein resulting from (9;22)(q34.1;q11.2). In 2009, it was individually identified by the two groups on the basis of gene expression profiling, COG-TARGET-St Jude consortium, and the Dutch COG.[48,49] This subgroup also harbor other recurrent genetic abnormality, the most common being IKZF1 genetic alteration and is associated with dismal prognosis. Like Ph+ ALL it is a genetically, clinically, and biologically heterogeneous subgroup of ALL with often MRD at remission induction and is associated with poor EFS when treated with standard chemotherapy alone. Patients with this subtype have a higher risk of relapse, lower 5-year EFS rates, and OS rates.

The Ph-like ALL is three to four times more common in children. Its prevalence varies with age, gender, race, and ethnicity. It accounts for nearly 12% of children, 21% of adolescents (16–20 years), 27% of young adults (21–39 years), and 20–24% of older adults (>40 years) patients with B-ALL, with a peak (27%) in young adults 21–39 years old.[50] It occur more frequently in males (2:1) and patients with Hispanic ethnicity, who have a particular preponderance of cytokine receptor-like factor 2 (CRLF2) rearrangements. This is in part explained by the higher frequency of germline Ph-like ALL risk variant in GATA3 (rs3824662) in Hispanics, which associated with high MRD at the end of remission induction and increased risk of relapse, a finding consistent with ancestry-related disparities in ALL treatment outcomes.[51-53]

We should look for it when the gene signature matches HR Ph+ ALL but BCR-ABL1 is negative.

20. What are the molecular characteristic of BCR/ABL1-like ALL?

On contrary to ALL with recurrent genetic alterations, the Ph-like ALL has a composite genomic landscape with varied genetic abnormalities affecting different classes of cytokine receptors and TKs. Like Ph+ ALL, a hallmark of Ph-like ALL is IKZF1 alterations (70–80%) as compared to non-Ph-like ALL (15%).[50,54,55]

Several classes of kinase-activating alterations have been described in Ph-like ALL. Only a small subset of patients did not have a kinase-activating alteration identified by transcriptome analysis. The major alterations involved include:
- *Kinase activating alterations activating JAK-STAT signaling:* Involving *CRLF2, JAK2, EPOR,* and other genes in this pathway.
- *ABL-class fusions:* ABL1, ABL2, CSF1R, PDGFRA, and PDGFRB
- *Ras pathway mutations:* KRAS, NRAS, NF1, PTPN11
- *Uncommon fusions:* NTRK3, PTK2B, BLNK.

Rearrangements of Cytokine Receptor CRLF2 and JAK Mutations

The majority of kinase-activating alterations results in activation of JAK-STAT signaling pathway. Most frequently seen are rearrangements or point mutations of CRLF2. These are described below.
- Rearrangement of the cytokine receptor CRLF2 occurs in approximately half of the Ph-like ALL cases. There are two mechanisms:
    1. Deletion of the pseudoautosomal region (PAR1) of chromosomes X or Y, which houses CRLF2 under control of the noncoding P2RY8 or CSF2RA promoters to drive fusion transcript expression and protein translation.

2. Translocation to the immunoglobulin heavy chain enhancer region (IGH-CRLF2). IGH-CRLF2 fusion results from t(X;14) or t(Y;14). IGH is noncoding in the fusions. It is associated with Hispanic ethnicity.

Both result in overexpression of full-length CRLF2 which heterodimerizes with interleukin 7 receptor alpha (IL7RA) to form the receptor for thymic stromal lymphopoietin (TSLP).

Children who harbor P2RY8-CRLF2 are younger (median age, 4 years) and have lower total leukocyte counts (TLCs) than those with IGH-CRLF2 (median age, 14 years) and are unlikely to be stratified as HR cases. IGH-CRLF2 has been reported to be two to four times more common than P2RY8-CRLF2 in adults and adolescents, whereas P2RY8-CRLF2 is marginally more common than IGH-CRLF2 in the children and adolescents, hence, emphasizing the variation in Ph-like ALL subtypes across the age spectrum.

- *Point mutations of CRLF2*: These are rare. The most common is p.Phe232Cys that results in homodimerization of CRLF2 and constitutive kinase signaling.

Janus Kinase Enzyme Mutations

Cytokine receptor-like factor 2 overexpression and JAK2 mutations work together and lead to constitutive activation of JAK-STAT signaling.

- JAK mutations are seen in approximately 50% of the childhood and adolescent ALL cases harboring CRLF2 rearrangement.
- They include activating JAK2 or JAK1 point mutations.
- Most common mutation is R683G in the JAK2 pseudokinase domain.
- JAK1 mutations are less common.

JAK2 Fusions and Truncating Rearrangements of the Erythropoietin Receptor

Rearrangements of JAK2 and EPOR (encoding the erythropoietin receptor), account for 7 and 5% of Ph-like ALL cases, respectively. At least 19 different JAK2 fusions have been identified, each of which result in expression of a chimeric fusion gene with preservation of the JAK2 kinase domain. The prevalence of JAK2 fusions is similar between the different age groups.

The EPOR rearrangements are more often seen in young adults (9%) as compared to children (5%), adolescents (3%), and older adults (1%), respectively. Four partner genes involved are IGH, immunoglobulin kappa (IGK), LAIR1, and THADA. Of these, most common is translocation of the *EPOR* gene to the enhancer regions of IGH or IGK, leading to the unrestricted expression of the truncated *EPOR* gene that triggers leukemogenesis. Other less common mechanism includes insertion and truncation of EPOR into the upstream region of LAIR1 or the THADA loci.

Janus kinase enzyme 2 rearrangements lead to constitutive activation of JAK-STAT signaling, whereas the EPOR rearrangements result in stabilized expression of the EPOR on the surface of B-cells, with failure of receptor downregulation and heightened JAK-STAT signaling in response to ligand (EPO) stimulation. In both contexts, the abnormal JAK-STAT signaling can be repealed by using JAK inhibitors such as ruxolitinib.

As compared to children adults have higher frequency of JAK2 fusions, EPOR-R, and, among CRFL2-R cases, more IGH-CRLF2 than P2RY8-CRLF2.

Other JAK/STAT Pathway-activating Alterations

In a subset of patients a myriad of structural mutations and DNA copy number alterations can be identified that can activate JAK-STAT pathway (JAK1, JAK3, IL7R, SH2B3, IL2RB, TYK2). These are twice as common as in children (14%) as compared to adolescents (5.0%), and adults (7.3%). This subset do not have any rearrangements of kinase or cytokine receptor genes, instead may have chromosomal rearrangements involving transcription factor genes (*EBF1*, *PAX5*) and/or epigenetic regulators (CREBBP, SETD2, ASXL1). Deletions of SH2B3 (encoding LNK, a negative regulator of JAKs) and IL7RA insertions/deletions can lead to activated JAK-STAT signaling that is sensitive to JAK inhibition.

They have lesser frequency of IKZF1 alteration, and a lower Ph-like gene expression coefficient on TLDA analysis, suggesting these may represent a distinct subset of Ph-like ALL.

ABL-class Fusions

Approximately 10% of the Ph-like patients (17% in children, 9% in adolescents, 10% young adults, and 9% older adults) have ABL-class (*ABL1, ABL2, CSF1R, PDGFRA, PDGFRB*) gene fusions resulting from translocations or inversions or deletion. The encoded chimeras include the carboxyl terminal portion of the ABL-class protein with its TKD intact joined in-frame to the amino terminal portion of the partner protein. The ABL1 inhibitors such as imatinib and dasatinib can inhibit the downstream signaling induced by each of the chimeric fusion proteins. Multiple fusion partners have been identified in each of the ABL-class genes, and in each instance the fusion involved the kinase as the downstream partner, thus preserving the kinase domain.

Uncommon Fusions Involving Kinase Genes

Uncommon Ras activating mutations of genes (*KRAS, NRAS, NF1, PTPN11*, and *CBL1*) are seen in 4% of Ph-like cases. These can also observed in hyperdiploid, hypodiploid, KMT2A-rearranged, and relapsed ALL. Other rare kinase alterations involving NTRK3, BLNK, PTK2B, and TYK2 have also been identified in Ph-like ALL. Identification of these is important as they are amenable to targeting with different TKI than JAK-STAT/ABL-class Ph-like ALL.

Other Genomic Alterations in Ph-like ALL

Although they usually accompany other genomic rearrangements, mutations, and/or deletions in IKZF1, PAX5, and EBF1 have been reported in isolation in Ph-like ALL. Isolated mutations in the Ras pathway also occur in a small number of Ph-like ALL cases, but have been reported in conjunction with CRLF2 overexpression with and without JAK alterations.

Germline Genomic Factors Linked to Ph-like ALL

Past studies have reported that Ph-like ALL is more common in persons of self-declared Hispanic/Latino ancestry. The risk of developing Ph-like ALL is high in persons with specific GATA3 polymorphisms, and with CRLF2-R. GATA3 risk alleles occur significantly more frequently in individuals with high Native American genetic ancestry and US Hispanics than in those of European descent.

21. What are the clinical features of Ph-like ALL?

The clinical features of Ph-like ALL are summarized in **Box 3**.[50,55]

> **BOX 3:** Clinical features of Philadelphia chromosome-like acute lymphoblastic leukemia (Ph-like ALL).
>
> *Clinical features of Ph-like ALL:*
> - More common in males
> - Older age at diagnosis. Peak prevalence appears to occur in adolescence and young adulthood
> - More likely to be associated with Downs syndrome
> - Associated with high-risk clinical features—elevated initial leukocyte count
> - Hyperdiploidy (same proportion as non-Ph-like B-ALL)
> - Poor treatment response—high end-induction minimal residual disease (MRD) rates, induction failure, and relapse

22. How to diagnose Ph-like ALL?

Due to the heterogeneous biology and several genetic targetable alterations the diagnosis of Ph-like ALL remains challenging. The goal is to improve outcome by identifying targetable kinase lesions, so that timely institution of TKIs can be done. Currently, there are two strategies. First is the St Jude approach, which emphasizes on performing comprehensive sequencing of all patients at diagnosis irrespective of Ph-like status. The second is COG approach, based on identifying Ph-like signature in all newly diagnosed HR B-ALL using TaqMan low-density microarray (LDA) followed by sequential genomic profiling and focused fusion/gene panel **(Flowchart 1)**.[6,7,50,55,56]

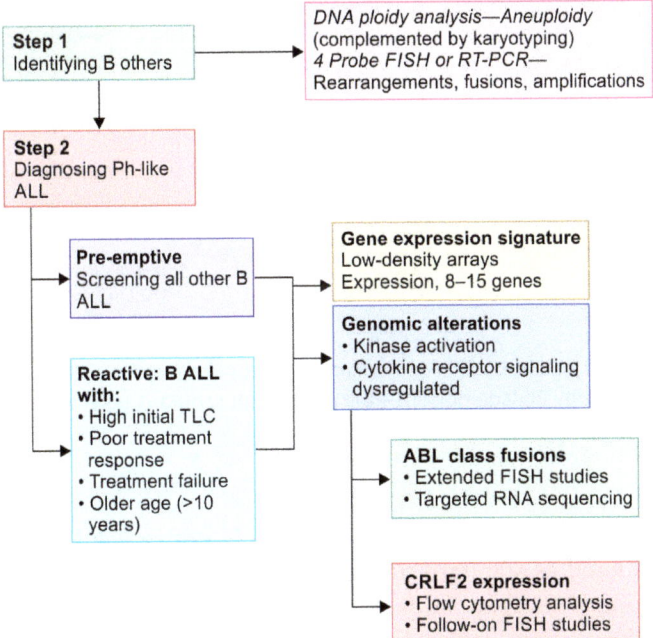

Flowchart 1: Schema for diagnosing Ph-like or BCR-ABL1-like ALL.

(CRLF2: cytokine receptor-like factor 2; FISH: fluorescence *in situ* hybridization; RT-PCR: reverse transcriptase-polymerase chain reaction; Ph-like ALL: Philadelphia chromosome-like acute lymphoblastic leukemia; RNA: ribonucleic acid; TLC: total leukocyte count)

23. What is the management of Ph-like ALL?

There is scant pediatric data available to make standard treatment protocols for Ph-like ALL in children. The management depends on the underlying genomic alteration identified. **Flowchart 2** summarizes the COG-defined diagnostic protocol and treatment options available as per the alteration identified.[50,55]

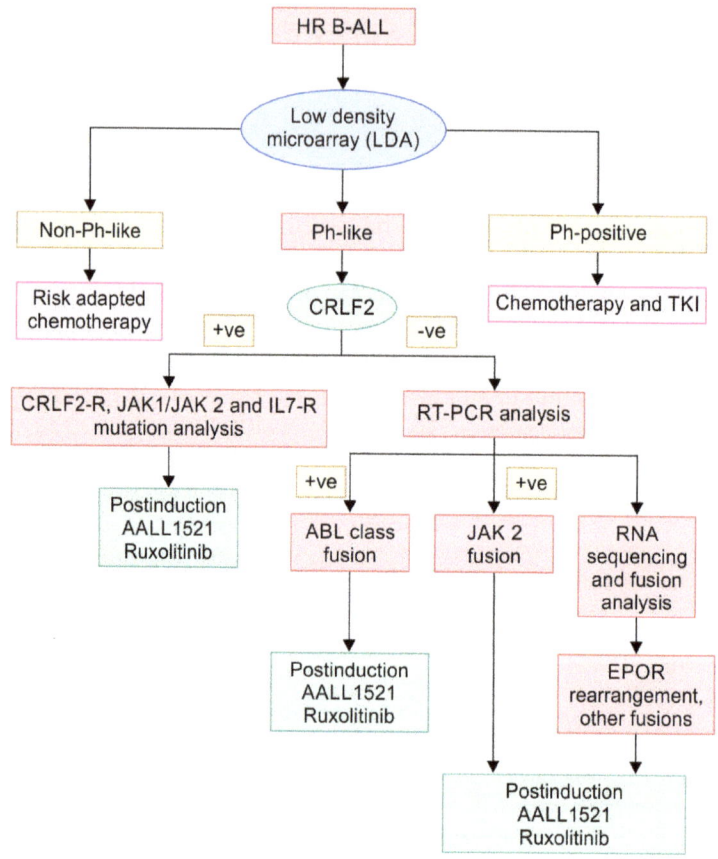

Flowchart 2: Current trials and treatment options available for Ph-like ALL.

(ALL: acute lymphoblastic leukemia; CRLF2: cytokine receptor-like factor 2; HR: high risk; IL: interleukin; JAK: Janus kinase enzyme; Ph: Philadelphia; RT-PCR: reverse transcriptase-polymerase chain reaction; RNA: ribonucleic acid; TKI: tyrosine kinase inhibitor)

SUMMARY

Philadelphia positive ALL is a distinct subtype of ALL. With advent of TKIs, HSCT in CR1 is no longer considered as standard therapy. The optimal treatment backbone includes chemotherapy along with TKs. To-date, pediatric data is limited and warrants more understanding of the genetics, molecular biology, and clinical profile of pediatric Ph+ ALL, which may further help to refine therapy and develop rational combinations of targeted agents that will further improve outcomes for this patient population.

REFERENCES

1. American Cancer Society. 2021. Cancer Facts & Figures 2021. [online] Available from https://www.cancer.org/content/dam/cancer-org/research/cancer-facts-and-statistics/annual-cancer-facts-and-figures/2021/cancer-facts-and-figures-2021.pdf [Last accessed October, 2022].
2. Bernt KM, Hunger SP. Current concepts in pediatric Philadelphia chromosome-positive acute lymphoblastic leukemia. Front Oncol. 2014;4:54.
3. Zawitkowska J, Lejman M, Płonowski M, Bulsa J, Szczepański T, Romiszewski M, et al. Clinical outcome in pediatric patients with Philadelphia chromosome positive ALL treated with tyrosine kinase inhibitors plus chemotherapy-the experience of a Polish Pediatric Leukemia and Lymphoma Study Group. Cancers (Basel). 2020;12(12):3751.
4. Pui CH, Pei D, Campana D, Cheng C, Sandlund JT, Bowman WP, et al. A revised definition for cure of childhood acute lymphoblastic leukemia. Leukemia. 2014;28(12):2336-43.
5. Fielding AK. Treatment of Philadelphia chromosome-positive acute lymphoblastic leukemia in adults: A broader range of options, improved outcomes, and more therapeutic dilemmas. Am Soc Clin Oncol Educ Book. 2015;e352-9.
6. Li S, Ilaria RL Jr, Million RP, Daley GQ, Van Etten RA. The P190, P210, and P230 forms of the BCR/ABL oncogene induce a similar chronic myeloid leukemia-like syndrome in mice but have different lymphoid leukemogenic activity. J Exp Med. 1999;189(9):1399-412.
7. Suryanarayan K, Hunger SP, Kohler S, Carroll AJ, Crist W, Link MP, et al. Consistent involvement of the bcr gene by 9;22 breakpoints in pediatric acute leukemias. Blood. 1991;77(2):324-30.
8. Lugo TG, Witte ON. The BCR-ABL oncogene transforms Rat-1 cells and cooperates with v-myc. Mol Cell Biol. 1989;9(3):1263-70.
9. Frank DA, Varticovski L. BCR/abl leads to the constitutive activation of Stat proteins, and shares an epitope with tyrosine phosphorylated Stats. Leukemia. 1996;10(11):1724-30.
10. Ilaria RL Jr, Van Etten RA. P210 and P190(BCR/ABL) induce the tyrosine phosphorylation and DNA binding activity of multiple specific STAT family members. J Biol Chem. 1996;271(49):31704-10.
11. Kaczmarska A, Śliwa P, Zawitkowska J, Lejman M. Genomic analyses of pediatric acute lymphoblastic leukemia Ph+ and Ph-like-recent progress in treatment. Int J Mol Sci. 2021;22(12):6411.
12. Mullighan CG, Miller CB, Radtke I, Phillips LA, Dalton J, Ma J, et al. BCR-ABL1 lymphoblastic leukaemia is characterized by the deletion of Ikaros. Nature. 2008;453(7191):110-4.
13. Iacobucci I, Storlazzi CT, Cilloni D, Lonetti A, Ottaviani E, Soverini S, et al. Identification and molecular characterization of recurrent genomic deletions on 7p12 in the IKZF1 gene in a large cohort of BCR-ABL1-positive acute lymphoblastic leukemia patients: On behalf of Gruppo Italiano Malattie Ematologiche dell'Adulto Acute Leukemia Working Party (GIMEMA AL WP). Blood. 2009;114(10):2159-67.
14. Martinelli G, Iacobucci I, Storlazzi CT, Vignetti M, Paoloni F, Cilloni D, et al. IKZF1 (Ikaros) deletions in BCR-ABL1-positive acute lymphoblastic leukemia are associated with short disease-free survival and high rate of cumulative incidence of relapse: A GIMEMA AL WP report. J Clin Oncol. 2009;27(31):5202-7.
15. Cobaleda C, Schebesta A, Delogu A, Busslinger M. Pax5: The guardian of B cell identity and function. Nat Immunol. 2007;8(5):463-70.
16. Urbanek P, Wang ZQ, Fetka I, Wagner EF, Busslinger M. Complete block of early B cell differentiation and altered patterning of the posterior midbrain in mice lacking Pax5/BSAP. Cell. 1994;79(5):901-12.
17. Nutt SL, Thevenin C, Busslinger M. Essential functions of Pax-5 (BSAP) in pro-B cell development. Immunobiology. 1997;198(1-3):227-35.
18. Schaniel C, Gottar M, Roosnek E, Melchers F, Rolink AG. Extensive in vivo self-renewal, long-term reconstitution capacity, and hematopoietic multipotency of Pax5-deficient precursor B-cell clones. Blood. 2002;99(8):2760-6.

19. Schaniel C, Bruno L, Melchers F, Rolink AG. Multiple hematopoietic cell lineages develop in vivo from transplanted Pax5-deficient pre-B I-cell clones. Blood. 2002;99(2):472-8.
20. Schultz KR, Carroll A, Heerema NA, Bowman WP, Aledo A, Slayton WB, et al. Long-term follow-up of imatinib in pediatric Philadelphia chromosome-positive acute lymphoblastic leukemia: Children's Oncology Group study AALL0031. Leukemia. 2014;28(7):1467-71.
21. Slayton WB, Schultz KR, Silverman LB, Hunger SP. How we approach Philadelphia chromosome-positive acute lymphoblastic leukemia in children and young adults. Pediatr Blood Cancer. 2020;67(10):e28543.
22. Arico M, Schrappe M, Hunger SP, Carroll WL, Conter V, Galimberti S, et al. Clinical outcome of children with newly diagnosed Philadelphia chromosome-positive acute lymphoblastic leukemia treated between 1995 and 2005. J Clin Oncol. 2010;28(31):4755-61.
23. Arico M, Valsecchi MG, Camitta B, Schrappe M, Chessells J, Baruchel A, et al. Outcome of treatment in children with Philadelphia chromosome-positive acute lymphoblastic leukemia. N Engl J Med. 2000;342(14):998-1006.
24. Biondi A, Schrappe M, De Lorenzo P, Castor A, Lucchini G, Gandemer V, et al. Imatinib after induction for treatment of children and adolescents with Philadelphia-chromosome-positive acute lymphoblastic leukaemia (EsPhALL): A randomised, open-label, intergroup study. Lancet Oncol. 2012;13(9):936-45.
25. Biondi A, Gandemer V, De Lorenzo P, Cario G, Campbell M, Castor A, et al. Imatinib treatment of paediatric Philadelphia chromosome-positive acute lymphoblastic leukaemia (EsPhALL2010): a prospective, intergroup, open-label, single-arm clinical trial. Lancet Haematol. 2018;5(12):e641-e652.
26. Rives S, Estella J, Gómez P, López-Duarte M, de Miguel PG, Verdeguer A, et al. Intermediate dose of imatinib in combination with chemotherapy followed by allogeneic stem cell transplantation improves early outcome in paediatric Philadelphia chromosome-positive acute lymphoblastic leukaemia (ALL): Results of the Spanish Cooperative Group SHOP studies ALL-94, ALL-99 and ALL-2005. Br J Haematol. 2011;154(5):600-11.
27. Manabe A, Kawasaki H, Shimada H, Kato I, Kodama Y, Sato A, et al. Imatinib use immediately before stem cell transplantation in children with Philadelphia chromosome-positive acute lymphoblastic leukemia: Results from Japanese Pediatric Leukemia/Lymphoma Study Group (JPLSG) Study Ph(+) ALL04. Cancer Med. 2015;4(5):682-9.
28. Omar AA, Basiouny L, Elnoby AS, Zaki A, Abouzid M. St. Jude Total Therapy studies from I to XVII for childhood acute lymphoblastic leukemia: a brief review. J Egypt Natl Canc Inst. 2022;34(1):25.
29. Hunger SP. Tyrosine kinase inhibitor use in pediatric Philadelphia chromosome-positive acute lymphoblastic anemia. Hematology Am Soc Hematol Educ Program. 2011;2011:361-5.
30. Liu-Dumlao T, Kantarjian H, Thomas DA, O'Brien S, Ravandi F. Philadelphia-positive acute lymphoblastic leukemia: Current treatment options. Curr Oncol Rep. 2012;14(5):387-94.
31. Zwaan CM, Rizzari C, Mechinaud F, Lancaster DL, Lehrnbecher T, van der Velden VHJ, et al. Dasatinib in children and adolescents with relapsed or refractory leukemia: Results of the CA180-018 phase I dose-escalation study of the Innovative Therapies for Children with Cancer Consortium. J Clin Oncol. 2013;31(19):2460-8.
32. Slayton WB, Schultz KR, Kairalla JA, Devidas M, Mi X, Pulsipher MA, et al. Dasatinib plus intensive chemotherapy in children, adolescents, and young adults with Philadelphia chromosome-positive acute lymphoblastic leukemia: Results of Children's Oncology Group Trial AALL0622. J Clin Oncol. 2018;36(22):2306-14.
33. Hunger S, Saha V, Devidas M, Valsecchi M, Gastier-Foster J, Cazzaniga G, et al. Final results of CA180-372/COG AALL1122 phase 2 trial of dasatinib and chemotherapy in pediatric patients with newly-diagnosed Philadelphia chromosome positive acute lymphoblastic leukemia (PH plus ALL). Pediatric Blood & Cancer. 2020;67:S15-S6.

34. Shen S, Chen X, Cai J, Yu J, Gao J, Hu S, et al. Effect of dasatinib vs imatinib in the treatment of pediatric Philadelphia chromosome-positive acute lymphoblastic leukemia: a randomized clinical trial. JAMA Oncol. 2020;6(3):358-66.
35. Kantarjian H, Giles F, Wunderle L, Bhalla K, O'Brien S, Wassmann B, et al. Nilotinib in imatinib-resistant CML and Philadelphia chromosome-positive ALL. N Engl J Med. 2006;354(24):2542-51.
36. Barr RD. Imatinib mesylate in children and adolescents with cancer. Pediatr Blood Cancer. 2010;55(1):18-25.
37. Carpenter PA, Snyder DS, Flowers MED, Sanders JE, Gooley TA, Martin PJ, et al. Prophylactic administration of imatinib after hematopoietic cell transplantation for high-risk Philadelphia chromosome-positive leukemia. Blood. 2007;109(7):2791-3.
38. Burke MJ, Trotz B, Luo X, Weisdorf DJ, Baker KS, Wagner JE, et al. Imatinib use either pre- or post-allogeneic hematopoietic cell transplantation (allo-HCT) does not increase cardiac toxicity in chronic myelogenous leukemia patients. Bone Marrow Transplant. 2009;44(3):169-74.
39. Burke MJ, Trotz B, Luo X, Baker KS, Weisdorf DJ, Wagner JE, et al. Allo-hematopoietic cell transplantation for Ph chromosome-positive ALL: impact of imatinib on relapse and survival. Bone Marrow Transplant. 2009;43(2):107-13.
40. Pfeifer H, Wassmann B, Bethge W, Dengler J, Bornhäuser M, Stadler M, et al. Randomized comparison of prophylactic and minimal residual disease-triggered imatinib after allogeneic stem cell transplantation for BCR-ABL1-positive acute lymphoblastic leukemia. Leukemia. 2013;27(6):1254-62.
41. Chen H, Liu KY, Xu LP, Liu DH, Chen YH, Zhao XY, et al. Administration of imatinib after allogeneic hematopoietic stem cell transplantation may improve disease-free survival for patients with Philadelphia chromosome-positive acute lymphoblastic leukemia. J Hematol Oncol. 2012;5:29.
42. Soverini S, De Benedittis C, Papayannidis C, Paolini S, Venturi C, Iacobucci I, et al. Drug resistance and BCR-ABL kinase domain mutations in Philadelphia chromosome-positive acute lymphoblastic leukemia from the imatinib to the second-generation tyrosine kinase inhibitor era: The main changes are in the type of mutations, but not in the frequency of mutation involvement. Cancer. 2014;120(7):1002-9.
43. Topp MS, Kufer P, Gökbuget N, Goebeler M, Klinger M, Neumann S, et al. Targeted therapy with the T-cell-engaging antibody blinatumomab of chemotherapy-refractory minimal residual disease in B-lineage acute lymphoblastic leukemia patients results in high response rate and prolonged leukemia-free survival. J Clin Oncol. 2011;29(18):2493-8.
44. Appelmann I, Rillahan CD, de Stanchina E, Carbonetti G, Chen C, Lowe SW, et al. Janus kinase inhibition by ruxolitinib extends dasatinib- and dexamethasone-induced remissions in a mouse model of Ph+ ALL. Blood. 2015;125(9):1444-51.
45. Jain N, Maiti A, Ravandi F, Konopleva M, Daver N, Kadia T, et al. Inotuzumab ozogamicin with bosutinib for relapsed or refractory Philadelphia chromosome positive acute lymphoblastic leukemia or lymphoid blast phase of chronic myeloid leukemia. Am J Hematol. 2021;96(8):1000-7.
46. Manabe A, Kawasaki H, Shimada H, Kato I, Kodama Y, Sato A, et al. Imatinib use immediately before stem cell transplantation in children with Philadelphia chromosome-positive acute lymphoblastic leukemia: results from Japanese Pediatric Leukemia/Lymphoma Study Group (JPLSG) Study Ph(+) ALL04. Cancer Med. 2015;4(5):682-9.
47. Zaliova M, Fronkova E, Krejcikova K, Muzikova K, Mejstrikova E, Stary J, et al. Quantification of fusion transcript reveals a subgroup with distinct biological properties and predicts relapse in BCR/ABL-positive ALL: implications for residual disease monitoring. Leukemia. 2009;23(5):944-51.
48. Den Boer ML, van Slegtenhorst M, De Menezes RX, Cheok MH, Buijs-Gladdines JGCAM, Peters STCJM, et al. A subtype of childhood acute lymphoblastic leukaemia with poor treatment outcome: a genome-wide classification study. Lancet Oncol. 2009;10(2):125-34.

49. Mullighan CG, Su X, Zhang J, Radtke I, Phillips LAA, Miller CB, et al.; Children's Oncology Group. Deletion of IKZF1 and prognosis in acute lymphoblastic leukemia. N Engl J Med. 2009;360(5):470-80.
50. Pui CH, Roberts KG, Yang JJ, Mullighan CG. Philadelphia chromosome-like acute lymphoblastic leukemia. Clin Lymphoma Myeloma Leuk. 2017;17(8):464-70.
51. Roberts KG, Gu Z, Payne-Turner D, McCastlain K, Harvey RC, Chen IM, et al. High frequency and poor outcome of Philadelphia chromosome-like acute lymphoblastic leukemia in adults. J Clin Oncol. 2017;35(4):394-401.
52. Jain N, Roberts KG, Jabbour E, Patel K, Eterovic AK, Chen K, et al. Ph-like acute lymphoblastic leukemia: a high-risk subtype in adults. Blood. 2017;129(5):572-81.
53. Roberts KG, Pei D, Campana D, Payne-Turner D, Li Y, Cheng C, et al. Outcomes of children with BCR-ABL1-like acute lymphoblastic leukemia treated with risk-directed therapy based on the levels of minimal residual disease. J Clin Oncol. 2014;32(27):3012-20.
54. Płotka A, Lewandowski K. BCR/ABL1-like acute lymphoblastic leukemia: from diagnostic approaches to molecularly targeted therapy. Acta Haematol. 2022;145(2):122-31.
55. Iacobucci I, Roberts KG. Genetic alterations and therapeutic targeting of Philadelphia-like acute lymphoblastic leukemia. Genes (Basel). 2021;12(5):687.
56. Conant JL, Czuchlewski DR. BCR-ABL1-like B-lymphoblastic leukemia/lymphoma: review of the entity and detection methodologies. Int J Lab Hematol. 2019;41 (Suppl 1):126-30.

EXPERT OPINION

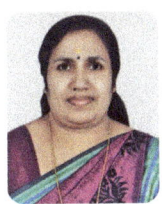

Priya Kumari T
Professor and Head, Department of Pediatric Oncology
Regional Cancer Centre, Thiruvananthapuram, Kerala, India

Philadelphia-positive Acute Lymphoblastic Leukemia

Targeted therapy with TKI has revolutionized the pediatric Ph+ ALL therapy and converted it from one of the least curable forms of childhood ALL subtypes in the pre-TKI era to one which has an OS rate closely reaching the other ALL subtypes.

Philadelphia-positive ALL is to be treated in the HR arm of the ALL chemotherapy protocol along with a TKI with close monitoring for treatment-related toxicities and adequate supportive care measures. We use BFM-based protocol in our institution. The TKI of choice can be either imatinib @ 300–340 mg/m^2/day or dasatinib @ 60–80 mg/m^2/day, considering their proven near equal efficacy and CNS control rates in various clinical trials. TKI is to be initiated by D15 of induction or earlier as soon as the Ph+ result is obtained and needs to be continued throughout the entire chemotherapy duration. Other ABL-TKIs like Nilotinib, bosutinib, and Ponatinib can be reserved for use in the relapsed setting with imatinib resistance.

Treatment response is monitored using MRD. EOI and end of consolidation (EOC) MRD helps in defining risk and guide further therapy. MRD by flow cytometry or PCR IgH/TCR MRD levels can identify HR patients who are EOI and EOC MRD +ve. These patients and patients who remain MRD +ve 3–4 months after therapy initiation are at HR of relapse and are candidates for HSCT in CR1. MRD levels based on quantitative assay qRT-PCR of BCR-ABL1 transcript were shown to be higher and less reliable in predicting outcome.

Imatinib and dasatinib are usually well tolerated in combination with chemotherapy and may be modified as necessary. In presence of myelosuppression, TKI may be continued for 2 weeks before stopping. During maintenance, mercaptopurine and methotrexate may be kept on hold initially prior to TKI in the setting of myelosuppression. TKI may also be held in the presence of serious infections, hepatic toxicity (transaminase >20 times normal, direct bilirubin >1.5 times Nl), and QTc prolongation (Gr 2 or higher). Both dasatinib and imatinib can cause serious effusions when TKI needs to be stopped to be restarted later @ 80% dose. Along with post bone marrow transplant (BMT) myelosuppression, TKI should be held until counts recover.

Central nervous system positivity in Ph+ ALL is reported to be higher (6–8%). The management includes intrathecal chemotherapy, CNS-directed systemic chemotherapy, and therapeutic cranial irradiation.

Philadelphia-positive ALL relapse treatment is not fully standardized. Many relapsed patients treated in the TKI era are salvaged successfully using reinduction, consolidation followed by allo-HSCT in second remission (CR2) by European and North American groups and this can be the relapse treatment option. A second remission is achievable in most relapsed patients using a TKI in combination with three-drug chemotherapy (eliminating anthracycline). At relapse it is essential to test for TKI mutation status (mutations can cause absolute/relative resistance to imatinib/dastinib, T315I being the most common) and BCR-ABL1 amplification (which can be overcome by using higher dosing with TKI). The same TKI (imatinib or dasatinib) may be restarted initially while awaiting the mutation report, since most patients will retain TKI sensitivity. Subsequently TKI may be modified based on the mutation status report (e.g., ponatinib if T315I mutation is detected). Once in CR2 these patients are further managed with consolidation and allo-HSCT. The French retrospective analysis (Lucie et al. PBC May 2021) is very promising. They reported that the TKI pretreated Ph+ pediatric patients in first relapse reinduced well with a second course of TKI along with either intensive or even nonintensive chemotherapy resulting in CR2 in 96% of patients. With further consolidation chemotherapy and allo-HSCT the 4-year EFS and OS were 60.9 and 76.1%. Allo-HSCT in CR2 was positively associated with the survival in this cohort.

Philadelphia Chromosome-like Acute Lymphoblastic Leukemia

Philadelphia chromosome-like ALL is defined as having a gene expression signature similar to *BCR-ABL1*-positive ALL, but lack the *BCR-ABL1* fusion gene. It accounts for 10–15% of NCI SR and NCI 22.6% of HR B-ALL cases in children and adolescents. These patients are at HR for poor treatment response or relapse.

Philadelphia chromosome-like ALL is not a single genetic lesion but a heterogeneous group of genetic alterations which predominantly affect either the JAK-STAT or the ABL kinase signaling pathways. The four genetically defined subsets of alterations are:
1. Alterations in JAK/STAT pathway genes (mainly CRLF2, JAK2, EPOR, IL7R, SH2B3)
   Cytokine receptor-like factor 2 rearrangements (50%): Include mutations involving IL7 receptor (JAK2 and JAK1). P2PY8-CRLF2 and IGH-CRLF2 are predominant translocations.
2. ABL class alterations (ABL1, ABL2, CSF1R, LYN, PDGFRA, PDGFRB)
3. Uncommon Ras pathway mutations (NRAS, KRAS, NF1 PTPN11, CBL)
4. Rare kinase fusions (NTRK3, PTK2B, BLNK).

There is no consensus approach to the diagnosis of Ph-like ALL. Optimal screening method and target population are still not fully defined. RNA sequencing enables identification of Ph-like phenotype and aberrant translocations but is unavailable in most centers. Hence routine screening of all patients for Ph-like ALL is impractical. A practical approach for Ph-like ALL screening especially in LMIC setting would be the following:

Patients to be screened: A child with B-cell other ALL (patients with high hyperdiploidy, *ETV6-RUNX1, BCR-ABL1, TCF3-PBX1,* and *MLL/KMT2A* rearrangements, are mutually exclusive with Ph-like ALL) who is MRD positive at the EOI is a highly likely candidate to have Ph-like ALL and requires screening.

An algorithm for Ph-like ALL screening:

Step 1: Screening for CRLF2 overexpression (most common abnormality, seen in up to 50% of cases)
    Screen for CRLF2 overexpression using qRT-PCR or flow cytometric immunophenotyping or FISH break-apart
    Categorizes as CRLF2 low/high

Step 2: Further testing if CRLF2 overexpressed/high: Ph-like ALL
    Identify partner
    P2YR8-CRLF2 using MLPA (multiplex ligation dependent probe analysis)
    IGH-CRLF2 with FISH
    Followed by JAK mutation analysis (JAK2 mutations are associated with 50% of CRLF2 rearranged ALL).

Step 3: Further testing if CRLF2 low/negative: Test for TK fusions
    FISH break-apart for ABL1, ABL2, PDGFRB, CSF1R, JAK2, EPOR
    If positive: Ph-like ALL
    If negative: Consider targeted mutation analysis, or RNA sequencing (for mutations in JAK, IL7R, FLT3, SH2B3, PTPN11, RAS).

5.4 ACUTE PROMYELOCYTIC LEUKEMIA

Debasish Sahoo, Jagdish P Meena

CASE VIGNETTE

A 12-year-old boy presented with complaints of left-sided weakness, progressive pallor, and skin bleeds. On examination, he had severe pallor, ecchymosis, and left-sided hemiplegia with facial nerve palsy. His bedside peripheral smear showed multiple promyelocytes. What are the distinguishing characteristics of promyelocytes in acute promyelocytic leukemia (APML)?

The hallmark of APML is the presence of the large atypical promyelocytes and other myeloid precursors in the peripheral blood, which are considered blast equivalents. The atypical promyelocytes in APML are characterized by large cells with a high nucleus-cytoplasmic ratio, folded, bilobed, creased, or reniform nuclei giving an "apple core appearance" prominent nucleoli. The cytoplasm is typically studded with coarse violet granules that may obscure the nuclear details (often coalescing to form Auer rods) **(Fig. 1)**. In the microgranular variant, these granules and Auer rods are less prominent in the microgranular variant of APML; the nucleus retains its characteristic bilobed, folded appearance. Other less common variants include hyperbasophilic variant.

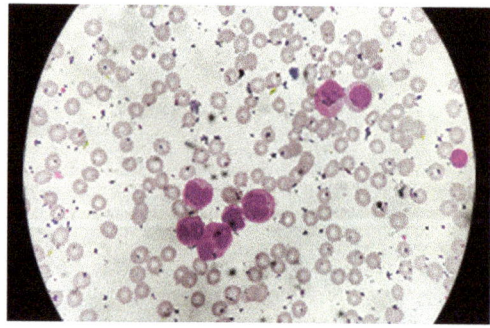

Fig. 1: Morphology of acute promyelocytic leukemia (APML): Abnormal large promyelocytes with nuclear folding giving an "apple core appearance" with abundant granules and Auer rods.

1. Flow cytometry showed high side scatter (SS), positivity for cMPO, CD13(br), CD33, CD117, CD11b (dim), CD64, CD9, CD25 (dim), and CD11c (dim het) and negativity for CD2, CD3, CD4, CD7, CD34, human leukocyte antigen (HLA)-DR, CD15, CD16, CD18, CD19, CD36, and CD56. What are the immunophenotypic features specific to APML?

The malignant atypical promyelocytes show bright positivity for cytoplasmic myeloperoxidase (cMPO) and early myeloid markers like CD13 and CD33 but are characteristically negative for CD11b, CD15, CD117 (expressed in mature myelocytes) and HLA-DR and CD34 (early myeloid progenitor cells—prematurity markers). CD9 expression is also a differentiating feature of APML from other non-M3 acute myeloid leukemia (AML).

Coexpression of CD2 is commonly observed in the microgranular variant of APML and is associated with a poorer outcome. A typical "teardrop pattern" is obtained on scatter plots on CD45 versus SS. In contrast, non-M3 AML consistently expresses the prematurity markers like HLA-DR and CD34.

2. Among AML subtypes, APML is one subtype with survival approaching that of acute lymphoid leukemia in children. However, the true survival rates of patients with APML may be lower than what is reported.[1] Why is it so?

The three main causes of early death in APML are hemorrhage, differentiation syndrome (DS), and infection. Many early deaths occur due to hemorrhages that happen before a child is enrolled into a protocol and often go unreported. Various cooperative group multicenter trials report a low early death rate (5–10%) within the first month of diagnosis. There is a paucity of data on the incidence of early death in unselected patients with APML outside of the clinical trial setting. A study using data from Surveillance, Epidemiology, and End Results (SEER) program found a significantly higher overall early death rate (17.3%).[2] Due to early deaths, in a study conducted in a real-world setting, 5-and 10-year OS were significantly worse than trial data.[3] The factors consistently associated with early deaths included baseline total leukocyte count $\geq 10 \times 10^9$/L, hypofibrinogenemia with plasma fibrinogen <1.5 g/L, and delay in all-trans-retinoic acid (ATRA) administration > 24 hours after hospital admission.[4] Therefore, prompt administration of ATRA and aggressive correction of hemostatic abnormalities, including hypofibrinogenemia and thrombocytopenia, are vital in reducing early deaths **(Fig. 2)**.

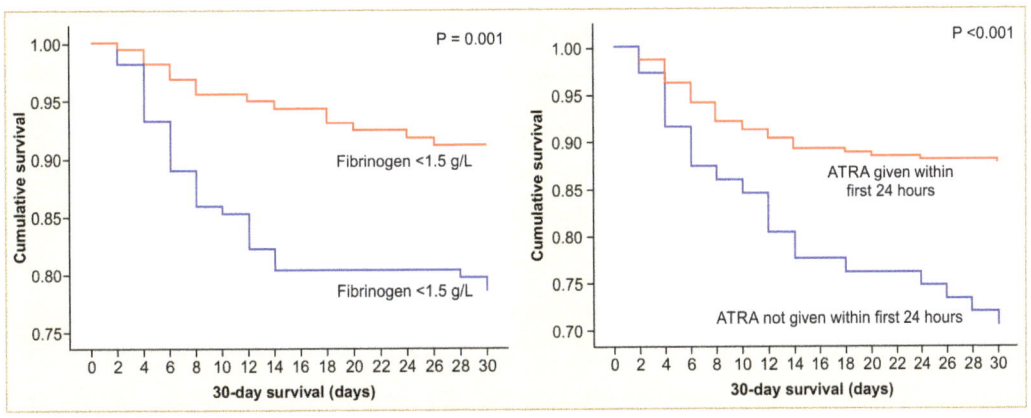

Fig. 2: Low fibrinogen and delay in all-trans-retinoic acid initiation were significantly associated with early deaths in the study by Gill et al.[3]

Recent evidence has shown that a comanagement strategy, including a simplified algorithm and partnership between experts, can significantly decrease early death to <10%.[5]

3. What is the mechanism of coagulopathy in APML?

The abnormal promyelocytes in APML have significantly higher expression of procoagulants like tissue factor (TF), annexin 2 and cysteine protease (CP), and fibrinolytic agents like tissue-plasminogen activator (t-PA) and urokinase-like plasminogen activator (u-PA) receptor. This results in the activation of coagulation cascade and fibrinolysis simultaneously.[1] In addition, exaggerated elastase activity causes depletion of α2 antiplasmin, and a decrease in thrombin activatable fibrinolysis inhibitor further promotes fibrinolysis **(Fig. 3)**.[6,7] Finally, inflammatory cytokines like interleukin-1 (IL-1) and tumor necrosis factor-α (TNF-α) promote the synthesis of TFs, contributing to the cascade.

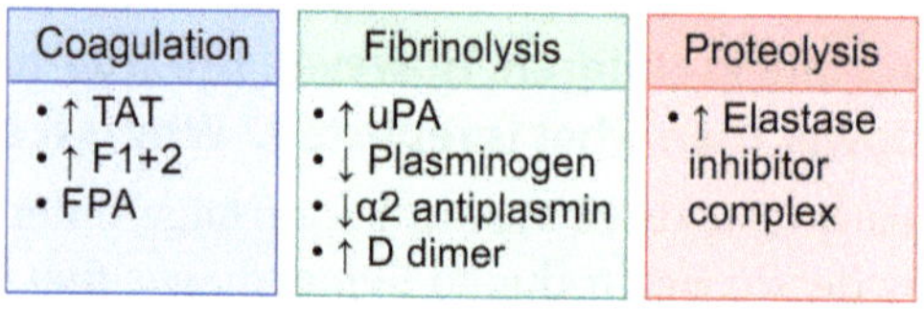

Coagulation	Fibrinolysis	Proteolysis
• ↑ TAT • ↑ F1+2 • FPA	• ↑ uPA • ↓ Plasminogen • ↓α2 antiplasmin • ↑ D dimer	• ↑ Elastase inhibitor complex

Fig. 3: Coagulopathy in acute promyelocytic leukemia (APML): The plasma levels of prothrombotic factors like thrombin-antithrombin complex (TAT), prothrombin fragment 1 + 2 (F1 + 2), and fibrinopeptide A (FPA) are elevated. Additionally, high levels of fibrin degradation products and urokinase-type plasminogen activator (uPA) along with low levels of plasminogen and α2-antiplasmin have been described, providing evidence for activation of fibrinolysis. Furthermore, elevated plasma levels of leukocyte elastase and fibrinogen split products of elastase demonstrate the activity of nonspecific proteases.

4. What are the differences between the coagulopathy of APML and disseminated intravascular coagulation (DIC) due to other causes?

Microvascular thrombosis, commonly described in the pathophysiology of DIC, is clinically uncommon in APML. In addition, thrombocytopenia seen in APML is compounded by decreased production of platelets due to bone marrow infiltration by the malignant cells. Furthermore, the maintained normal levels of physiological anticoagulants in APML suggest that they are not being utilized for the neutralization of activated coagulation proteins as there is lesser activation of the coagulation cascade. Additionally, plasma levels of fibrinogen and factor V are found to be lower, and levels of d-dimer fibrin degradation products are significantly higher in APML when compared with DIC, strongly suggesting primary fibrinolytic activation leading to hyperfibrinolysis rather than an excessive expression of procoagulants like TF and annexin V is the main driver of bleeding diathesis in APML **(Table 1)**.[8]

TABLE 1: Comparison of parameters of hemostasis in APML and DIC.

Markers	APML	DIC
Prothrombin time	↔ (usually ↑↑)	↔ (usually ↑)
aPTT	↔ (usually ↑↑)	↔ (usually ↑)
Fibrinogen	↓ (↓↓ if hyperfibrinolysis)	↓↓
FDP	↑↑	↑
D-dimer	↑↑	↑
Protein-C	↔	↓
Protein-S	↔	↓
Antithrombin	↔	↓
Platelets	↓	↓↓
Annexin II	↑↑	↑↑

Contd...

Contd...

Markers	APML	DIC
Rotational thromboelastometry:		
• Clot formation time	↑↑	↑/Variable
• Maximal clot firmness	↓	↓/Variable

(APML: acute promyelocytic leukemia; aPTT: activated partial thromboplastin time; DIC: disseminated intravascular coagulation; FDP: fibrinogen degradation product)

5. How do various therapeutic agents affect coagulopathy in APML?

All-trans-retinoic acid is known to decrease the expression of TF, CP, annexin II, and other inflammatory cytokines in the abnormal promyelocytes, thereby preventing excessive activation of both coagulation cascade and fibrinolytic events in children with APML. It also reduces the amount of fibrinolytic events by promoting the expression of plasminogen activator inhibitor 1 (PAI-1) and thrombomodulin in endothelial cells, resulting in a reduction in the synthesis of active plasmin **(Fig. 4)**.[9]

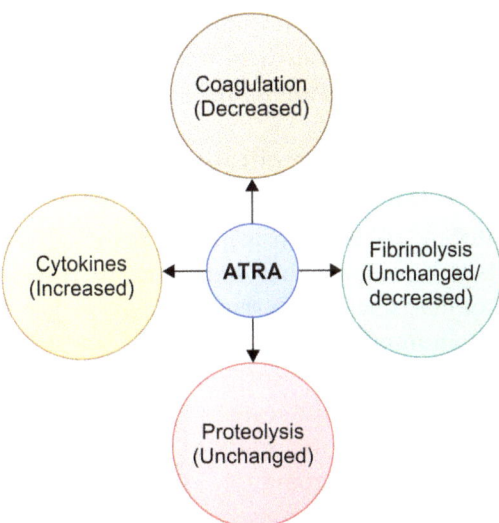

Fig. 4: Effect of all-trans-retinoic acid (ATRA) on coagulopathy in acute promyelocytic leukemia (APML) (a) ATRA causes a reduction in expression of both TF and CP, resulting in a reduction of procoagulant activity; (b) ATRA increases levels of both plasminogen activators as well as inhibitors, thus, resulting in unaltered or reduced fibrinolytic activity; (c) nonspecific proteases: no effect; (d) ATRA increases production of cytokines, including IL-1β and TNF-α, that induce the endothelium thrombogenicity.
(*Source:* Modified from Barbui T, Finazzi G, Falanga A. The impact of all-trans-retinoic acid on the coagulopathy of acute promyelocytic leukemia. Blood. 1998;91(9):3093-102.)[4]

Paradoxically, ATRA may promote thrombosis. It may induce ETosis,[5] a novel cell death pathway, in APML cells. ETosis, meaning cell death by the release of extracellular traps (ETs), is characterized by fragmentation of the nuclear and granule membranes within the cell leading to the interaction of decondensed nuclear chromatin with various antimicrobial peptides and enzymes (such as elastases and cathepsin G). The cell membrane subsequently undergoes fragmentation leading to the release of ETs, which are essentially web of peptides and enzymes trapped over the scaffolding of extracellular decondensed chromatin and histone proteins which forms a sticky mesh. These ETs can activate the coagulation cascade by the binding of decondensed chromatin to various procoagulant proteins along with the exposed and the activated surface of cell membrane of the cell, forming a backbone for coagulation and fibrinolysis. Additionally, cell-free DNA released during the process can activate the coagulation pathway by contact activation. The extracellular chromatin of the abnormal promyelocytes exerts cytotoxic effects on the endothelial cells, which explains the increased risk of life-threatening bleeds like pulmonary hemorrhage, and intracranial hemorrhage seen after initiation of therapy and increased susceptibility to bleeding manifestations even in the presence of apparently adequate hemostatic levels of platelets and other coagulation factors.[10]

In the pre-ATRA era, it was observed that initiation of cytotoxic chemotherapy could worsen the coagulopathy by elevated expression of TF and formation of TF microparticles which can activate and accelerate the coagulation cascade. It was also seen that red blood cells (RBCs) expose the phosphatidylserine moiety on their plasma membrane upon exposure to anthracyclines, where platelets and TF bearing microparticles can bind to them, initiating the coagulation cascade. Anthracyclines can also cause endothelial damage and dysfunction, thus contributing to coagulation in patients with APML.

6. Thrombosis is an underrated complication of APML, often overshadowed by hemorrhage. What are its pathogenesis and management?

A number of factors contribute to thrombosis in APML, though the incidence of clinically significant thrombosis is less common than hemorrhage. The malignant promyelocytes directly contribute to thrombosis by overexpression of factors like TF, CP, and annexin V. A DIC-like state is activated, promoting thrombosis. ATRA is also thought to upregulate the expression of various adhesion molecules such as very late antigen-4 (VLA4) and lymphocyte function-associated 1 (LFA1) on the cell membrane of the leukemic clones, leading to increased adhesion to the endothelium and thus endothelial damage and activation. It also increases the procoagulant characters of the endothelium. Anthracycline-induced apoptosis of the leukemic clones results in an increase in cellular TF activity and the release of TF-bearing microparticles from leukemic blasts.[6] In cerebral venous thrombosis, as in the index child **(Fig. 5)**, anticoagulation was started in the absence of other contraindications while maintaining platelet count above the target range. Central venous catheterization was avoided in view of this increased risk of thrombosis.

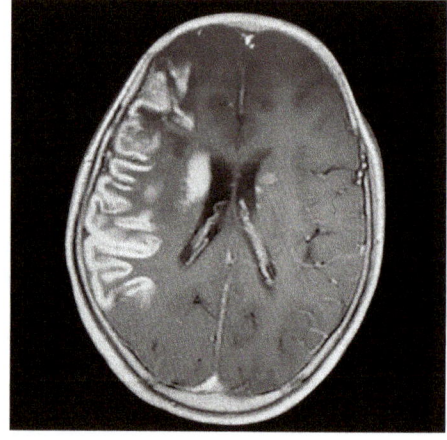

Fig. 5: Magnetic resonance imaging (MRI) of the index child showing cerebral venous thrombosis and venous infarct.

7. After starting ATRA, the index child developed weight gain, edema, mild pleural effusion, and respiratory distress, with X-ray showing bilateral infiltrates. A diagnosis of DS was made. Elucidate the pathophysiology and manifestations of DS. How will you prevent and treat DS?

The pathophysiology of DS and the resultant clinical manifestations are contributed by a systemic inflammatory response, endothelial damage, and microcirculation obstruction, and finally, tissue infiltration, mediated by the release of various mediators including ILs and proteases, and expression of endothelial adhesion molecules. It can be observed in up to 20% of children with APML, typically occurring in the second week of therapy. ATRA removes the differentiation block caused by PML-retinoic acid receptor alpha (RARA). This results in increased maturation of promyelocytes and increased cytokine release. The symptomatology may include unexplained fever, weight gain, breathlessness, edema, pleuropericardial effusion, pulmonary infiltrates, hypotension, and renal failure, which may be fatal. It should be suspected in the presence of any of the symptoms with a low threshold for starting steroids. Temporary discontinuation of the differentiating agent may be required in a few selected patients with significant pulmonary or renal impairment. In view of the higher incidence of DS in high-risk patients [total leukocyte count (TLC) > 10,000/ mm^3], the standard of care includes prophylactic dexamethasone and early initiation of chemotherapy in this group of patients.

8. Elaborate on the leukemogenic effects of PML-RARA. What are the available methods to detect PML-RARA?

The PML/RARA oncoprotein binds to the corepressor complex with a very high affinity resulting in repression of various RARA target genes, which are involved in cellular differentiation and maturation. PML/RARA also causes disruption of PML nuclear bodies (NBs) structure. These result in a differentiation block, proliferation of the leukemic promyelocytes, and lack of apoptosis. Differentiating agents like ATRA and ATO promote ubiquitin-proteasome pathway-mediated degradation of the PML/RARA oncoprotein. This results in transcriptional reactivation of RARA target genes and reformation of NBs, thus inducing terminal differentiation of leukemic clones.[11]

Various methods available for PML-RARA detection are conventional karyotyping, fluorescent in situ hybridization (FISH), PML immunostaining with specific antibodies, and RT-PCR detection, among which RT-PCR has the highest sensitivity. Because of the high sensitivity, it is also the preferred modality for minimal residual disease (MRD) monitoring.

9. What are the various RARA rearrangements in variant APML and their significance?

Retinoic acid receptor alpha is a highly promiscuous gene, with more than 15 identified atypical fusion partners like ZBTB16, NPM1, STAT5B, BCOR, FIP1L1, PRKAR1A, and NABP1.[12,13] Patients with these atypical RARA fusion partners often differ from traditional APML as many lack Auer rods, have a younger age at presentation, and are often less responsive to differentiation therapy. Other cases of APML, which lack RARA rearrangement, but are diagnosed on the basis of morphological examination alone, demonstrate fusions with other members of the retinoid signaling family. However, most cooperative groups exclude patients with atypical or absent RARA rearrangements from the clinical trials, and thus the outcomes in this subgroup are available from small case series and case reports. One of the series reported that 9 of 18 patients with atypical APML showed superior EFS with AML therapy compared to APML therapy.[14]

10. What is the incidence of FMS-like tyrosine kinase gene (FLT3) mutations in pediatric APML? What does it indicate in terms of prognosis?

Mutations in *FLT3* have been reported in up to 40% of pediatric cases. *FLT3* mutations include internal tandem duplications (*FLT3-ITD*) and a missense mutation at amino acid 835, both of which lead to the constitutional activation of the tyrosine kinase receptor.[15] Studies in both pediatric patients and adults have shown that *FLT3* mutations are associated with a higher WBC count at presentation and thus a higher risk of mortality.[16] However, its use as an independent prognostic marker and role in risk stratification are controversial. Most cooperative group trials except the CCLG-APL 2016 study don't consider *FLT3* mutations for risk stratification.

11. Summarize the major trials in APML conducted in the pediatric population.

The summary of various trials in pediatric APML is given in **Table 2**.

TABLE 2: The summary of various trials in pediatric APML.

Group	BFM 94, 98, 2004	APL 94, 2000	AESOP-GIMEMA 2005	PEMA 2006	COG AAML 1331 (2022)
Number of children	81	31	124	66	154
Drugs	ATRA + cytarabine + etoposide + idarubicin/ daunorubicin, and mitoxantrone	ATRA + cytarabine + daunorubicin	ATRA + idarubicin, mitoxantrone	ATRA + idarubicin, mitoxantrone	ATRA + ATO + IDA (in HR patients)
ATRA dosage (mg/m²)	25	45	25	25	25
CR rate (%)	95	97	96	92	100
5 years EFS (%)	76	71	76	77	2 years: HR: 96.4% SR 98%
5 years OS (%)	87	90	89	87	100%
Cumulative anthracycline dose (doxorubicin equivalent in mg/m²)	350	495	650	650	180 (high risk only)

(CR: complete response; HR: high risk; SR: standard risk; EFS: event-free survival; OS: overall survival)

12. How do ATRA and ATO act synergistically?

Acute promyelocytic leukemia is characterized by PML-RARA-induced transcriptional inhibition of retinoic acid receptor target genes and many epigenetic changes. Transglutaminase 2 (TGM2) and retinoic acid receptor beta (RARβ) are two genes closely involved in retinoic acid-mediated maturation and differentiation. Both of them have been proven to be heavily methylated in the presence of PML-RARA oncoprotein and undergo extensive histone modification, thus altering the expression of many genes. A combination of ATRA and ATO leads to a sustained expression of these target genes (TGM2 and RARβ), resulting in maturation and terminal differentiation of the abnormal promyelocytes.[17] ATO also promotes apoptosis of the malignant promyelocytes. It has been suggested that ATO additionally causes ETosis of leukemia-initiating cells (LIC), thus resulting in deeper remission and reduction in relapses.

13. What dose of ATRA is the standard of care in pediatric APML? Substantiate

Due to the correlation of ATRA-related side-effects like DS and pseudotumor cerebri with the dose of ATRA, dose reduction from 45–25 mg/m^2 was first studied by AML-Berlin-Frankfurt-Münster (BFM) group. Though, it was found that the reduced dose was equally effective, there were still high rates of central nervous system (CNS) adverse effects like headache and raised intracranial pressure.[18] The CALGB C9710 trial used a higher dose but demonstrated no additional benefit.[19] Hence 25 mg/m^2 is being used from AAML0631 onward and is the current standard of care.[20]

14. Should we start ATRA alone, chemotherapy alone, or ATRA and chemotherapy simultaneously for a patient with APML in an emergency?

Acute promyelocytic leukemia is a medical emergency, and ATRA should be administered as soon as the diagnosis of APML is suspected. Concomitant therapy with ATRA and chemotherapy has been associated with improved outcomes as compared to sequential therapy. Chemotherapy can be started at 48 hours of ATRA in children with standard risk APML (TLC < 10,000/ mm^3), whereas it has to be initiated simultaneously in high-risk APML to prevent the development of DS. ATRA may later be stopped if a diagnosis of non-M3 AML or ATRA-resistant APML is established.

15. What specific monitoring is required for a child on ATRA and ATO?

Serum electrolytes (including calcium and magnesium), 12-lead ECG, and creatinine should be assessed at baseline prior to initiation of therapy. During induction, additional monitoring includes CBC, hepatic function, blood glucose, and coagulation at least twice weekly. During consolidation, weekly monitoring is recommended.

16. Are there clear guidelines regarding CNS prophylaxis in APML?

Central nervous system involvement in APML is less common, and thus CNS prophylaxis is not routinely recommended in all patients. The BFM practice of prophylactic cranial irradiation has been abandoned. The European Leukemia Net[21] recommends the use of CNS prophylaxis using intrathecal therapy only in high-risk patients (presenting TLC >10,000/ mm^3) or patients with intracranial hemorrhage. Lumbar puncture and intrathecal therapy should also be postponed till the resolution of coagulopathy in view of the risk of bleeding. There is no clear evidence supporting or refuting the use of CNS prophylaxis in the ATO era.

17. What are the risk factors associated with CNS involvement in APML? How will you manage?

Factors like high TLC (>10 × 10^9/L) at initial diagnosis, intracranial hemorrhage, CD2, and/or CD56 expression in the abnormal promyelocytes, PML-RARA bcr3 isoform, DS, and use of single-agent chemotherapy are associated with CNS involvement and CNS relapse of APML. CNS involvement appears to respond well to triple intrathecal chemotherapy and craniospinal irradiation, but ATRA and ATO do not cross the blood-brain barrier.[22] Use of cranial irradiation is currently limited to those patients who do not respond to intrathecal therapy.

18. What are optimal time points for MRD monitoring in APML?

In view of virtually absent resistance at onset and persistence of late maturing promyelocytes at the end of induction, postinduction MRD need not be done. A positive postinduction MRD is not associated with a poorer outcome. This is particularly true for patients treated with a combination of ATRA and ATO without chemotherapy. However, postconsolidation MRD is crucial in decisions, especially in high-risk patients. MRD positivity in two consecutive bone marrow samples or serial increase in copy number of PML-RARA transcripts is associated with relapses and thus provides the reason for MRD monitoring and treatment of MRD relapses.

19. What is the evidence for and against maintenance therapy in APML?

The initial results were conflicting: North American Intergroup Study I0129[23] and the European APML Group APML 93 trial[24] suggested a reduction in relapses with the use of maintenance therapy, while a GIMEMA trial[25] and Japanese Leukemia Study Group APML 97 trial[26] found no benefit. A Cochrane review showed no significant differences in overall survival with or without maintenance therapy or between different types of maintenance therapy regimens, though the use of any maintenance therapy did result in improvement in event-free survival.[27] However, with the integration of ATO in frontline treatment, the benefit of maintenance therapy has become questionable. The recent COG AAML1331 has validated the removal of maintenance in both standard and high risks with an excellent survival even without maintenance therapy.[28]

20. What is the chemotherapy-free approach in APML?

Traditionally, APML has been treated with a combination of differentiating agents (ATRA with/without ATO) and chemotherapy (anthracyclines with/without cytarabine). However, due to the synergistic activity of ATRA and ATO, their combination has been employed successfully in adults with APML, restricting the use of chemotherapy only to the induction phase in high-risk patients. The same approach has been recently validated in pediatric patients in COG AAML 1,331 successfully eliminating the use of chemotherapy, except in induction in high-risk patients. Thus, the chemotherapy-free approach (ATRA + ATO) has become the new standard of care in pediatric APML patients as well.

21. Describe management strategy in APML with CNS involvement.

There are currently no well-defined guidelines for the management of APML with CNS involvement in view of the rarity of CNS involvement. Various strategies like cranial radiotherapy, intrathecal chemotherapy, and combinations of agents used to treat primary APML have been used to treat CNS disease. Hence, the evidence is based on small case series and reports. In patients with CNS relapse, autologous or allogeneic stem cell transplants have been used as consolidative therapy, depending on the clinical situation and molecular status.[29]

22. Has resistance to ATRA/ATO been described? Are there any alternative agents in the pipeline? Explain the mechanism.

Mutations leading to amino acid substitution in the ligand-binding domain (LBD) and the PML-B2 domain of PML-RARA oncoprotein have been proposed as molecular mechanisms causing resistance to ATRA and arsenic trioxide (ATO), respectively. In mutation involving LBD, ATRA binding with LBD is inhibited. Thus, ATRA-dependent dissociation of corepressor, degradation of PML-RARA oncoprotein by proteasome pathway, and reformation of NB, leading to cell differentiation, are inhibited. In the presence of PML-B2 mutation, binding of ATO with PML-B2 is prevented, and SUMOylation of PML-RARA, followed by multimerization and degradation, is impaired, leading to ATO resistance.[30]

Arsenic trioxide forms an integral component of the treatment of relapsed/refractory patients treated with ATRA/chemotherapy. Am80 is a synthetic retinoid having a higher binding affinity with PML-RARA than ATRA and is currently experimental. Since epigenetic modification forms an important component in the pathogenesis of the disease, histone deacetylase inhibitors, like sodium butyrate, valproic acid, and trichostatin A, have been utilized in combination with ATRA to inhibit corepressors complexes that contain histone deacetylases (HDACs). Considering the high level of expression of CD 33, gemtuzumab ozogamicin (GO), a monoclonal antibody against CD 33, has been successfully employed in the setting of relapsed or refractory disease.

23. How are molecular persistence and molecular relapse managed?

Persistence of disease or MRD at the end of consolidation, and more commonly molecular relapse (defined as persisting or rising *PML-RARA* transcript levels in two consecutive bone marrow samples), is associated with a higher risk of relapse. A combination of ATRA and ATO can be employed in patients with molecular persistence or molecular relapse who were initially treated with ATRA plus chemotherapy. Conversely, ATRA plus chemotherapy can be employed when molecular persistence occurs after treatment with ATRA and ATO. Gemtuzumab ozogamicin can also be used for salvage as a bridge to hematopoietic stem cell transplantation (HSCT). Consolidative HSCT (autologous or allogeneic) is recommended after salvage therapy.

24. How will you approach hematological relapse?

Treatment includes the use of ATO, GO, and HSCT. ATO, in combination with chemotherapy and/or ATRA, is the most common regime for initial therapy. Consolidative HSCT may be essential based on the timing of relapse, the initial treatment used, and response to salvage therapy. The choice of type of HSCT, allogeneic or autologous, is based on treatment-related mortality (TRM) and MRD monitoring for PML-RARA. Though associated with higher TRM, an allogeneic transplant is preferred in patients who continue to have detectable MRD after savage therapy.

REFERENCES

1. Alizadeh AA, McClellan JS, Gotlib JR, Coutre S, Majeti R, Kohrt HE, et al. Early mortality in acute promyelocytic leukemia may be higher than previously reported. Blood. 2009;114(22):1015.
2. Park JH, Qiao B, Panageas KS, Schymura MJ, Jurcic JG, Rosenblat TL, et al. Early death rate in acute promyelocytic leukemia remains high despite all-trans retinoic acid. Blood. 2011;118(5):1248-54.
3. Gill H, Yung Y, Chu H, Au WY, Yip PK, Lee E, et al. Characteristics and predictors of early hospital deaths in newly diagnosed acute promyelocytic leukemia: a 13-year population-wide study. Blood Adv. 2021;5(14):2829-38.
4. Altman JK, Rademaker A, Cull E, Weitner BB, Ofran Y, Rosenblat TL, et al. Administration of ATRA to newly diagnosed patients with acute promyelocytic leukemia is delayed contributing to early hemorrhagic death. Leuk Res. 2013;37(9):1004-9.
5. Jillella AP, Arellano ML, Gaddh M, Langston AA, Heffner LT, Winton EF, et al. Comanagement strategy between academic institutions and community practices to reduce induction mortality in acute promyelocytic leukemia. J Oncol Pract. 2021;17(4):e497-e505.
6. Breen KA, Grimwade D, Hunt BJ. The pathogenesis and management of the coagulopathy of acute promyelocytic leukaemia. Br J Haematol. 2012;156:24-36.
7. Oudijk EJ, Nieuwenhuis HK, Bos R, Fijnheer R. Elastase mediated fibrinolysis in acute promyelocytic leukemia. Thromb Haemost. 2000;83:906-8.
8. Falanga A, Barbui T. Coagulopathy of acute promyelocytic leukemia. Acta Haematol. 2001;106:43-51.
9. Barbui T, Finazzi G, Falanga A. The impact of all-trans-retinoic acid on the coagulopathy of acute promyelocytic leukemia. Blood. 1998;91:3093-102.
10. Wartha F, Henriques-Normark B. ETosis: a novel cell death pathway. Sci Signal. 2008;1(21)pe25.
11. de Thé H, Zhu J, Nasr R, Ablain J, Lallemand-Breittenbach V. PML/RARA as the master driver of apl pathogenesis and therapy response. In: Andreeff M (Ed). Targeted Therapy of Acute Myeloid Leukemia. Current Cancer Research. New York: Springer; 2015.
12. Zhang X, Sun J, Yu W, Jin J. Current views on the genetic landscape and management of variant acute promyelocytic leukemia. Biomark Res. 2021;9:33.
13. de Braekeleer E, Douet-Guilbert N, de Braekeleer. RARA fusion genes in acute promyelocytic leukemia: a review. Expert Rev. Hematol. 2014;7:347-57.
14. Zhao J, Liang JW, Xue HL, Shen SH, Chen J, Tang YJ, et al. The genetics and clinical characteristics of children morphologically diagnosed as acute promyelocytic leukemia. Leukemia 2019;33:1387-99.
15. Kuchenbauer F, Schoch C, Kern W, Hiddemann W, Haferlach T, Schnittger S. Impact of FLT3 mutations and promyelocytic leukemia-breakpoint on clinical characteristics and prognosis in acute promyelocytic leukemia. Br J Haematol. 2005;130:196-202.
16. Kutny MA, Moser BK, Laumann K, Feusner JH, Gamis A, Gregory J, et al. FLT3 mutation status is a predictor of early death in pediatric acute promyelocytic leukemia: a report from the Children's Oncology Group. Pediatr Blood Cancer. 2012;59:662-7.
17. Huynh TT, Sultan M, Vidovic D, Dean CA, Cruickshank BM, Lee K, et al. Retinoic acid and arsenic trioxide induce lasting differentiation and demethylation of target genes in APML cells. Sci Rep. 2019;9:9414.
18. de Botton S, Coiteux V, Chevret S, Rayon C, Vilmer E, Sanz M, et al. Outcome of childhood acute promyelocytic leukemia with all-trans retinoic acid and chemotherapy. J Clin Oncol. 2004;22(8):1404-12.

19. Powell BL, Moser B, Stock W, Gallagher RE, Willman CL, Stone RS, et al. Preliminary Results from the North American Acute Promyelocytic Leukemia (APL) Study C9710. Blood. 2006;108 (11):566.
20. Kutny MA, Alonzo TA, Gerbing RB, Wang YC, Raimondi SC, Hirsch BA, et al. Arsenic trioxide consolidation allows anthracycline dose reduction for pediatric patients with acute promyelocytic leukemia: report from the Children's Oncology Group Phase III Historically Controlled Trial AAML0631. J Clin Oncol. 2017;35(26):3021-9.
21. Sanz MA, Fenaux P, Tallman MS, Estey EH, Löwenberg B, Naoe T, et al. Management of acute promyelocytic leukemia: updated recommendations from an expert panel of the European Leukemia Net. Blood. 2019;133 (15):1630-43.
22. Furuya A, Kawahara M, Kumode M, Ohira Y, Usui A, Nagai S, et al. Central nervous system involvement of acute promyelocytic leukemia, three case reports. Clin Case Rep. 2017;5(5):645-53.
23. Douer D, Zickl LN, Schiffer CA, Appelbaum FR, Feusner JH, Shepherd L, et al. All-trans retinoic acid and late relapses in acute promyelocytic leukemia: very long-term follow-up of the North American Intergroup Study I0129. Leuk Res. 2013;37(7):795-801.
24. Kelaidi C, Chevret S, De Botton S, Raffoux E, Guerci A, Thomas X, et al. Improved outcome of acute promyelocytic leukemia with high WBC counts over the last 15 years: the European APL Group experience. J Clin Oncol. 2009;27(16):2668-76.
25. Avvisati G, Petti M, Lo Coco F, Testi A, Fazi P. AIDA: the Italian way of treating acute promyelocytic leukemia. Blood. 2003;102(11):142a.
26. Asou N, Kishimoto Y, Kiyoi H, Okada M, Kawai Y, Tsuzuki M, et al. A randomized study with or without intensified maintenance chemotherapy in patients with acute promyelocytic leukemia who have become negative for PML-RARA transcript after consolidation therapy: the Japan Adult Leukemia Study Group (JALSG) APL97 study. Blood. 2007;110(1):59-66.
27. Muchtar E, Vidal L, Ram R, Gafter-Gvili A, Shpilberg O, Raanani P. The role of maintenance therapy in acute promyelocytic leukemia in the first complete remission. Cochrane Database Syst Rev. 2013;(3):CD009594.
28. Kutny MA, Alonzo TA, Abla O, Rajpurkar M, Gerbing RB, Wang YC, et al. Assessment of Arsenic Trioxide and All-trans Retinoic Acid for the Treatment of Pediatric Acute Promyelocytic Leukemia: A Report From the Children's Oncology Group AAML1331 Trial. JAMA Oncol. 2022;8(1):79-87.
29. Vega-Ruiz A, Faderl S, Estrov Z, Pierce S, Cortes J, Kantarjian H, et al. Incidence of extramedullary disease in patients with acute promyelocytic leukemia: a single-institution experience. Int J Hematol. 2009;89(4):489-96.
30. Tomita A, Kiyoi H, Naoe T. Mechanisms of action and resistance to all-trans retinoic acid (ATRA) and arsenic trioxide (As_2O_3) in acute promyelocytic leukemia. Int J Hematol. 2013;97:717-25.

EXPERT OPINION

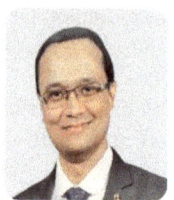

Nirmalya Roy Moulik MD PhD MRCPCH
Associate Professor, Pediatric Oncology
Tata Memorial Hospital, Dr. E Borges Road,
Parel, Mumbai 400012

1. Should we start ATRA alone, chemotherapy alone, or ATRA and chemotherapy for a patient with APML in an emergency?

It depends on the institutional policy, generally, people prefer starting unstable patients on a single differentiating agent rather than two to minimize the chances and complications arising out of DS due to the use of two agents simultaneously. Our institutional protocol mandates starting of ATO whenever a child with suspected APML comes in. I would not prefer starting only chemotherapy as the use of differentiating agents has significantly reduced the initial morbidity and mortality in APML. In current practice, chemotherapy in the form of anthracyclines is an add-on agent in patients with high-risk APML with high baseline white cell counts.

2. Do you prefer ATRA or ATO in APML? What is your take on the anthracyclines-free regimen?

In current protocols, ATO and ATRA are used together in view of their synergistic action on the abnormal proliferation of the APML clones by inducing differentiation and apoptosis; hence, once cannot be used in preference to the other. Though initially found useful in adult studies, chemotherapy (anthracycline)-free regimens are now proven to be safe and efficacious in non-HR APML and are the current standard of care in most of the pediatric protocols used worldwide. However, in HR, APML anthracyclines are still used for initial control of leukocytosis and reduction in chances of relapse.

3. Is there any role in doing PML-RARA break apart in all patients?

Though in our institution, we use RARA break-apart probe in all suspected APML samples undergoing FISH, it is of clear benefit only in samples which are FISH negative but have morphological features of APML as well as strong clinical suspicion. FISH with break-apart RARA probe on metaphase cells was found to be a very efficient strategy to detect unknown RARA variant translocations and can facilitate diagnosis in a minor proportion of cases harboring atypical/cryptic translocations. Therefore, I would not recommend RARA break apart in all cases of APML.

4. Do you recommend CNS prophylaxis in APML? What do you follow at your center? Describe management strategy in APML with CNS involvement at your center.

The indication for CNS prophylaxis is unclear in APML. In the initial period, due to the presence of an active coagulopathy, the risks clearly outweigh the benefits. Following adult guidelines, many pediatric APML protocols are now free of any CNS prophylaxis, CNS disease being exceedingly rare in APML. However, our institutional protocol has five doses of triple intrathecal starting postinduction. APML with CNS involvement is a rare occurrence and can be managed with intrathecal chemotherapy only without any clear advantage of using cranial radiation. Similarly, our institutional policy is to treat APMLs with CSF blasts with weekly TITs till clearance or five intrathecal in total whichever is more. Other patients with CNS involvement in view of CNS bleed, etc., are managed with the five-scheduled triple intrathecal.

5. What are the optimal time points for MRD/qPCR PML-RARA monitoring in APML?

Molecular MRD monitoring is an important prognosticating tool for APML, and the most important time-point is post first cycle of consolidation. Many protocols also advocate mMRD at the end of induction, but the cost-benefit ratio is not favorable in a resource-constrained setting. We repeat mMRD in bone marrow after every cycle of chemotherapy until negative and once again at the end of treatment, following which we prefer peripheral blood mMRD monitoring for 3 years.

6. What is the evidence for and against maintenance therapy in APML? What do you follow at your center?

Maintenance therapy has been shown to be of no added benefit in many randomized studies in adult APML as well as some single-arm pediatric studies. Maintenance therapy is therefore unnecessary in the current era, especially when patients are being treated with ATO/ATRA combination. Our institutional protocol had maintenance until recently. However, maintenance therapy has been removed from the currently updated protocol.

CHAPTER 6

Chronic Myeloid Leukemia

Prashant Prabhakar, Jagdish P Meena

CASE VIGNETTE

A 4-year-old male child presented with complaints of:
- Progressive abdominal distension for the past 2 months
- Abdominal pain localized to left side of abdomen for 1 month
- Low-grade fever on and off for 1 month.

There was no history of rash, bone pain, or transfusion of blood products.

On general examination, there was the presence of pallor. There were no petechiae and no lymphadenopathy. On systemic examination, there was massive splenohepatomegaly (liver 7 cm, spleen 9 cm below costal margin).

Lab investigations: Hemoglobin (Hb) 7.1 g/dL, total lymphocyte count (TLC) 2.5 lakhs/mm^3, and platelets 2 lakhs/mm^3.

Peripheral smear: Blasts 3%, basophils 12% with 5% promyelocytes and metamyelocytes.

So, a clinical possibility of chronic myeloid leukemia (CML) was considered.

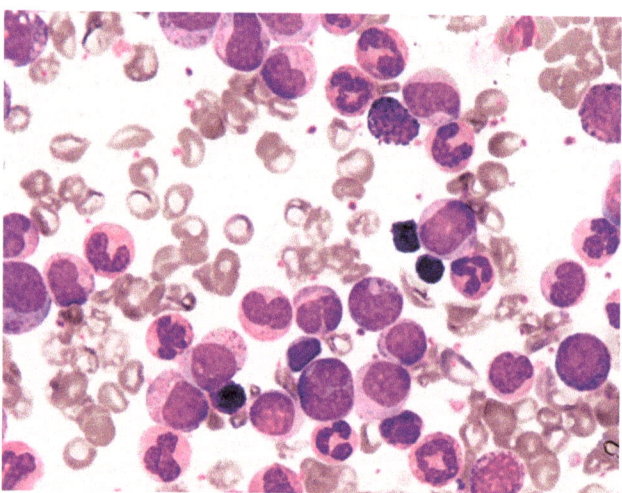

Fig. 1: Peripheral blood smear of patient showing marked leukocytosis with a spectrum of maturing granulocytic elements—increased promyelocytes, metamyelocytes and basophilia; features suggestive of Chronic Myeloid Leukemia—Chronic Phase.
Courtesy: Dr Smeeta Gajendra, Department of Laboratory Oncology, BRA-IRCH, AIIMS, New Delhi.

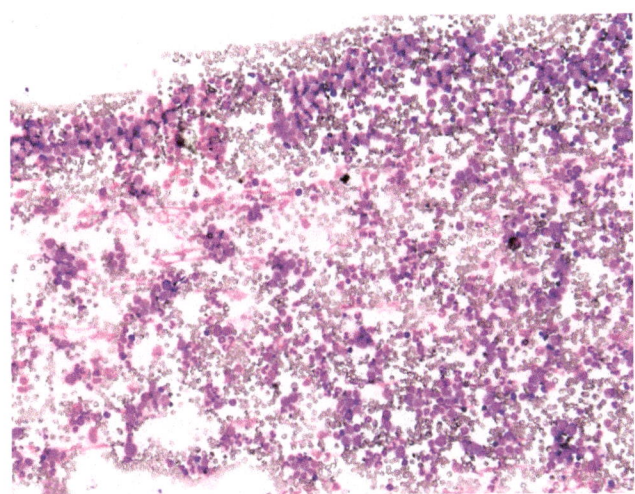

Fig. 2: Bone marrow trephine biopsy—markedly hypercellular with an increased myeloid/erythroid ratio and numerous band and segmented granulocytes.
Courtesy: Dr Smeeta Gajendra, Department of Laboratory Oncology, BRA-IRCH, AIIMS, New Delhi.

1. What is CML? What is the incidence of CML in children?

Chronic myeloid leukemia (CML) is a type of myeloproliferative neoplasm which is characterized by uncontrolled proliferation of granulocytes with preserved maturation. It accounts for 2–3% of leukemias in children <15 years, 9% of leukemias in adolescents between 15 and 19 years, and is extremely rare in infancy.[1]

2. How is pediatric CML different from adult CML?

Chronic myeloid leukemia in pediatric and adolescents is not only about the age distribution. It is biologically and clinically different from adults.

Clinically, as per the CML IV study, the adolescent and young adult (AYA) has a more aggressive disease with high total leucocyte counts, huge splenomegaly in proportion to their body surface area, and a high incidence of advanced phases of the disease. The median white blood cell (WBC) count is around 2.5 lakh, while it ranges from 80,000 to 1.5 lakh in adults.[2]

Biologically, adult CML has a single breakpoint cluster within the first centromeric 1.5 kb of BCR. At the same time, in the pediatric age group, there is a bimodal breakpoint cluster which is similar to Ph+ acute lymphoblastic leukemia (ALL) in adults.

The other features unique to the pediatric population are the long-term side effects, resistance, and compliance issues of tyrosine kinase inhibitor (TKI).[3]

3. What is the clinical presentation of CML?

The common clinical presentation is malaise, fatigue, on and off fever, generalized weakness, and dragging pain abdomen, mainly in the left hypochondrium (due to splenomegaly).[1] Rarely, there can be symptoms of hyperleukocytosis like—headache, dizziness, blurring of vision, and priapism. The symptoms of CML-accelerated phase (AP) are also similar except for additional features of lymphadenopathy, rapid worsening of systemic symptoms, and splenomegaly. Patients with BC present with clinical features of acute leukemia. Splenomegaly is an important clinical finding in CML, and it is present in 70–90% of cases.[4]

4. What are the differential diagnoses to be considered in a case of CML?

The symptoms of CML are nonspecific, although the findings of splenomegaly, and high TLC count in a well-preserved child raise a high suspicion of CML. The close mimickers of CML that must be kept in mind are:[5]

- *Leukemoid reaction:* Most important differential of those presenting with TLC counts of around 50,000. It can occur in various conditions like infections, especially *Staphylococcus aureus* and *Streptococcus pneumonia*, inflammatory conditions, and steroid intake. The findings of shift-to-left, toxic granules, Dohle's body in leukocytes, and absence of basophilia in the peripheral smear with a high LAP (leukocyte alkaline phosphatase) score help to differentiate it from CML. Splenomegaly is also an uncommon feature.
- *Juvenile myelomonocytic leukemia (JMML):* The common clinical findings are splenomegaly, fever, rashes, and lung involvement. The features that separate it from CML are younger age of onset (median 2 years), thrombocytopenia, and absence of Ph translocation (BCR-ABL).
- *Ph+ ALL:* It is a close differential for the CML blast crisis (BC). It is very difficult to distinguish the two, especially if CML presents as a de-novo BC and there is no history to suggest chronic myeloproliferation. The peripheral smear finding of myelocyte bulge (more myelocyte than metamyelocyte), basophilia, and eosinophilia with marked splenomegaly point more toward CML. The type and pattern of the Ph chromosome also give a clue; in CML, it is seen in lymphoblast and neutrophils but presents only in lymphoblasts in the case of Ph+ ALL.

5. The TLC of our index case is 250,000/cumm. Does the child require leukapheresis? What are the indications of leukapheresis in CML?

Indications of leukapheresis in CML are based on symptoms rather than counts as in cases of acute leukemia. In fact, most of the patients presenting with very high TLC don't require leukapheresis. This is because the majority of the circulating cells in CML are maturing WBCs (contrary to the immature cells seen in acute leukemias), which has a very low risk of thrombosis and leukostasis. In most of the cases, starting early hydroxyurea (@ 25–100 mg/kg/day orally in three-four divided doses, maximum dose 6 g) leads to the reduction in TLC and reduce the risk of leukostasis without requiring leukapheresis. Leukapheresis is only to be considered in special scenarios where there are signs and symptoms of leukostasis and end-organ damage like respiratory distress with pulmonary infiltrates, central nervous system (CNS) symptoms suggestive of ischemic or hemorrhagic stroke, severe retinopathy/papilledema, and priapism.[6,7]

The index case had no signs and symptoms suggestive of hyperleukocytosis, so he was started on hydroxyurea and allopurinol with an advise of liberal fluid intake and samples were sent for further work up.

6. What is the baseline diagnostic evaluation required in this case?

The baseline work-up for establishing the diagnosis in the pediatric age group is the same as in adults, and it includes:
- Complete blood counts (CBC) with differential counts show high TLC counts with basophilia in almost all cases and eosinophilia in 90% of cases. Platelets are normal or high, and in <5% cases, it can be low, and then a BC should be suspected.
- Viral markers—human immunodeficiency virus (HIV), hepatitis B surface antigen (HbsAg), and hepatitis C virus (HCV)
- Metabolic profile—liver function test (LFT), kidney function test (KFT), and lipid profile
- Thyroid function test
- Spleen and liver size—measured and documented as below costal margin
- Bone marrow aspiration—morphology including the percentage of blasts, promyelocytes, and basophils
- Peripheral blood or bone marrow—for qualitative and quantitative reverse transcription polymerase chain reaction (RT-PCR) using an international scale (IS) for BCR-ABL1. At our institute, we do qualitative at baseline followed by quantitative for the remainder of the treatment part.
- Karyotype for additional chromosomal abnormalities (ACA) in Ph + cells which are known as clonal cytogenetic evolution. Fluorescence in situ hybridization (FISH) is not an adequate substitute for karyotyping because it will not detect additional chromosomal abnormality (ACA).
- *Fluorescence in situ hybridization:* It should be performed when Ph is not detected by karyotype.
- Bone marrow biopsy—to look for fibrosis which has prognostic significance, focal areas of blasts.

CASE (Continued)

The child underwent a bone marrow aspiration, and all the baseline investigations from bone marrow aspiration (BMA) and peripheral blood were sent. BMA showed hematopoietic cells of all series with a myeloid: erythroid ratio of 8:1, 8% basophils, promyelocytes, and myelocytes with 7% blasts. The molecular study for qualitative RT PCR for BCR-ABL1 fusion transcript was positive—e13/14a2 (p210 type).

7. According to the definition, this child falls in which phase of CML?

This child was diagnosed as a case of CML-chronic phase (CP) as per World Health Organization (WHO) and European LeukemiaNet (ELN) criteria. The latest definition as per WHO and ELN has been charted further; it also shows the differences between the two:
- *Accelerated phase* (**Table 1**):

TABLE 1: Accelerated phase.

WHO criteria (presence of 1 or more criteria)	ELN criteria (presence of 1 or more criteria)
Blasts in peripheral blood or bone marrow 10–19%	Blasts in peripheral blood or bone marrow 15–29% Blasts plus promyelocytes in blood/bone marrow >30%, but the blasts should be <30%
Basophils ≥20% in blood	Basophils ≥20% in blood
Persistent thrombocytopenia (<1 lakh/dL), which is unrelated to therapy	Persistent thrombocytopenia (<1 lakh/dL) which is unrelated to therapy
Thrombocytosis (>10 lakh/dL) which is unrelated to therapy	Not included
Increasing TLC count and increase in spleen size unresponsive to therapy	Not included
The appearance of a new or additional clonal genetic abnormalities by cytogenetics that were originally not present at the time of diagnosis (second Ph clone, trisomy 8 or 19, isochromosome 17q) is also known as clonal evolution	Not included

(ELN: European LeukemiaNet; TLC: total lymphocyte count; WHO: World Health Organization)

- *Blast crisis* **(Table 2)**:

TABLE 2: Blast crisis.

WHO criteria (presence of 1 or more criteria)	ELN criteria (presence of 1 or more criteria)
Peripheral blood or BM blasts ≥20% of nucleated BM cells	Peripheral blood or BM blasts ≥ 30% of nucleated BM cells
Blast proliferation at extra medullary sites, except spleen	Blast proliferation at extra medullary sites, except the spleen
Bone marrow biopsy: Large, clusters/foci of blasts (even if rest of the marrow shows chronic phase)	Not included

(BM: bone marrow; TLC: total lymphocyte count; WHO: World Health Organization)

- *Chronic phase* **(Table 3)**:

TABLE 3: Chronic phase.

WHO criteria (presence of all of the following criteria)	ELN criteria (presence of all of the following criteria)
<10% blasts in peripheral blood and BM	<15% blasts in peripheral blood and BM
Does not meet any criteria for AP or BC	Does not meet any criteria for AP or BC

(AP: accelerated phase; BC: blast crisis; BM: bone marrow; TLC: total lymphocyte count; WHO: World Health Organization)

Children's Oncology Group (COG) working group has recently recommended using WHO criteria for definition.[6]

WHO 2022 Classification of Hematolymphoid tumors, however has removed accelerated phase from the recent classification. The idea is to put emphasis on high risk features associated with resistance to TKI and progression of chronic phase.

The criteria for BC also has been slightly changed:
i. ≥ 20% myeloid blasts
ii. Any increase in lymphoblast in PB/BM (cut-off not defined).

8. Now that we have the diagnosis of CML-CP, What is the first line TKI that should be started in this child?

The first TKI approved for pediatric use was imatinib in 2003, followed by second generation (2G) TKIs—dasatinib and nilotinib which were approved in 2017 and 2018, respectively as first- and second-line therapy for pediatric CML.[1] Nilotinib is approved only for children >1 year of age. Bosutinib has recently been tried in the pediatric age group showing a similar response as compared to other TKI. While the availability of multiple drugs gives different treatment options, especially in the case of a suboptimal response, it also makes the task of choosing the best first-line drug difficult. The various factors that we must keep in mind while starting a child on TKI are efficacy, toxicity profile, drug availability, ease of administration, financial constraints, and comorbidities. There is more experience in children with the oldest drug—imatinib as far as the efficacy and toxicities are concerned. So, it is the first-line TKI which is used in our unit. There are certain issues with other agents, like the cost of 2G, TKIs are significantly higher as compared with imatinib. In the case of drugs like nilotinib, food delays the absorption, and so concomitant administration with meals should be avoided, which is practically not always feasible in children. Moreover, it has to be taken twice a day, thus requiring good compliance.

CASE *(Continued)*

After counseling the family regarding the nature and details about the disease, the child was started on imatinib and was advised regular follow-up for monitoring the response to treatment and the toxicity associated with imatinib. What are the routine investigations recommended in a case of CML and what should be the frequency of monitoring the same?

9. What are the routine tests required and the frequency with which it has to be done for monitoring the treatment response and toxicity?

- Kidney function tests, LFT, calcium and phosphate, Lipase, glucose, uric acid, lipid profile, glycated hemoglobin (HbA1c), and thyroid function test—3 monthly
- Vitamin D and parathyroid hormone (PTH)—Yearly
- Spleen size to be noted below costal margin—every visit
- Height, weight, and body mass index (BMI)—3 monthly
- Echo and electrocardiogram (ECG) for QT interval—annually
- Dual-energy X-ray absorptiometry (DEXA) scan—5 yearly

- *Monitoring for disease response:*
  - Peripheral blood qRT-PCR for BCR-ABL1 transcript ration IS—monthly for initial 3 months followed by every 3 monthly thereafter
  - Bone marrow aspirate for differential and karyotype—every 3 months (some recommend 6 monthly) till complete cytogenetic response and then only if there is loss of response.
  - Complete blood counts with differential counts—weekly for first 4 weeks, followed by every 2 weeks till 3 months followed by 3 monthly.

10. What are the different prognostic scores in CML and what will be the most applicable prognostic score in this child? Is the use of prognostic score recommended in pediatric age group for deciding the first line therapy?

The three baseline prognostic scores that are used in CML are Sokal, Euro, and EUTOS. These scores have been devised based on baseline clinical (age, spleen size) and hematological parameters (platelet count and peripheral blast percentage) at diagnosis. These risk scores were designed to evaluate the difference in survival and response rate based on baseline features. Sokal and EUTOS scores were developed during pre-imatinib era, in patients (children and adults both) who received hydroxyurea, busulfan, and interferon, respectively. A Sokal score for patients <45 years was established which is still useful in TKI era. Subsequently, the EUTOS score was devised for adult patients treated with imatinib. The use of TKI resulted in improved life expectancy of CML patients which was comparable to that of the general population.

The comorbidities, rather than the disease per se, are the most common cause of death in CML patients in TKI era. Therefore, a new scoring system has been devised—ELTS (EUTOS Long Term Survival Score), which predicts the probability of leukemia-related death (LRD). A recent study in adults has shown that ELTS score better predicted the probability of dying from CML than previous prognostic scores. The I-CML-Ped Study tested the ELTS score in 350 children and adolescents diagnosed with CML CP and treated with imatinib. The children were allocated to low ($n = 199$), intermediate ($n = 68$), and high ($n = 42$) risk groups as per ELTS score. The 5-year progression-free survival (PFS) rates were 96% for low risk, 88% for intermediate risk, and 67% for high risk. These differences in PFS were significantly different according to risk groups. Therefore, ELTS score is considered best for baseline risk stratification in children and adolescents with CML compared to the other three scores.[8] COG recommends not to use Sokal, EUTOS scores for risk assessment or taking decisions regarding treatment of pediatric CML. As far as ELTS score is concerned, more data is required to confirm its use for prognostication in adolescents and children with CML.[6] The current recommendation is against using any prognostic score for deciding the first line therapy in pediatric and adolescents due to scarcity of data, which we follow in our unit.

CASE *(Continued)*

At 3 months of starting imatinib, there was no hepatosplenomegaly. CBC–Hb—10.1, TLC—9,450/mm^3, differential leukocyte count (DLC)–N—55%, L—40%, basophils—1%, peripheral smear—no abnormal like promyelocytes, myelocytes, and platelets—2.25 lakhs/mm^3. Peripheral blood—qBCR-ABL1 IS ratio was 1.77%.

11. Is the molecular response adequate as per treatment milestones for the child? What are the different criteria for monitoring treatment response?

The use of targeted therapy and gradual understanding of using minimal residual disease (MRD) for prognostication have shifted the treatment of CML, from the era of hematopoietic stem cell transplantation (HSCT) to all the patients to individualized treatment based on molecular response. There are no pediatric-specific criteria for response milestones, and we use adult guidelines for the same. The two major groups—National Comprehensive Cancer Network (NCCN) and ELN have slight differences in their cut off for response milestones.

The various cut offs for hematological, cytogenetic, and molecular response are given in **Table 4**.

TABLE 4: Various cut offs for hematological, cytogenetic, and molecular response.

Response/relapse	Definition
Complete hematologic response (CHR)	• Complete normalization of peripheral blood counts with leukocyte count <10 × 10^9/L • Platelet count <450 × 10^9/L • No immature cells, such as myelocytes, promyelocytes, or blasts in peripheral blood • No signs and symptoms of disease with resolution of palpable splenomegaly
Cytogenetic response	• Complete cytogenetic response (CCyR): No Ph-positive metaphases • Partial cytogenetic response (PCyR): 1–35% Ph-positive metaphases • Major cytogenetic response (MCyR): 0–35% Ph-positive metaphases (includes complete + partial response) • Minor cytogenetic response: >35–65% Ph-positive metaphases
Molecular response	• Early molecular response (EMR): BCR-ABL1 (IS) ≤10% at 3 and 6 months • Major molecular response (MMR): BCR-ABL1 (IS) ≤0.1% or ≥3-log reduction in BCR-ABL1 transcripts from the standardized baseline, if qPCR (IS) is not available • Deep molecular response (DMR): MR4.0: BCR-ABL1 (IS) ≤0.01% or MR4.5: BCR-ABL1 (IS) ≤0.0032% • Complete molecular response—no detectable BCR-ABL1
Relapse	• Any sign of loss of hematologic response • Any sign of loss of CCyR or its molecular response correlate defined as an increase in BCR-ABL1 transcript to >1% • 1-log increase in BCR-ABL1 transcript levels with loss of MMR

Therefore, this patient is currently in complete hematological response and has also achieved early molecular response.

12. How is the response of imatinib in this case as per "response milestones criteria" by ELN and NCCN? What is the next step to be done in this child?

As there are no pediatric guidelines available for response milestone assessment, so we use modified response assessment criteria which is recommended by various studies. There is some difference in the cut off values of BCR-ABL1 for defining response according to ELN and NCCN guidelines.

The chart below shows response milestones for CML patients on TKI as per NCCN and ELN guidelines **(Tables 5 and 6)**.

TABLE 5: NCCN criteria for response milestones.

Early treatment response milestones			
BCR-ABL 1 (IS)	3 months	6 months	12 months
>10%	YELLOW		RED
>1–10%	GREEN		YELLOW
>0.1–1%	GREEN		LIGHT GREEN
≤0.1%	GREEN		

Color	Concern	Clinical considerations	Recommendations
RED	TKI-resistant disease	• Evaluate patient compliance and drug interactions • Consider mutational analysis	Switch to alternate TKI and evaluate for allogeneic HCT
YELLOW	Possible TKI resistance	• Evaluate patient compliance and drug interactions • Consider mutational analysis • Consider bone marrow cytogenetic analysis to assess for MCyR at 3 months or CCyR at 12 months	Switch to alternate TKI or continue same TKI (other than imatinib) or increase imatinib dose to a max of 800 mg and consider evaluation for allogeneic HCT
LIGHT GREEN	TKI-sensitive disease	• If treatment goal is long-term survival: ≤1% optimal • If treatment goal is treatment-free remission survival: ≤0.1% optimal	• If optimal: Continue same TKI • If not optimal: Shared decision-making with patient
GREEN	TKI-sensitive disease	Monitor response and side effects	Continue same TKI

(CML: chronic myeloid leukemia; CCyR: complete cytogenetic response; HCT: hematopoietic cell transplant; MCyR: major cytogenetic response; TKI: tyrosine kinase inhibitor)

TABLE 6: ELN 2020 criteria.

	Optimal	Warning	Failure
Baseline	NA	High-risk ACA, high-risk ELTS score	NA
3 months	BCR-ABL1 ≤10% IS	>10%	>10% if confirmed within 1-3 months
6 months	BCR-ABL1 ≤1% IS	>1–10%	>10%
12 months	BCR-ABL1 ≤ 0.1% IS	>0.1–1%	>1%
Any time	BCR-ABL1 ≤0.1% IS	>0.1–1%, loss of ≤0.1% (MMR)[a]	>1%, resistance mutations, high-risk ACA

(ACA: additional chromosome abnormalities in Ph+ cells; ELTS EUTOS: long-term survival score; NA: not applicable)
For patients aiming at treatment-free remission (TFR), the optimal response (at any time) is BCR-ABL1 ≤ 0.01%.
-A change of treatment may be considered if MMR is not reached by 36–48 months.
[a]Loss of MMR (BCR-ABL1 >0.1%) indicates failure after TFR.

Our index case has optimal response as per both the guidelines and therefore there is no need to change treatment or do any additional investigations except for doing routine investigations as mentioned above. Monitor quantitative BCR-ABL IS transcript ratio every 3 monthly.

CASE (Continued)

The patient was under regular follow-up and was doing well. After around 9 months from diagnosis, in a regular visit, qBCR-ABL1 was 0.66%. Clinically, there was no hepatosplenomegaly and routine CBC showed Hb 9.8 g/dL, TLC 8,000, DLC—basophils was 1%, and platelets 2.5 lakhs. There was no history suggestive of infection and compliance was good.

13. **There is a slight difference in the response milestone criteria between NCCN and ELN as highlighted in previous question, while suboptimal response cut off for BCR-ABL1 at 9 months is >0.1% as per ELN, it is >1% as per NCCN. So, this child is under green zone as per NCCN and in warning zone as per ELN criteria. So, can we individualize further steps based on other factors?**

Our index case has no other features of disease progression so we can follow the child as per NCCN guideline and therefore no further work-up is required and child was continued on same dose.

CASE (Continued)

The patient was under regular follow-up and was doing well. After around 18 months from diagnosis, there was an increase in spleen size (5 cm) which was detected on examination and routine CBC showed Hb 9.8 g/dL, TLC 31,930, and DLC—basophils was 5%, blasts 2%, and qBCR-ABL1 was 32%. There was no history suggestive of infection and compliance was good.

14. **How to monitor compliance to TKI therapy?**

Noncompliance is the main cause of loss of initial good response especially in adolescents and young adults especially during the first year of therapy and even afterwards. Counseling and emphasizing on the importance of taking TKIs should be discussed with parents and the patients in detail. They should be asked about their compliance to medication in each visit and various steps should be taken to ensure the same. Patients should be instructed to take the medicine at a specific time each day like after dinner, maintain a diary or set reminders on smart phone every day to take medicines. Therapeutic drug monitoring of TKI is not recommended.

15. **What is the possible etiology of increased spleen and worsening CBC parameters? What are the next steps to be taken in this case? What is the characteristic of advanced stage of CML?**

The index case has progressed to AP as per definition by WHO, there is splenomegaly and rising TLC not responding to therapy although this criterion is not included in defining AP as per NCCN guideline.

Patients in advanced stage of CML (AP and BC) can present in two ways:
1. Patients in de-novo BC/AP
2. Patients who progress from CP to advanced phase during treatment.

A total of 3.5% of pediatric CML patients present with BC, while 4% present in AP.[9] This proportion is similar to adult patients.[10] In the I-CML-Ped Study,[9] majority of de-novo BC was of lymphoid type (76%), though the possibility of some being Ph+ ALL could not be excluded. 35% of these children also had extramedullary disease. The 5-year OS was 94% in patients presenting with AP and 74% for patients presenting with de-novo BC.

The cumulative incidence of progression to AP or BC was 3% at 1 year and 7% at 3 years. The most common blast phase was of lymphoid type (70%) which is in contrast to adults who have myeloid blast phase (70–80%) as the predominant BC. The median age at diagnosis of AP/BC was 13.2 years. There was some difference in baseline clinical profile of those patients who progressed to advanced phase (AP/BC) compared to those who remained in CP. These patients had more aggressive clinical features like massive splenomegaly, high TLC, and lower platelets counts. Almost 60% of the patients had received hydroxyurea before starting TKI. The early cytogenetic and molecular responses are considered to the best predictor of favorable outcome.[11] The same was reflected in this study. The OS was poor with 5-year OS < 50%. At the time of AP/BC, 90% of the patients had acquired ACA and 50% had acquired tyrosine kinase domain (TKD) mutations.[12]

A study comparing the clinical and genomic profile of patients with de-novo and secondary BC has shown different characteristics among both the groups, although the proportion of patients in both groups was same.[13] The children with de-novo BC presented at a younger age (median age 5.5 years) as compared to secondary BC (median age 16 years). There was a marked difference in the cytogenetic profile between the two groups. Complex karyotype was more prevalent in secondary blast phase (88 vs. 20%). The most common chromosomal anomaly was monosomy 7. Most of the patients with acquired BC had only BCR-ABL1 translocation at baseline. This reflects that these patients have acquired clonal evolutions leading to the crisis. The percentage of TKD mutation was almost same in both the groups. The striking difference of this study with that of Meyran et al.[12] was, that the OS of patients with secondary BC was similar to that of de-novo BC. This can be attributed to early transplant (within 4 months) done in this study.[13]

16. What is the next step in managing this child—changing or adjusting TKI or continuing similar chemotherapy? What are the indications of changing TKIs?

The common indications of changing TKIs are **Flowchart 1**.[6]
- Intolerance due to toxicity
- Tyrosine kinase domain mutation that leads to resistance of a particular TKI.
- Failure to achieve treatment milestones as per guidelines stated above.

Flowchart 1: When to switch-tyrosine kinase inhibitor (TKI).

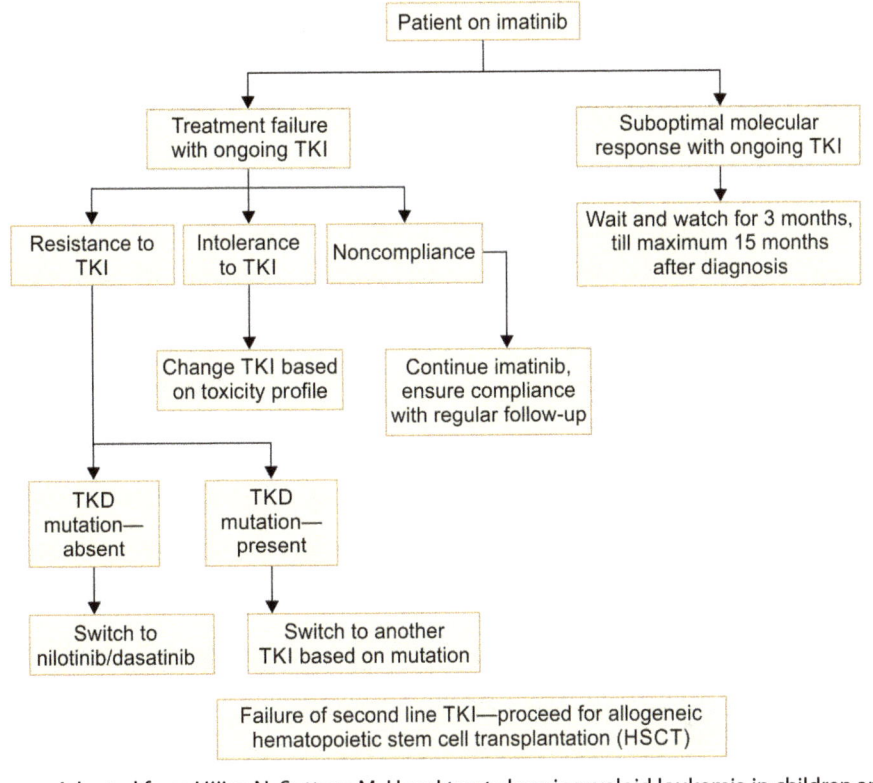

Source: Adapted from Hijiya N, Suttorp M. How I treat chronic myeloid leukemia in children and adolescents. Blood. 2019;133(22):2374-84.

17. What are the investigations to be sent in this case? How do you treat advanced phase (AP/BC) of CML?

The median time of transformation from AP to BC is 6–18 months. The rate of transformation to blast phase per year has decreased from 20 to 35% in pre-TKI era to 1–1.5% in TKI era. There are two types of AP—de-novo and transformed. The treatment for both the groups is different. De-novo APs are those patients who present at baseline with AP and are treatment naive. While the transformed AP refers to the patients who progressed from CP to AP, the prognosis of transformed AP is less favorable than de-novo AP.

Treatment of de-novo advanced phase CML (AP/BC) **(Flowchart 2):**
- Send TKD mutation
- Start treatment with 2G TKI as it attains a deeper and faster molecular response with comparable toxicity with imatinib. However, imatinib may also be considered as first line as the frequency of TKD mutation in de novo advance disease is very less compared to transformed AP as shown in a study.

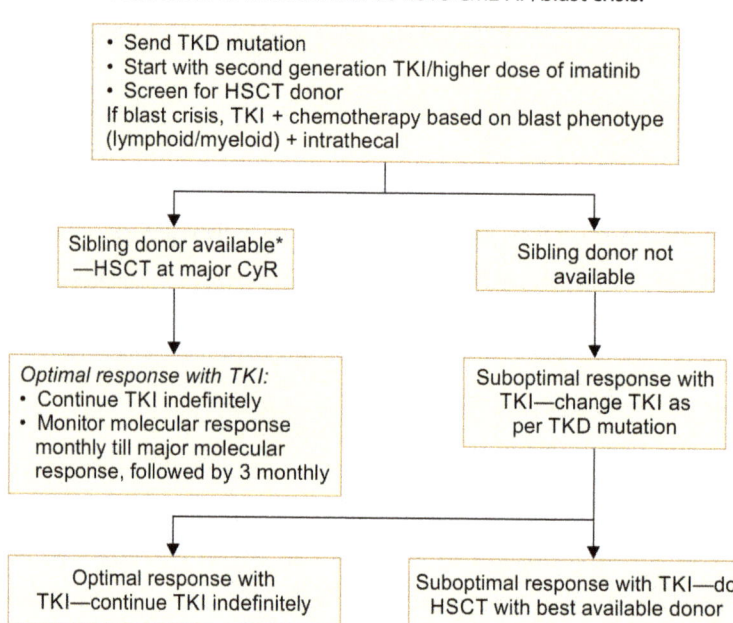

Flowchart 2: Treatment of de novo CML-AP/blast crisis.

*If there is optimal response to TKI—patient can be continued on the same and HSCT may be deferred with close monitoring,
(CyR: cytogenetic response; HSCT: hematopoietic stem cell transplantation; TKD: tyrosine kinase domain; TKI: tyrosine kinase inhibitor)

- *Role of HSCT:* The current recommendation as per COG and BFM group is to do HSCT once MMR has been achieved, if a matched sibling donor (MSD) is available. There is no prospective head-to-head trial comparing long-term TKI with HSCT in these patients. Recently data from the International Registry for CML in children and adolescents has been published, which included 20 patients with de novo AP, with only six patients undergoing HSCT and still achieving an excellent 5-year OS of 94%. As a starting therapy, 17 patients received only TKI and three patients received TKI and chemotherapy.[9] This data although very small but has shown the possibility of using only TKI for de novo AP. The toxicity and transplant-related mortality (TRM) associated with HSCT outweighs its benefit when compared with the TKIs alone. Moreover, the options of 2G-TKI help in attaining a deeper and rapid MMR with acceptable toxicity.

Therefore, a reasonable approach to treat these patients which we follow in our unit includes—starting on 2G-TKI (imatinib can also be considered) and to continue on TKI only if the treatment milestones are achieved under close follow-up with quantitative RT-PCR.

Treatment of transformed advanced phase (Flowchart 3):
- Noncompliance is one of the most common causes of treatment failure in CML. Therefore, the first step is to check drug compliance, dose and use of any herbal medications which leads to low levels of TKI in blood.

Flowchart 3: Treatment of CML-CP progressing to accelerated phase/blast crisis.

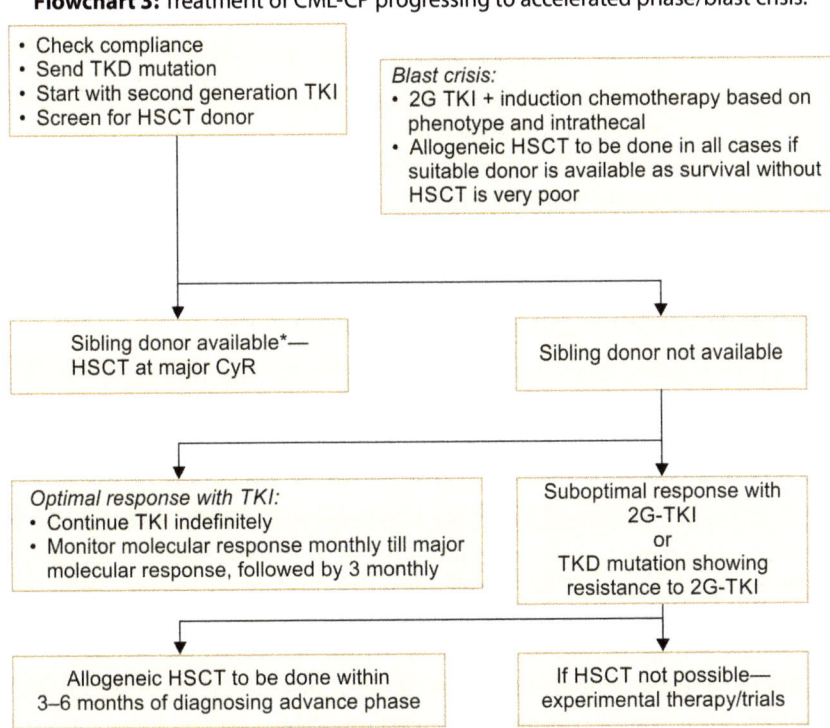

*If there is optimal response to TKI—patient can be continued on the same and HSCT may be deferred with close monitoring till there is evidence of failure to 2G-TKI
(CML: chronic myeloid leukemia; CP: chronic phase; CyR: cytogenetic response; HSCT: hematopoietic stem cell transplantation; TKD: tyrosine kinase domain; TKI: tyrosine kinase inhibitor)

- Send TKD mutations and cytogenetics for ACA as most of the patients have acquired these changes during conversion to advanced phase.[12]
- Switch to 2G-dasatinib. It will be prudent to start 2G-TKI as the patient has high chance of TKD mutation and they achieve a deeper and faster molecular remission.
- Hematopoietic stem cell transplantation work-up and donor search—these patients will require HSCT as the outcome is poor without HSCT at least as per I-CML study.[6] However, the lack of data comparing HSCT versus long-term TKI makes it difficult to recommend one particular treatment. Few studies recommend that if optimal treatment response is achieved on 2G-TKI then HSCT can be postponed till the time there is no failure to second line treatment.

18. What are the indications of doing TKD mutation in CML?

Primary resistance to TKI in patients presenting in CP is very rare, so routine testing for mutations is not indicated. The various indications of doing TKD mutations as per various pediatric CML guidelines are treatment failure or suboptimal response:[6]
- Patients showing suboptimal response (failure to achieve treatment milestones) on starting treatment.

- There is evidence for loss of response that was achieved like—loss of MMR or 1-log increase in BCR-ABL1 transcript ratio.
- Patients in CP progressing to accelerated or blast phase
- Patients presenting with de novo accelerated or blast phase—as per I-BFM group.[7]

So, our case in discussion has progression to AP while on TKI with good compliance to medicine as suggested by history. The TKD mutation was sent and the child was started on 2G-TKI—dasatinib. Furthermore, the family was counseled regarding the need for HSCT and the transplant work-up including HLA matching was sent. The child was called every 4 weekly with q RT-PCR BCR-ABL reports.

19. How to differentiate de-novo CML BC from Ph+ ALL?

A recent study has shown the use of FISH for BCR-ABL rearrangement neutrophils to differentiate de-novo CML BC from Ph+ ALL.[14]

20. Should we have offered fertility preservation to this child? What is the current recommendation regarding fertility preservation in newly diagnosed CML?

Although fertility preservation is not well developed in India but there are recommendations from BFM and COG group to discuss regarding the options of sperm cryopreservation. While there is very low risk of teratogenicity for males on imatinib and recommendation is to continue the drug while planning conception, the data on 2G-TKIs are lacking. The two main reasons for doing sperm cryopreservation in all boys are—firstly, the patients may anytime require switching from imatinib to higher generation TKI and secondly, some experimental data have shown that long term use of imatinib decreases the sperm motility and testicular size.

The ideal timing for sperm preservation is before starting on any therapy. However, if this is not feasible then it should be as soon as the patient is off hydroxyurea for 3 months. The recommendation in female is to do oocyte preservation for all postmenarche females who are undergoing HSCT.[7]

21. What are the doses and adverse effects of TKIs?

Name of TKI	Doses	Side effects
Imatinib	260–340 mg/m^2/dose once daily	Side effects in children are milder than in adults:[15,16] • *Hematological:* Neutropenia (33%) and thrombocytopenia (20%) • *GI:* Nausea (13%), diarrhea, local esophageal irritation (to avoid this, imatinib should be taken in a sitting position, with a glass of water) • Infection (17%) • Growth delay (this effect is more pronounced when imatinib is started in the pre-pubertal phase[17] • Muscle cramps • Bone pain • Fluid retention (3%), weight gain • Skin rash (13%) • Hepatotoxicity (7%)

Contd...

Contd...

Name of TKI	Doses	Side effects
Dasatinib	60 mg/m²/dose once daily	• Similar side effect profile as imatinib • Pleural effusion is common in adults treated with dasatinib (28%); however, it is rarely seen in pediatric patients[18]
Nilotinib	230 mg/m²/dose twice daily	The common adverse effects are:[19] • Liver dysfunction (62.1%)—raised bilirubin, elevated ALT • Headache (46.6%) • Pyrexia (37.9%) • Rash (53.4%) *Others*: • Thrombocytopenia (16%) • QT prolongation (13.8%) (monitor electrolytes, ECG at baseline, after 1 week, and after any dose modification) • Fluid retention (10.3%) • Growth retardation (5.2%)
Ponatinib[20,21]		• *Most common grade 3 toxicity:* Hematological toxicity (29%)—neutropenia, thrombocytopenia • *Nonhematological toxicity:* Rare, e.g., pancreatitis, hepatotoxicity, and PRES • Skin rash • Arterial thrombotic events (ATE)—not seen in children in contrast to adults
Bosutinib[22]		• Grade 3/4 toxicity observed in 43% patients • Most common—GI toxicity (87%), followed by rash (39%) and hepatotoxicity

(ALT: alanine aminotransferase; GI: gastrointestinal; PRES: posterior reversible encephalopathy syndrome; TKI: tyrosine kinase inhibitor)

22. What are the indications of HSCT? What is the preferred donor source and conditioning regime?

The morbidity and TRM associated with HSCT make TKI more advantageous. But, in children and adolescents, as the treatment is started at a growing age, long-term toxicity is an important concern. Therefore, a balance between toxicity and cure has to be achieved while deciding treatment.

The indications of HSCT in pediatric CML are:[6]
 (i) Progression to BC from CP
 (ii) Progression to AP from CP—patients can be managed on TKI alone if they attain optimal treatment milestones
 (iii) Accelerated phase/BC at diagnosis—patients can be managed on TKI +/- chemotherapy if they attain optimal treatment milestones
 (iv) Failure of two or more TKIs
 (v) Intolerable toxicity to TKIs
 (vi) Poor compliance to TKI (controversial)

The overall survival (OS) for those undergoing HSCT with MSD was 91 versus 69% for matched unrelated donor (MUD).[23]

23. Can we consider stopping imatinib if a patient is in complete molecular remission >2 years?

There are various studies in adults supporting the stoppage of TKI once a deep and sustained molecular remission has been maintained for >2 years. Recent NCCN guidelines recommend stopping TKIs in adults (age >18 years) who fulfill the following criteria:

(i) CML-CP on TKI for at least 3 years
(ii) Stable deep molecular response (Q-RT-PCR <0.01% IS) maintained for >2 years.
(iii) No history of TKI resistance
(iv) Accessibility to Q-RT-PCR testing as close monitoring of the BCR-ABL transcript ratio every 3–4 weeks is mandatory after stopping the medication.

However, currently there is not enough evidence in pediatric population to stop TKI even after sustained MMR. Therefore, it is currently not recommended in pediatric CML.[6]

REFERENCES

1. Hijiya N, Suttorp M. How I treat chronic myeloid leukemia in children and adolescents. Blood. 2019;133(22):2374-84.
2. Hehlmann R, Lauseker M, Saußele S, Pfirrmann M, Krause S, Kolb HJ, et al. Assessment of imatinib as first-line treatment of chronic myeloid leukemia: 10-year survival results of the randomized CML study IV and impact of non-CML determinants. Leukemia. 2017;31(11):2398-406.
3. Krumbholz M, Karl M, Tauer JT, Thiede C, Rascher W, Suttorp M, et al. Genomic BCR-ABL1 breakpoints in pediatric chronic myeloid leukemia. Genes Chromosomes Cancer. 2012;51(11):1045-53.
4. Millot F, Suttorp M, Guilhot J, Sedlacek P, de Bont ES, Li CK, et al. The International Registry for Chronic Myeloid Leukemia (CML) in Children and Adolescents (I-CML-Ped-Study): Objectives and preliminary results. Blood. 2012;120(21):3741.
5. Suttorp M, Millot F, Sembill S, Deutsch H, Metzler M. Definition, epidemiology, pathophysiology, and essential criteria for diagnosis of pediatric chronic myeloid leukemia. Cancers (Basel). 2021;13(4):798.
6. Athale U, Hijiya N, Patterson BC, Bergsagel J, Andolina JR, Bittencourt H, et al. Management of chronic myeloid leukemia in children and adolescents: recommendations from the Children's Oncology Group CML Working Group. Pediatr Blood Cancer. 2019;66(9):e27827.
7. de la Fuente J, Baruchel A, Biondi A, de Bont E, Dresse MF, Suttorp M, et al. Managing children with chronic myeloid leukaemia (CML): recommendations for the management of CML in children and young people up to the age of 18 years. Br J Haematol. 2014;167(1):33-47.
8. Millot F, Guilhot J, Suttorp M, Güneş AM, Sedlacek P, de Bont E, et al. Prognostic discrimination based on the EUTOS long-term survival score within the International Registry for Chronic Myeloid Leukemia in children and adolescents. Haematologica. 2017;102(10):1704-8.
9. Millot F, Maledon N, Guilhot J, Güneş AM, Kalwak K, Suttorp M. Favourable outcome of de novo advanced phases of childhood chronic myeloid leukaemia. Eur J Cancer. 2019;115:17-23.
10. Hoffmann VS, Baccarani M, Hasford J, Lindoerfer D, Burgstaller S, Sertic D, et al. The EUTOS population-based registry: incidence and clinical characteristics of 2904 CML patients in 20 European Countries. Leukemia. 2015;29(6):1336-43.
11. Baccarani M, Deininger MW, Rosti G, Hochhaus A, Soverini S, Apperley JF, et al. European LeukemiaNet recommendations for the management of chronic myeloid leukemia: 2013. Blood. 2013;122(6):872-84.

12. Meyran D, Petit A, Guilhot J, Suttorp M, Sedlacek P, de Bont E, et al. Lymphoblastic predominance of blastic phase in children with chronic myeloid leukaemia treated with imatinib: a report from the I-CML-Ped Study. Eur J Cancer. 2020;137:224-34.
13. Sembill S, Göhring G, Schirmer E, Lutterloh F, Suttorp M, Metzler M, et al. Paediatric chronic myeloid leukaemia presenting in de novo or secondary blast phase—a comparison of clinical and genetic characteristics. Br J Haematol. 2021;193(3):613-8.
14. Balducci E, Loosveld M, Rahal I, Boudjarane J, Alazard E, Missirian C, et al. Interphase FISH for BCR-ABL1 rearrangement on neutrophils: a decisive tool to discriminate a lymphoid blast crisis of chronic myeloid leukemia from a de novo BCR-ABL1 positive acute lymphoblastic leukemia. Hematol Oncol. 2018;36(1):344-8.
15. Bond M, Bernstein ML, Pappo A, Schultz KR, Krailo M, Blaney SM, et al. A phase II study of imatinib mesylate in children with refractory or relapsed solid tumors: a Children's Oncology Group study. Pediatr Blood Cancer. 2008;50(2):254-8.
16. Millot F, Guilhot J, Nelken B, Leblanc T, de Bont ES, Békassy AN, et al. Imatinib mesylate is effective in children with chronic myelogenous leukemia in late chronic and advanced phase and in relapse after stem cell transplantation. Leukemia. 2006;20(2):187-92.
17. Bansal D, Shava U, Varma N, Trehan A, Marwaha RK. Imatinib has adverse effect on growth in children with chronic myeloid leukemia. Pediatr Blood Cancer. 2012;59(3):481-4.
18. Gore L, Kearns PR, de Martino ML, Lee, de Souza CA, Bertrand Y, et al. Dasatinib in Pediatric patients with chronic myeloid leukemia in chronic phase: results from a phase II trial. J Clin Oncol. 2018;36(13):1330-8.
19. Hijiya N, Maschan A, Rizzari C, Shimada H, Dufour C, Goto H, et al. A phase 2 study of nilotinib in pediatric patients with CML: long-term update on growth retardation and safety. Blood Advances. 2021;5(14):2925-34.
20. Rossoff J, Huynh V, Rau RE, Macy ME, Sulis ML, Schultz KR, et al. Experience with ponatinib in paediatric patients with leukaemia. Br J Haematol. 2020;189(2):363-8.
21. Millot F, Suttorp M, Versluys AB, Kalwak K, Nelken B, Ducassou S, et al. Ponatinib in childhood Philadelphia chromosome-positive leukaemias: an international registry of childhood chronic myeloid leukaemia study. Eur J Cancer. 2020;136:107-12.
22. Pennesi E, Brivio E, Willemse ME, Huitema ADR, Chandra S, Vijayakumar A, et al. A Phase I/II Study of Bosutinib in Pediatric Patients with Resistant/Intolerant or Newly Diagnosed Philadelphia Chromosome-Positive Chronic Myeloid Leukemia, Study ITCC (Innovative Therapies for Children with Cancer European Consortium) 054 and COG (Children's Oncology Group Consortium) AAML1921: Results from the Phase I Trial in Resistant/Intolerant Patients. Blood. 2021;138(Supplement 1):2558.
23. Cwynarski K, Roberts IAG, Iacobelli S, van Biezen A, Brand R, Devergie A, et al. Stem cell transplantation for chronic myeloid leukemia in children. Blood. 2003;102(4):1224-31.

EXPERT OPINION

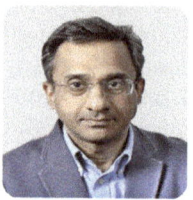

Deepak Bansal MD DNB FIAP FAMS
Professor, Hematology-Oncology Unit, Department of Pediatrics, Advanced Pediatrics Center
Postgraduate Institute of Medical Education and Research
Chandigarh, India. Email: deepakbansaldr@gmail.com

1. Is it recommended to do cytogenetics at diagnosis and follow-up? Is it from peripheral blood or bone marrow? What do you follow at your center?

Bone marrow is typically always performed at diagnosis to confirm the phase at diagnosis. Therefore, the *BCR: ABL1* fusion gene is conveniently demonstrated at diagnosis either by conventional cytogenetics (chromosome banding analysis of marrow cell metaphases), FISH analysis, or qualitative PCR from the bone marrow sample. However, each of these studies can also be done on peripheral blood. The laboratory at the Postgraduate Institute of Medical Education and Research (PGIMER), Chandigarh, offers FISH at diagnosis. Subsequently, quantitative real-time PCR (RQ-PCR) for determining *BCR-ABL1* transcripts level is performed from the peripheral blood during follow-up.

2. What is the first-line TKI that should be started in a child with CML?

Three Food and Drug Administration (FDA)-approved TKIs are available for first-line use in pediatrics for CML: Imatinib (approved: 2003), dasatinib (approved: 2017), and nilotinib (approved: 2018). Imatinib and dasatinib are administered once a day with or without food. Nilotinib is administered twice a day without food 2 hours prior and 1 hour after administration, rendering it potentially difficult for a young child or adolescent.

Imatinib has several generic formulations; it is the most cost-effective and financially viable option in the long term.

Second-generation TKIs (dasatinib and nilotinib) have been shown to induce a faster and deeper molecular response (DMR) in adults. Data from small pediatric series have shown a similar trend. A faster DMR has NOT been shown to have a survival benefit. It may be helpful to accelerate the achievement of DMR and, therefore, the number of eligible patients for attempting discontinuation of TKI therapy to achieve treatment-free remission (TFR). Nevertheless, the evidence for stopping TKI in pediatric CML is limited to small series or case reports in children.

Therefore, imatinib continues to be the most popular first-line choice for CP CML in children because of its cost-effectiveness, proven efficacy, and years of experience. However, one may elect to start with a second-generation TKI on a case-by-case basis.

Imatinib is administered as the first-line TKI in PGIMER, Chandigarh, for CP CML in children.

3. What are the indications of changing TKIs? What do you follow at your center?

The question of changing TKIs arises when target PCR goals are not achieved at the desired time points or when there is serial evidence of loss of molecular response or progression to blast or AP. Suboptimal compliance is often a common culprit and should be excluded by gentle and persistent history. If compliance is confirmed, a practical option is an increase in the dose of imatinib, particularly in the past when access to dasatinib was limited. With relatively easy access to TKD mutations and dasatinib, mutation-directed TKI can now be administered.

For patients who progress on first- and second-generation TKIs, there are no additional TKIs currently approved in pediatrics. However, there is substantial experience treating adults with the third-generation TKI ponatinib, which has activity against the T315I mutation.

4. When do you do TKD mutation in CML at your center?

The NCCN guidelines recommend that mutational analysis be sent after initiating TKI therapy if there is a suboptimal response to therapy, failure of prior response, or escalation to advanced stage CML. We request TKD mutations for the listed indications as well.

5. How to differentiate between de novo and transformed blastic crises? Share your experience of treating these two entities.

The clinical characteristics of CML in lymphoid BC resemble those of ALL. The question is whether a patient with newly diagnosed Ph-positive leukemia has Ph-positive ALL or CML in lymphoid BC. The B-lymphoblasts of CML BC have a phenotype indistinguishable from de novo B-lineage ALL.

The fusion protein in CML is characteristically the slightly longer p210 variant, whereas the p190 variant is more frequent in B-lineage ALL.

Additional factors supporting a diagnosis of CML in lymphoid BC include persistence of cells with only the t(9;22) without secondary cytogenetic abnormalities present at diagnosis and a significant ongoing discrepancy between MRD as assessed by BCR-ABL1 PCR and other methods such as flow cytometry.

In everyday practice, it is arduous to distinguish the two.

6. When do you recommend HSCT in CML?

Hematopoietic stem cell transplantation is indicated for patients: (1) resistant to or intolerant of all approved TKIs; (2) presenting with de novo blast phase; or (3) who progress to advanced phase during treatment. However, a 2019 analysis from the I-CML-Ped registry suggests that some patients with de-novo advanced-phase CML may be treated with frontline TKI, with or without chemotherapy, with reservation of HSCT for those with a suboptimal initial response.

7. Can we consider stopping imatinib if a patient is in complete molecular remission?

There is limited data on discontinuing TKIs in pediatric/adolescent patients following the attainment of deep and sustained molecular remission. The NCCN guidelines for discontinuing TKIs in adults include: (1) age ≥18 years, (2) CP CML, (3) no history of advanced stage CML, (4) TKI therapy for ≥3 years, (5) stable molecular response (MR4: ≤0.01% IS or better) for ≥2 years, and (6) access to reliable and frequent qPCR testing.

In adults, within 6 months of stopping TKI, 50–60% have a disease recurrence. A Children's Oncology Group study is ongoing to assess the feasibility of TFR. As per "western" literature, routine discontinuation of TKI outside of a clinical trial is not recommended as the data is limited in pediatrics. Having said that the author feels that one may attempt to stop TKI on a case-by-case basis in a reliable and compliant pediatric patient/family. All the above-listed NCCN criteria should be fulfilled (except, of course, age). Frequent monitoring with PCR is indicated while attempting TFR, which is a financial concern.

8. Share your experience of the late effects of TKIs in CML. Do you recommend fertility preservation to children with CML, and what do you follow at your center?

There are several publications on the adverse effects of imatinib on growth. A recent analysis of the cohort of CML patients in PGIMER, Chandigarh, has shown that the growth spurt is delayed. However, the final height is not affected. We have not experienced hypothyroidism in our patients.

Imatinib results in fairer skin in the majority of children. It is reversible on stopping imatinib. Immunoglobulin levels are often reduced; however, immunoglobulin levels are suggested to be checked in patients with CML receiving imatinib only with recurrent/unusual infections.

TKIs are teratogenic. There are reports of fetal abnormalities or spontaneous abortions, particularly in the first trimester with TKI. Females should be counseled to avoid pregnancy while receiving TKI. Before attempting to conceive, there should be a prolonged washout period after TKI discontinuation. The therapy with TKI should be held throughout the pregnancy. If treatment is needed during pregnancy, interferon therapy can be considered, particularly during the second trimester or beyond. TKI therapy can be resumed after pregnancy. However, mothers are advised not to breastfeed as imatinib, and likely other TKIs can be transmitted through breast milk. There have been no reported adverse effects or congenital abnormalities in the offspring of males receiving TKI during conception.

There is scarce literature on fertility and the ability to reproduce after prolonged TKI administration. Oligospermia in men on chronic TKIs has been reported.

CHAPTER 7

Juvenile Myelomonocytic Leukemia

Aditya Gupta, Aditya Kumar Gupta

CASE VIGNETTE

At 1 year of age, a child was referred from a hospital to our center with history of on and off fever, progressive abdominal distension, and cough and coryza for a duration of 6 months. He had history of recurrent blood transfusion [packed red blood cell (pRBC)] before presentation.

There was no history of bleeding from any site, jaundice. No history of any lump over the body, any pathological fracture, no preceding viral exanthem, no neurodevelopmental delay, regression, or early morning seizure. Child was immunized to date and the bacille Calmette-Guérin (BCG) scar was present. Child was fifth born child of a nonconsanguinous marriage. There was no family history of tuberculosis (TB), malignancy, repeated blood transfusions, or early deaths in siblings. Child was suspected outside to have juvenile myelomonocytic leukemia (JMML) in view of hepatosplenomegaly on examination and monocytosis on the peripheral blood smear.

Investigations done revealed the following: Complete blood count (CBC) hemoglobin (Hb) 9.4 g%, total leukocyte count (TLC) 58,000/cumm, platelet 32,000/cumm. Absolute monocyte count was 6,700/cumm. Peripheral smear showed leukocytosis with 2% blasts, 9% monocytes and thrombocytopenia **(Fig. 1)**. Bone marrow aspiration (BMA) showed hematopoietic cells of all series (M:E = 1.5:1) along with 10% blasts and 2% basophils. Work-up for viral mimickers was negative [parvovirus/cytomegalovirus (CMV)/Ebstein-Barr virus (EBV)], cytogenetics for t(9;22) was negative, and next-generation sequencing (NGS) from peripheral blood and buccal swab was sent which showed somatic *PTPN11* mutation and absence of germline mutation in the same.

The child was diagnosed to have JMML.

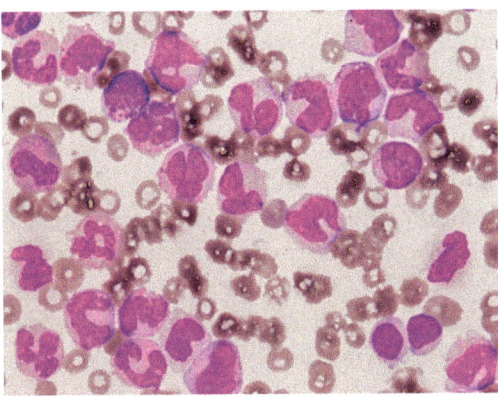

Fig. 1: Peripheral blood smear of patient showing leukocytosis with monocytosis and thrombocytopenia.

1. How does a child with JMML present and when should a child be suspected to have JMML?

Juvenile myelomonocytic leukemia is a rare disorder accounting for around 1% of pediatric leukemias with an estimated incidence of 1.2 per million.[1] The clinical presentation is varied—most children are aged <3 years at the time of diagnosis and there is a slight male preponderance (M:F 2.5:1).[2] Most children initially have nonspecific complaints—fever, cough, rash, abdominal distention, diarrhea, etc. along with hepatomegaly and splenomegaly on examination. Other signs and symptoms are due to bone marrow (BM) involvement, i.e., history of blood transfusions, pallor, minor or major bleeds, and recurrent infections.

However, there are two features which should prompt a clinician to suspect JMML—presence of monocytosis on peripheral blood smear and a large spleen—both of which are also essential for diagnosis.[2-4]

Other findings on history/physical examination include café au lait spots/xanthoma—particularly in patients with a family history of neurofibromatosis, lymphadenopathy, and sometimes central nervous system (CNS) findings such as facial palsy or excessive urination secondary to diabetes insipidus.[5]

Laboratory findings commonly include a high TLC although counts <10,000/cumm are common in children with JMML having monosomy 7.[2]

Peripheral smear findings include a striking monocytosis with absolute monocyte count >1,000/mm³, myeloid shift toward left, blasts usually are around 2-5% along with thrombocytopenia.[3,6]

Bone marrow examination is not very specific for JMML—there is myeloid preponderance noted with left shift along with increased monocytic precursors.

2. What is the diagnostic criteria of JMML and which differential diagnosis should be considered and ruled out in a case with suspected JMML?

The 2016 World Health Organization (WHO) classification of myeloid neoplasms and acute leukemia laid out the following diagnostic criteria for JMML **(Box 1)**.[7]

Since the presentation of JMML is not specific and its clinical presentation can be mimicked by a large variety of nonmalignant and malignant disorders, it is imperative to keep certain other differential diagnosis and rule them out.[8]

The essential diagnostic criteria itself requires blast percentage <20% and absence of t(9:22) to distinguish JMML from two common childhood hematolymphoid malignancies—namely, acute leukemia and chronic myeloid leukemia.

Infections which can mimic and have a similar presentation as that of JMML include disseminated CMV, EBV, HHV6, and parvovirus infections—hence should be ruled out in a case of suspected JMML.[9,10]

Other disorders which can have similar presentation include immunodeficiencies such as Wiskott–Aldrich syndrome, leukocyte adhesion defect, etc. and other diseases like infantile ostepetrosis.[8,11]

The following diagnostic work-up algorithm given in **Flowchart 1** can be followed for diagnosis of JMML:[12]

Juvenile Myelomonocytic Leukemia

BOX 1: Diagnostic criteria for JMML.

Clinical/hematological features (all are mandatory):
- Peripheral blood monocyte count >1 × 10^9/L
- Blast percentage in peripheral blood and bone marrow <20%
- Splenomegaly
- Absence of Philadelphia chromosome (BCR/ABL rearrangement)

Genetic studies (any 1):
- Somatic mutation in *PTPN11* or *K-RAS* or *N-RAS*
- Clinical diagnosis of NF-1 or germline *NF1* mutation
- Germline *CBL* mutation and loss of heterozygosity of *CBL*

If no criteria in genetic studies is met—any two of the following:
- Monosomy 7 or any other chromosomal abnormality
- HbF increased for age
- Myeloid precursors on peripheral blood smear
- Spontaneous growth or GM-CSF hypersensitivity in colony assay
- Hyperphosphorylation of STAT5

(ABL: Abelson murine leukemia virus homolog; BCR: breakpoint cluster region; GM-CSF: granulocyte macrophage colony-stimulating factor; HbF: fetal hemoglobin; JMML: juvenile myelomonocytic leukemia)

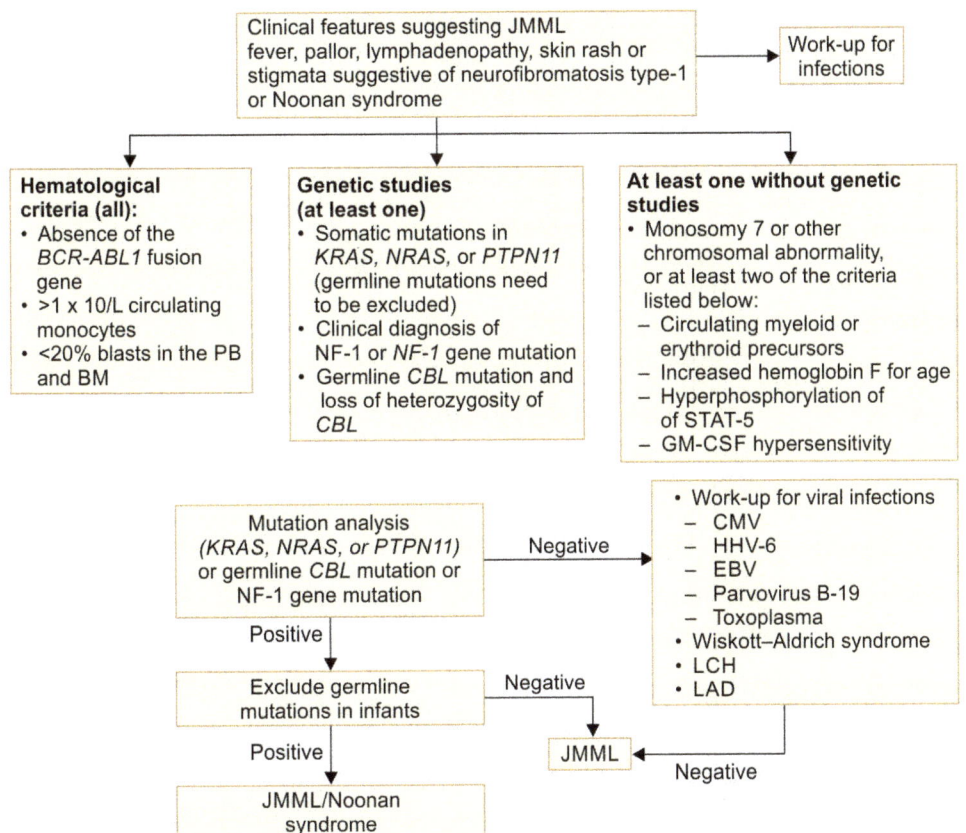

Flowchart 1: Diagnostic work-up algorithm for diagnosis of JMML.

(BCR-ABL: breakpoint cluster region-Abelson proto-oncogene; BM: bone marrow; CMV: cytomegalovirus; EBV: Ebstein-Barr virus; GM-CSF: granulocyte macrophage colony-stimulating factor; JMML: juvenile myelomonocytic leukemia; LCH: langerhans cell histiocytosis; LAD: leukocyte adhesion defect; PB: peripheral blood)

3. What underlies the pathogenesis of JMML and how does it affect the management?

Juvenile myelomonocytic leukemia is a type of RASopathy[13]—a disease whose pathogenesis involves a pathological upregulation and activation of RAS-RAF-MAPK (mitogen-activated protein kinase) pathway. Another characteristic is the hypersensitivity of myeloid precursors to granulocyte macrophage colony-stimulating factor (GM-CSF)—which in fact has been used as a diagnostic criteria as outlined above and is one of the hallmarks of the disease.[14]

The mutations described so far in JMML occur in genes and affects those proteins which are integral part of RAS pathway and these mutations result in its upregulation.

These genes include *PTPN11, KRAS, NRAS, NF,* and *CBL*. >90% of children diagnosed with JMML have a mutation in the above mentioned genes.[13]

However, the clinical profile and features vary dramatically depending upon whether the mutation is somatic or germline.

Patients with germline mutations in *PTPN11* have Noonan syndrome—such individuals develop a transient myeloproliferative disorder—which tends to ameliorate by itself.[15]

Similarly while somatic mutations in *KRAS/NRAS/CBL* portend a poor prognosis and need for urgent hematopoetic stem cell transplant (HSCT)[16-18]—germline mutations in the same genes results in a milder phenotype and wait and watch strategy might be appropriate. A broad outline on how to approach a child with JMML depending upon whether the mutation is germline or somatic can be made out from **Table 1**.[19]

TABLE 1: Clinical course and its relation to type of mutations in JMML.

Mutation	Type	Clinical course	Action
NF 1	Germline	Clinical features of neurofibromatosis tend to have higher platelet count, higher blast percentage, and a rapidly fatal course	Urgent HSCT
PTPN11	• Germline • Somatic	• Noonan's phenotype—mild disease/transient myeloproliferation • Higher TLC/blast percentage, younger age of presentation, rapidly fatal	• Wait and watch/mild chemotherapy • Urgent HSCT
NRAS	• Germline • Somatic	• Mild disease/transient myeloproliferation • Maximum clinical diversity: Many are clinically well; tendency to relapse post-HSCT	• Wait and watch/mild chemotherapy • Follow-up for spontaneous regression in mild disease • Urgent HSCT in aggressive cases
KRAS	• Germline • Somatic	• Mild disease/transient myeloproliferation • Aggressive disease, lower age/monosomy 7	• Wait and watch/mild chemotherapy • Urgent HSCT
CBL	Germline	Self-limiting in many cases—clinical progression in few	Wait and watch/mild chemotherapy followed by HSCT if disease progresses

(HSCT: hematopoetic stem cell transplant; TLC: total leukocyte count)

4. Which other genetic aberrations and cytogenetic abnormalities are found in JMML and how do they impact prognosis?

Genetic Aberrations

Apart from the mutations in the above mentioned five genes—other genetic aberrations found frequently in JMML include mutations in *SETB2* and *JAK3* which are found in around 15% of the patients.[20]

Activating mutations in *ALK* and *ROS1* genes are also reported along with mutations in epigenetic modifiers and spliceosome complex such *EZH2*, *ASXL1*, and *DNMT3A*.[21]

Juvenile myelomonocytic leukemia as a disorder is known to have paucity of mutations (apart from the five mutations included in its definition) and additional mutations are involved in tumor progression and associated with particularly poor outcomes especially patients which harbor *SETBP1* mutations tend to have a dismal prognosis.[22]

Aberrant methylation of certain genes also affects prognosis of patients with JMML with genes such as *BMP4*, *CALCA*, *CDKN2B*, and *RARB* found to be hypermethylated and associated with a poorer outcome.[23]

Depending upon the methylation pattern JMML can be classified into three broad subtypes.[23]

1. *High methylation group:* Associated with somatic *PTPN11* mutations; poorer prognosis
2. *Low methylation:* Associated with somatic *NRAS* and *CBL* mutations—favorable prognosis
3. *Intermediate methylation group:* Somatic *KRAS* mutations and monosomy 7.

Cytogenetic Abnormalities

Most common cytogenetic abnormality seen in patient with JMML is monosomy of chromosome 7 present in about 25% of the patients. Around 10% patients also harbor another cytogenetic abnormality which includes deletion of chromosome 5q/7q.[2,8,19]

These karyotypic abnormalities usually get acquired during management and treatment or when the child progresses to have a blast crisis. Monitoring of them is hence important as far as response assessment is concerned.[24]

Children having JMML with monosomy 7 have lower counts, fetal hemoglobin (HbF) which is near normal and an erythroid predominance on BM examination. Patients harboring this cytogenetic abnormality are usually classified as having standard risk if no other high-risk features are present.

The above child was started on chemotherapy and given two cycles of Ara-C/6MP serving as a bridge till HSCT.

5. What is the role of chemotherapy in management of JMML?

The only curative option for JMML is an allogeneic HSCT which results in cure of about 60% of the patients. In such a scenario where the only curative therapy is allo-HSCT, role of both pre- and post-transplant chemotherapy is controversial.

In the absence of transplantation, most children succumb to their disease within 10–12 months—mostly due to respiratory involvement and infiltration of lung with leukemic cells. A proportion of patients progress to have a blastic transformation.[2]

Abdul Wajid et al. in retrospective analysis of 33 patients treated at a tertiary care center showed that sequential chemotherapy with 6MP +Ara-C-based regimen resulted in response in subset of patients—while the response to chemotherapy might be prolonged and sustained in a subset of patients with good prognostic factors—it is however temporary and chemotherapy is not curative.[25]

Intensive chemotherapeutic agents, however, do not have any proven efficacy and can result in treatment-related morbidity and mortality.

In some patients especially those with high-leukemic burden or aggressive disease or pulmonary involvement, salvage regimens with fludarabine and high-dose cytarabine combinations maybe used to achieve remission as the child awaits transplant.[19]

6. What is the role of azacitidine as pre-/post-transplant chemotherapy in JMML?

Azacitidine which is a DNA hypomethylating agent is known to induce stable long-term remissions in a subset of patients with JMML. While it is not a curative option, it is an attractive option to consider during the window period to transplantation for disease control and decreasing the leukemic burden.[26]

Many case reports and series have reported and concluded that low-dose azacitidine is well tolerated and effective in JMML and can induce a complete clinical, cytogenetic, and/or molecular remissions before Allo-HSCT.[27-29]

But its use is associated with good outcome mostly in patients who already had a good molecular/clinical profile such as those with germline mutations of *KRAS*, *NRAS* or *PTPN11* and mildly symptomatic patients having *CBL* mutations.

7. What is the role of splenectomy in patient with JMML?

In the past with lack of availability of centers for allo-HSCT, splenectomy was either used to control disease symptoms or for palliation. It decreases pRBC and platelet transfusion requirement albeit at the risk of increased rate of infection. It also has been done to promote engraftment post-allo-HSCT, however, its routine use, however, is not recommended and spleen size/splenectomy does not have any effect on outcome of JMML post-HSCT.[30]

Since the child had a matched sibling donor—was taken up for allogeneic HSCT postbusulfan, fludarabine, and melphalan-based conditioning was used along with cyclosporine (CSA)/methotrexate (MTX) for graft versus host disease (GvHD) prophylaxis. Child had 100% donor chimerism after 4 weeks, however, child developed a skin rash along with persistent diarrhea as a manifestation of GvHD—which was steroid refractory but improved postruxolitinib.

8. What are the outcomes following HSCT in JMML and which factors affect the prognosis?

Allo-HSCT is the only known curative option in patients with JMML.[31,32] However, only about 50% patients are known to have long-term survival post-Allo-HSCT with relapse following transplant being the most common cause of mortality. A second transplant can salvage a subset of patients experiencing relapse.[33]

Either matched sibling donor or matched unrelated donor is considered as the first choice in patients with transplant. Umbilical cord blood (UCB) can considered as an option in those patients which lack a matched donor and have an aggressive disease requiring urgent HSCT. Due to the low weight of patients, UCB unit and the stem cells in it are sufficient usually.[34,35]

While earlier total body irradiation (TBI)-based conditioning was considered and used, it has slowly fallen out of favor due to its toxicity profile to high-dose alkylating agents with a cell nonspecific action. Bu-Cy-Mel-based conditioning is used most frequently including its use by the European Society for Blood and Marrow Transplantation (EBMT) group which reported an event-free survival of matched sibling and matched unrelated donor as 55 and 49%, respectively.[31]

Factors which predict a poorer outcome included age >2 years, female donor to male recipient, matched unrelated donor or mismatched noncord donor as compared to matched sibling donor, use of TBI as conditioning and no use of serotherapy in conditioning regimen. Busulfan, cyclophosphamide, and melphalan conditioning regimen was shown to have risk of relapse while serotherapy was associated with lower nonrelapse mortality. These factors were reported from a 25-year series from 1986 to 2011 in 91 patients with JMML who underwent a HSCT in France.[36]

In another study of 121 patients by Yoshida et al. also, Bu-Cy-Mel as conditioning regimen had lowered risk of relapse. Chronic GvHD was associated with a lower risk of relapse.[37]

For GvHD prophylaxis, CSA and MTX are the two most commonly used drugs in patients having a matched sibling donor while thymoglobulin (ATG) is added in those having matched unrelated donor. ATG is not known to increase relapse risk though it can attenuate the graft versus leukemia effect.

Juvenile myelomonocytic leukemia patients undergoing HSCT usually have a lower risk for GvHD probably owing to their young age and in those patients not having acute GvHD manifestation, GvHD prophylaxis should be tapered between D+60 and D+180.[19]

9. How to manage a child who relapses post-transplant and what factors predict relapse?

Donor-recipient chimerism helps to identify the children who can and are at a higher risk of relapse. If there is a fall in donor chimerism rapid tapering of immunosuppression can be tried which if fails can be supplanted by donor lymphocyte transfusions.[38]

Factors which predict an increased risk of relapse include age >4 years, acute myeloid leukemia (AML)-like molecular signature, high methylation of CpG islands in some genes, *PTPN11/NF1* mutations, and initial blast count of 20% or more.[39]

In all around 30–40% of children with JMML who receive a HSCT will relapse. A second allogeneic HSCT using the same donor with less intense GvHD prophylaxis or a different donor can salvage about 30% of the patients which undergo a relapse.[40]

There are different approaches to conditioning with Patel et al.[39] using mitoxantrone and high-dose Ara-C while TBI-based conditioning being used by EBMT group in patients relapsing post-HSCT.[31] Both approaches however involve a tapered down GvHD prophylaxis if same donor is used. Allo-HSCT remains the only modality offering a cure even in setting of relapse and remains the treatment of choice.

10. What are the newer therapeutic options and novel drugs which are being explored for the management of JMML?

Since, JMML involves RAS hyperactivation, researchers have attempted post-translational modification of RAS protein through inhibition of the enzyme farnesyltransferase. While a response was demonstrated in vivo, such drugs like R115777 (Zarnestra) failed clinical trials.[41]

Inhibition of Src kinase and JAK kinase by dasatinib and ruxolitinib respectively is also being explored in JMML. Use of ruxolitinib has stabilized the disease in a few patients.[42]

Another novel approach is the use of bisphosphonates via the suppression of farnesylation and geranylgeranylation. Zoledronic acid can inhibit the colony-forming activity of JMML precursor cells. This approach though has not been tried clinically.[43]

Since JMML is a RASopathy which involves RAF/MEK/ERK and PI3K/Akt/mammalian target of rapamycin (mTOR) pathways downstream—MEK inhibitors and mTOR inhibitors use is being explored with promising results in preclinical studies.[40,44]

REFERENCES

1. Hasle H, Kerndrup G, Jacobsen BB. Childhood myelodysplastic syndrome in Denmark: incidence and predisposing conditions. Leukemia. 1995;9(9):1569-72.
2. Niemeyer CM, Arico M, Basso G, Biondi A, Rajnoldi AC, Creutzig U, et al. Chronic myelomonocytic leukemia in childhood: a retrospective analysis of 110 cases. European Working Group on Myelodysplastic Syndromes in Childhood (EWOG-MDS). Blood. 1997;89(10):3534-43.
3. Loh ML. Recent advances in the pathogenesis and treatment of juvenile myelomonocytic leukaemia. Br J Haematol. 2011;152(6):677-87.
4. Aricò M, Biondi A, Pui CH. Juvenile myelomonocytic leukemia. Blood. 1997;90(2):479-88.
5. Stiller CA, Chessells JM, Fitchett M. Neurofibromatosis and childhood leukaemia/lymphoma: a population-based UKCCSG study. Br J Cancer. 1994;70(5):969-72.
6. Passmore SJ, Hann IM, Stiller CA, Ramani P, Swansbury GJ, Gibbons B, et al. Pediatric myelodysplasia: a study of 68 children and a new prognostic scoring system. Blood. 1995;85(7):1742-50.
7. Swerdlow SH, Campo E, Harris NL, Jaffe ES, Pileri SA, Stein H, et al. (Eds). WHO Classification of Tumours of Haematopoietic and Lymphoid Tissues, 4th edition. Lyon: International Agency for Research on Cancer; 2017.
8. Loh ML. Childhood myelodysplastic syndrome: focus on the approach to diagnosis and treatment of juvenile myelomonocytic leukemia. Hematology. 2010;2010(1):357-62.
9. Karow A, Baumann I, Niemeyer CM. Morphologic differential diagnosis of juvenile myelomonocytic leukemia–pitfalls apart from viral infection. J Pediatr Hematol Oncol. 2009;31(5):380.
10. Pinkel D. Differentiating juvenile myelomonocytic leukemia from infectious disease. Blood. 1998;91(1):365-7.
11. Yoshimi A, Kamachi Y, Imai K, Watanabe N, Nakadate H, Kanazawa T, et al. Wiskott-Aldrich syndrome presenting with a clinical picture mimicking juvenile myelomonocytic leukaemia. Pediatr Blood Cancer. 2013;60(5):836-41.
12. Gupta AK, Meena JP, Chopra A, Tanwar P, Seth R. Juvenile myelomonocytic leukemia- a comprehensive review and recent advances in management. Am J Blood Res. 2021;11(1):1-21.
13. Lasho T, Patnaik MM. Juvenile myelomonocytic leukemia - a bona fide RASopathy syndrome. Best Pract Res Clin Haematol. 2020;33(2):101171.
14. Emanuel PD, Bates LJ, Castleberry RP, Gualtieri RJ, Zuckerman KS. Selective hypersensitivity to granulocyte-macrophage colony-stimulating factor by juvenile chronic myeloid leukemia hematopoietic progenitors. Blood. 1991;77(5):925-9.

15. Bader-Meunier B, Tchernia G, Miélot F, Fontaine JL, Thomas C, Lyonnet S, et al. Occurrence of myeloproliferative disorder in patients with Noonan syndrome. J Pediatr. 1997;130(6):885-9.
16. Shannon KM, O'Connell P, Martin GA, Paderanga D, Olson K, Dinndorf P, et al. Loss of the normal NF1 allele from the bone marrow of children with type 1 neurofibromatosis and malignant myeloid disorders. N Engl J Med. 1994;330(9):597-601.
17. Niemeyer CM, Kang MW, Shin DH, Furlan I, Erlacher M, Bunin NJ, et al. Germline *CBL* mutations cause developmental abnormalities and predispose to juvenile myelomonocytic leukemia. Nat Genet. 2010;42(9):794-800.
18. De Filippi P, Zecca M, Lisini D, Rosti V, Cagioni C, Carlo-Stella C, et al. Germ-line mutation of the NRAS gene may be responsible for the development of juvenile myelomonocytic leukaemia. Br J Haematol. 2009;147(5):706-9.
19. Locatelli F, Niemeyer CM. How I treat juvenile myelomonocytic leukemia. Blood. 2015;125(7):1083-90.
20. Bresolin S, De Filippi P, Vendemini F, D'Alia M, Zecca M, Meyer LH, et al. Mutations of SETBP1 and JAK3 in juvenile myelomonocytic leukemia: a report from the Italian AIEOP study group. Oncotarget. 2016;7(20):28914-9.
21. Murakami N, Okuno Y, Yoshida K, Shiraishi Y, Nagae G, Suzuki K, et al. Integrated molecular profiling of juvenile myelomonocytic leukemia. Blood. 2018;131(14):1576-86.
22. Stieglitz E, Troup CB, Gelston LC, Haliburton J, Chow ED, Yu KB, et al. Subclonal mutations in SETBP1 confer a poor prognosis in juvenile myelomonocytic leukemia. Blood. 2015;125(3):516-24.
23. Lipka DB, Witte T, Toth R, Yang J, Wiesenfarth M, Nöllke P, et al. RAS-pathway mutation patterns define epigenetic subclasses in juvenile myelomonocytic leukemia. Nat Commun. 2017;8(1):2126.
24. Honda Y, Tsuchida M, Zaike Y, Masunaga A, Yoshimi A, Kojima S, et al. Clinical characteristics of 15 children with juvenile myelomonocytic leukaemia who developed blast crisis: MDS Committee of Japanese Society of Paediatric Haematology/Oncology. Br J Haematol. 2014;165(5):682-7.
25. Wajid MA, Gupta AK, Das G, Sahoo D, Meena JP, Seth R. Outcomes of juvenile myelomonocytic leukemia patients after sequential therapy with cytarabine and 6-mercaptopurine. Pediatr Hematol Oncol. 2020;37(7):573-81.
26. Cseh A, Niemeyer CM, Yoshimi A, Dworzak M, Hasle H, van den Heuvel-Eibrink MM, et al. Bridging to transplant with azacitidine in juvenile myelomonocytic leukemia: a retrospective analysis of the EWOG-MDS study group. Blood. 2015;125(14):2311-3.
27. Furlan I, Batz C, Flotho C, Mohr B, Lübbert M, Suttorp M, et al. Intriguing response to azacitidine in a patient with juvenile myelomonocytic leukemia and monosomy 7. Blood. 2009;113(12):2867-8.
28. Hashmi SK, Punia JN, Marcogliese AN, Gaikwad AS, Fisher KE, Roy A, et al. Sustained remission with azacitidine monotherapy and an aberrant precursor B-lymphoblast population in juvenile myelomonocytic leukemia. Pediatr Blood Cancer. 2019;66(10):e27905.
29. Fabri O, Horakova J, Bodova I, Svec P, Striezencova ZL, Bubanska E, et al. Diagnosis and treatment of juvenile myelomonocytic leukemia in Slovak Republic: novel approaches. Neoplasma. 2019;66(5):818-24.
30. Ozyürek E, Cetin M, Tuncer M, Hiçsönmez G. The role of splenectomy in children with juvenile myelomonocytic leukemia. Turk J Pediatr. 2007;49(2):154-7.
31. Locatelli F, Nöllke P, Zecca M, Korthof E, Lanino E, Peters C, et al. Hematopoietic stem cell transplantation (HSCT) in children with juvenile myelomonocytic leukemia (JMML): results of the EWOG-MDS/EBMT trial. Blood. 2005;105(1):410-9.
32. Locatelli F, Niemeyer C, Angelucci E, Bender-Götze C, Burdach S, Ebell W, et al. Allogeneic bone marrow transplantation for chronic myelomonocytic leukemia in childhood: a report

from the European Working Group on myelodysplastic syndrome in childhood. J Clin Oncol. 1997;15(2):566-73.
33. Chan RJ, Cooper T, Kratz CP, Weiss B, Loh ML. Juvenile myelomonocytic leukemia: a report from the 2nd International JMML Symposium. Leuk Res. 2009;33(3):355-62.
34. Locatelli F, Crotta A, Ruggeri A, Eapen M, Wagner JE, Macmillan ML, et al. Analysis of risk factors influencing outcomes after cord blood transplantation in children with juvenile myelomonocytic leukemia: a EUROCORD, EBMT, EWOG-MDS, CIBMTR study. Blood. 2013;122(12):2135-41.
35. Smith FO, King R, Nelson G, Wagner JE, Robertson KA, Sanders JE, et al. Unrelated donor bone marrow transplantation for children with juvenile myelomonocytic leukaemia. Br J Haematol. 2002;116(3):716-24.
36. Meyran D, Porcher R, Raus N, Strullu M, Ouache M, Yakouben K, et al. Allogeneic hematopoietic stem cell transplantation (HSCT) for juvenile myelomonocytic leukemia (JMML) in France: a Retrospective Study of Société Française De Greffe De Moelle Et De Thérapie Cellulaire. Biol Blood Marrow Transplant. 2013;19(2):S163.
37. Yoshida N, Sakaguchi H, Yabe M, Hasegawa D, Hama A, Hasegawa D, et al. Clinical outcomes after allogeneic hematopoietic stem cell transplantation in children with juvenile myelomonocytic leukemia: a report from the Japan Society for Hematopoietic Cell Transplantation. Biol Blood Marrow Transplant. 2020;26(5):902-10.
38. Yoshimi A, Bader P, Matthes-Martin S, Starý J, Sedlacek P, Duffner U, et al. Donor leukocyte infusion after hematopoietic stem cell transplantation in patients with juvenile myelomonocytic leukemia. Leukemia. 2005;19(6):971-7.
39. Patel SA, Coulter DW, Grovas AC, Gordon BG, Harper JL, Warkentin PI, et al. Cytosine arabinoside and mitoxantrone followed by second allogeneic transplant for the treatment of children with refractory juvenile myelomonocytic leukemia. J Pediatr Hematol Oncol. 2014;36(6):491-4.
40. Locatelli F, Algeri M, Merli P, Strocchio L. Novel approaches to diagnosis and treatment of juvenile myelomonocytic leukemia. Expert Rev Hematol. 2018;11(2):129-43.
41. Castleberry RP, Loh ML, Jayaprakash N, Peterson A, Casey V, Chang M, et al. Phase II Window Study of the farnesyltransferase inhibitor R115777 (Zarnestra®) in untreated juvenile myelomonocytic leukemia (JMML): a Children's Oncology Group Study. Blood. 2005;106(11):2587.
42. Loh ML, Tasian SK, Rabin KR, Brown P, Magoon D, Reid JM, et al. A phase 1 dosing study of ruxolitinib in children with relapsed or refractory solid tumors, leukemias, or myeloproliferative neoplasms: a Children's Oncology Group phase 1 consortium study (ADVL1011). Pediatr Blood Cancer. 2015;62(10):1717-24.
43. Ohtsuka Y, Manabe A, Kawasaki H, Hasegawa D, Zaike Y, Watanabe S, et al. RAS-blocking bisphosphonate zoledronic acid inhibits the abnormal proliferation and differentiation of juvenile myelomonocytic leukemia cells in vitro. Blood. 2005;106(9):3134-41.
44. Liu W, Yu WM, Zhang J, Chan RJ, Loh ML, Zhang Z, et al. Inhibition of the Gab2/PI3K/mTOR signaling ameliorates myeloid malignancy caused by Ptpn11 (Shp2) gain-of-function mutations. Leukemia. 2017;31(6):1415-22.

EXPERT OPINION

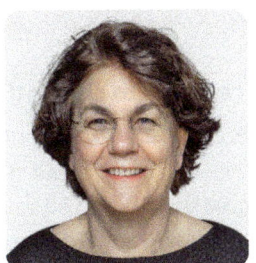

Charlotte Niemeyer MD
Medical Director
Division of Pediatric Oncology and Hematology
Center for Pediatrics and Adolescent Medicine, University of Freiburg, Germany

1. Over the past two decades, how have we improved in the understanding of the disease biology?

In the last two decades, we discovered germline *CBL* mutations and learned that biallelic inactivation of the *CBL* locus can give rise to JMML. We appreciated that about 90% of patients harbor molecular alterations in one of five genes (*PTPN11*, *NRAS*, *KRAS*, *NF1*, or *CBL*), which define genetically and clinically distinct subtypes. In addition, we learned that mutation in *JAK3*, *SETBP*1, and *RAS* double mutations were the most common secondary somatic changes. Lastly, we recognized that the DNA hypermethylation predicts poor outcome.

At the same time, we understood the importance of a rational diagnostic approach. Presence of myeloid or erythroid precursors (with or without blasts) on blood smear is noted in 90% of JMML patients and probably more characteristic for JMML than monocytosis. Also, we learned to stress the importance of HbF as a crucial diagnostic and prognostic parameter. A very high HbF may immediately help to guide further diagnostic efforts (and spare tests for viral mimics, Ph+ disease, etc.). In addition, the predictive value of HbF (high risk defined as HbF >15%, for infants less than 12 months of age: > the upper limit of age-adjusted normal) is excellent and almost as good than DNA hypermethylation.

2. Is there a subset of JMML patients who we can observe and follow without giving chemotherapy?

The important question is whether there are JMML patients who can be cured without HSCT. First, JMML patients with *CBL* germline mutation generally have self-limiting disease; leukocytosis and splenomegaly regress during childhood. Some of these *CBL*-mutated JMML patients have, however, gross splenomegaly resulting in developmental delay; the splenomegaly is difficult to treat and does not respond well to chemotherapy. Second, some young *NRAS*-mutated JMML patients are clinically very well despite a full-blown JMML picture. They show low-risk features (age <2 years, HbF <15% or for infants >9 months of age within age-adjusted normal limits), a low-blast count (<10% in the BM). These patients can be subjected to a long-term watch and wait strategy. Some of them may benefit from a short course of 6-MP when the white blood cell (WBC) is very high or the platelet count quite low. However, enough data indicate these patients can normalize their clinical and hematological picture over the years while keeping the NRAS clone with same high variant allelic frequency.

3. Which patients of JMML can respond to chemotherapy only?

As discussed under 2. and 4., there are some patients who may not require stem cell transplantation. Even if some of the watch and wait *NRAS*-mutated JMML patients may intermittently receive 6-MP to improve their blood counts, it is important to understand that in JMML chemotherapy cannot substitute for stem cell transplantation.

4. What chemotherapy would you use as a bridge to HSCT in JMML and why?

Our standard of care prior to HSCT is azacitidine therapy. Based on our study (Niemeyer et al. Blood Advances 2021), the Food and Drug Administration (FDA) approved azacitidine for newly diagnosed JMML. In patients who do not respond to azacitidine and cannot be subjected to HSCT timely, an intensive regimen with high-dose Ara-C and fludarabine, first described in JMML by the Children's Oncology Group (COG) in the US, can be helpful. There is a small group of *KRAS*-mutated patients, who exhibit an extraordinary response to azacitidine by reaching a molecular remission; these children may be cured in the absence of HSCT as well.

5. Do you make any modifications to the conditioning for HSCT in JMML specifically for the disease?

We generally apply a conditioning regimen with busulfan, cyclophosphamide, and melphalan. In patients with *KRAS*-mutated JMML, the incidence of relapse was very low; we therefore changed to a preparative regimen with treosulfan, thiotepa, and melphalan (see https://ewog-mds.org). For patients with very high risk of relapse (age >2 years and *PTPN11* mutation) we currently pilot post-HSCT azacitidine + DLI.

6. Do you use granulocyte colony-stimulating factor (GCSF) post-HSCT for your JMML patients post–HSCT?

We do not use GCSF post-HSCT, because it may stimulate a malignant stem/progenitor cell and increase the risk of relapse.

CHAPTER 8

Anaplastic Large Cell Lymphoma

Prashant Prabhakar, Aditya Kumar Gupta

CASE VIGNETTE

A 12-year-old male child presented with the complaints of:
- Exertional breathlessness for 6 months
- Fever on and off for 4 months
- Recurrent dry cough, chest pain for 4 months
- Weight loss for 4 months

After initial evaluation, based on clinical and radiological findings, at a peripheral healthcare center, a suspicion of pulmonary tuberculosis was kept and he was started on antitubercular treatment (ATT). There was no symptomatic improvement even after 2 months of ATT. Therefore, he was referred and reevaluated at our center. The chest X-ray **(Fig. 1A)** showed completely opacified left hemithorax and the CT chest **(Fig. 2A)** revealed a mass encircling the left main bronchus with collapse consolidation of the left lung. Fiberoptic bronchoscopy **(Fig. 3)** showed a left endobronchial mass and biopsy for histopathology from the mass was sent. The biopsy report **(Figs. 4A to 4F)** confirmed it to be a case of anaplastic large cell lymphoma (ALCL). Metastatic workup done with a bone marrow (BM) aspirate and biopsy and a positron emission tomography (PET) scan **(Fig. 5A)** showed a localized nonmetastatic disease. The **Figs. 1B, 2B and 5B** show the complete resolution of mass after completing treatment.

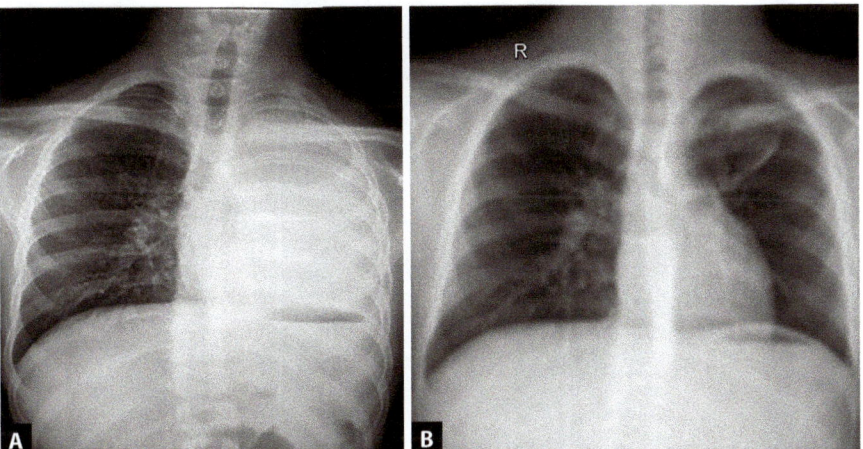

Figs. 1A and B: (A) Chest X-ray image showing complete white-out appearance of left lung with ipsilateral mediastinal shift. Also note left main bronchus is not separately visible; (B) Chest X-ray showing disappearance of left sided mass lesion and complete expansion of left lung after treatment completion.

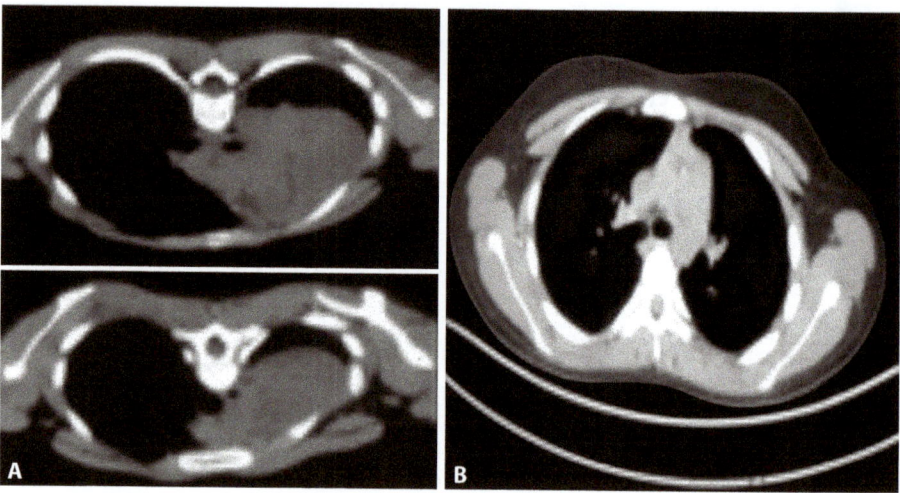

Figs. 2A and B: (A) Computed tomography scan image showing mass encircling left main bronchus with collapse-consolidation of left lung; (B) Computed tomography scan image showing disappearance of left-sided mass lesion and complete expansion of left lung after treatment completion.

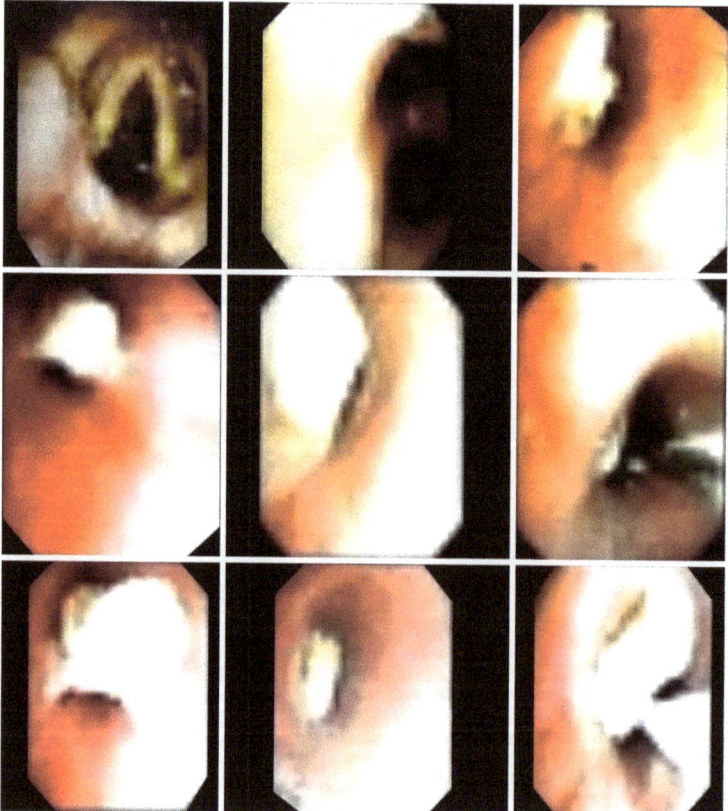

Fig. 3: Bronchoscopic images of tumor: the left main bronchus is filled with an adherent caseous material almost completely obstructing it. Bronchoalveolar lavage and biopsy being taken.

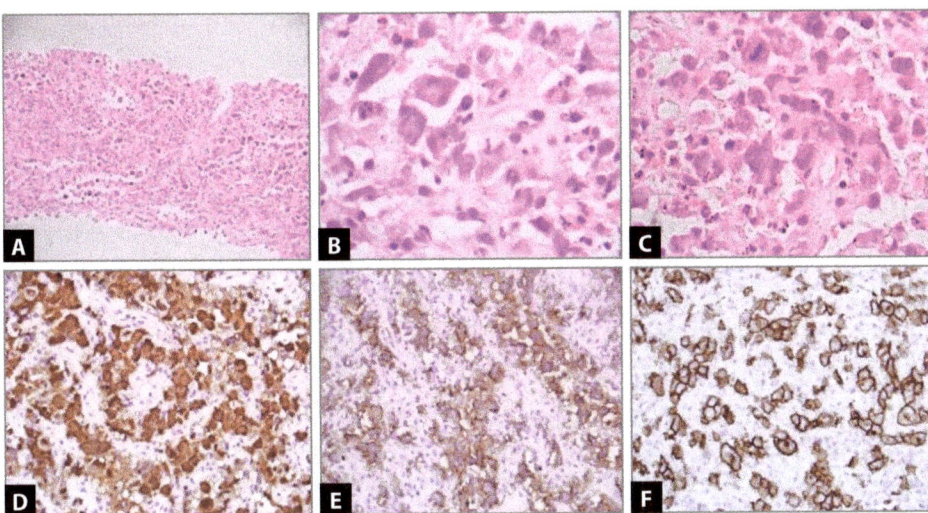

Figs. 4A to F: Core needle biopsy shows atypical large lymphoid cells (A) with moderate to abundant cytoplasm and enlarged vesicular nuclei (B); mitoses were frequent (C). The large cells show immunopositivity for ALK (D), EMA (E) and CD30 (F).

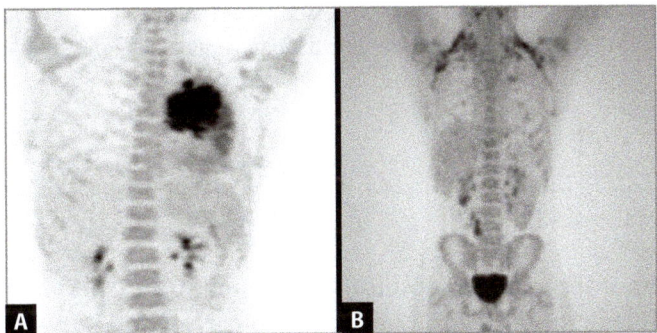

Figs. 5A and B: (A) Maximum intensity projection of FDG-PET image showing left lung mass. No lesions were found elsewhere; (B) FDG PET-CT images after completion of 6 cycles of chemotherapy showing resolution of left-sided mass lesion and metabolic activity. (FDG: fluorodeoxyglucose; PET: positron emission tomography)

1. **This patient who was finally diagnosed with ALCL presented with an endobronchial mass. ALCL is known to be a mimicker of many common diagnoses. What are the common presentations of ALCL in pediatric and young adults?**

Anaplastic large cell lymphoma is a unique subtype of peripheral T-cell lymphoma. It constitutes 10–15% of pediatric and young adults non-Hodgkin lymphoma (NHL).[1] The mean age of presentation is 12 years and is rare in children <1 year of age.[2] It is more common in boys (M:F—6.5:1). The most common presenting features are peripheral, intra-abdominal, and mediastinal lymphadenopathy often associated with systemic B symptoms such as fever and weight loss. B symptoms are a very common feature of ALCL among all NHL. It may present rarely with waxing and waning lymphadenopathy or other nonspecific symptoms which makes the diagnosis often challenging.[1] The involvement of extranodal organs such as skin, lung, bones, liver, and soft tissue is a very distinct feature of ALCL and almost one-third cases present with extranodal disease due to which the diagnosis can often be missed initially. However, bone marrow (BM), central nervous system (CNS) and gastrointestinal system are rarely involved. Gross involvement of BM is seen in <15% cases but reverse transcriptase polymerase chain reaction (RT-PCR) for NPM1-anaplastic lymphoma kinase (ALK) can detect minimal disease in around 50% cases of ALK+ ALCL. ALCL can present with concomitant hemophagocytic lymphohistiocytosis (HLH) in 10–12% of cases. BM involvement is more common in small cell (SC) variant.

2. What are the differences between ALK-positive (ALK+) versus ALK-negative (ALK–) ALCL?

The World Health Organization classification in 2016 classifies ALCL into: (1) ALK-positive nodal/systemic; (2) ALK-negative nodal/systemic; (3) primary cutaneous; and (4) breast implant-associated ALCL–.[3] Morphologically and phenotypically both ALK+ and ALK– types are similar, but they have prognostic importance. ALK positivity is more associated with younger age group. Pediatric ALCLs are ALK-positive in greater than 90% cases while only 5–10% adult cases are ALK+.[4]

Anaplastic lymphoma kinase-positive has excellent prognosis as compared to ALK-negative. However, the presence of some chromosomal rearrangements has significant effect on the overall survival (OS) in the later one. These common genetic associations with ALCL are:
- *DUSP-22* rearranged
- *TP63* rearranged
- Triple negative ALCL

5-year OS for *DUSP*-22 rearranged ALCL is 90%, *TP63* rearranged ALCL is 17%, and that of triple negative ALCL is 42%.[5]

3. What are the unique histopathological examination (HPE) and immunohistochemical (IHC) features of ALCL? What is the correlation between ALK positivity by IHC and ALK translocation? Can the pattern of ALK positivity on IHC give a clue to the type of ALK translocation?

Anaplastic large cell lymphoma is an aggressive NHL which morphologically shows malignant histiocytes, and on the IHC can be confused with Hodgkin lymphoma (HL). Immunophenotypic and *TCR* gene studies confirmed its origin from T cell and led to the recognition that it is a special subtype of peripheral T-cell lymphoma lacking expression of T-cell protein. There are various morphological subtypes based on variability of cell size and histological architecture, but all types are characterized by the presence of large cells with abundant cytoplasm and horseshoe-shaped nucleus known as *Hallmark cells*. The diagnosis mainly relies on morphology with IHC showing CD30 and ALK positivity along with negative B-cell markers.

The different subtypes of ALCL are:
- *C ALCL (common variant of ALCL):* This is the most frequent morphological subtype accounting for 60% of all cases and they have abundant Hallmark cells. There is characteristic invasion of lymph node (LN) sinus with perivascular distribution of malignant cells.

- **S ALCL (small cell variant):** This subtype mainly contains predominantly small to medium-sized tumor cells with a smaller number of Hallmark cells.
- **LH ALCL (lymphohistiocytic variant):** This subtype contributes to around 10% cases. The dominant cells in this subtype are reactive histiocytes. These cells mask the small population of actual hallmark cells.

The other two subtypes are: Hodgkin-like and composite-type.
Anaplastic lymphoma kinase positivity by IHC shows a strong correlation with ALK rearrangement in more than 98% cases, so there is no need for fluorescence in situ hybridization (FISH) to confirm ALK translocation. The pattern of ALK immunostaining positivity also gives a clue to the type of rearrangement, because the localization of the ALK fusion protein is dependent on the ALK fusion partner. The nuclear and cytoplasmic ALK positivity is seen in NPM-ALK translocation, while the non-NPM partner shows either nuclear or cytoplasmic staining.

4. What is the role of ALK rearrangement, especially NPM-ALK rearrangement in the pathogenesis of ALCL? Is there association of ALK with some other pediatric tumor?

NPM-ALK is the most common ALK fusion in ALK positive ALCL (70–80%) with t(2;5) (p23;q35) (6). ALK, also known as CD246, is a classical *Receptor Tyrosine Kinase of Insulin receptor superfamily*. The *ALK* gene is located at chromosome 2p23 and is normally expressed in nervous system during embryonic development. As per studies in mice and drosophila, *ALK* gene has been postulated to play a role in the development of nervous system and gut; however, it gets downregulated after birth. The *NPM* gene is located at 5q35. NPM is a universally expressed phosphoprotein. Its function is transfer of ribonucleoproteins between nucleus and cytoplasm. NPM carries oligomer units, which lead to the joining of two identical subunits of NPM-ALK to form a single unit. This homodimerization results in constitutive activation of ALK tyrosine kinase.

Activation of ALK stimulates many signal pathways, including JAK/STAT, PI3K/AKT, RAS/RAF/MEK/ERK, and PLCγ pathways.

JAK/STAT pathway has been studied in-depth in the pathogenesis of ALCL. This pathway keeps a strict regulation over activation of STATs which keeps a balance between activation and inhibition pathway. This in turn has a crucial role in normal development and differentiation of cells. NPM-ALK fusion leads to the activation of STAT3 by phosphorylation, JAK3 activation, and Shp1 downregulation. STAT3 activation leads to uncontrolled proliferation and tumorigenesis.[6]

The other pediatric malignancies associated with ALK rearrangement are neuroblastoma, rhabdomyosarcoma, and inflammatory myofibroblastic tumor (IMT).

CASE *(Continued)*

The patient had B-symptoms and the HPE revealed it to be a *common* variant of ALK+ ALCL.

5. What are the poor prognostic factors in ALCL? There are certain controversies in poor prognostic factors like B-symptoms, time of relapse, ALK positivity, histopathological type, and minimal disseminated disease (MDD), do they have prognostic significance?

Mediastinal, skin, and visceral (lung, liver, spleen) involvement were poor prognostic factors according to a large European intergroup study which analyzed 225 children enrolled between 1987 and 1997 in Berlin-Frankfurt-Münster (BFM) and UK Children's cancer study group. 5-year progression-free survival (PFS) for those patients with at least one risk factor was 61%, against 89% for those without these risk factors. However, 10-year follow-up results of 420 patients enrolled in ALCL99 trial showed that SC or LH histology and MDD were poor prognostic factors.

Minimal residual disease (MRD) in BM was supposed to be a biological marker for prognosis in hematological malignancy only till few years back. However, it is turning out to be an important factor in solid tumor, especially NHL like Burkitt lymphoma (BL) and ALCL. The detection of blasts in BM or peripheral blood by routine microscopy is very rare in ALCL because of the submicroscopic nature of involvement of BM. This submicroscopic involvement of BM at baseline which cannot be detected by conventional microscopy, but can be detected by more sensitive methods like flow cytometry or PCR is known as minimal disseminated disease. The target protein for detecting MDD in case of ALCL is NPM-ALK fusion protein by PCR. The detection of MDD and its impact on disease prognosis have been studied and it has been found to be an independent poor prognostic factor for relapse/refractory disease. Patients with both these poor factors did worse in long-term follow-up with 10-year PFS as low as 40% against 86% for those without these features. The other factors such as mediastinal, skin, visceral, and peripheral LN involvement lost significance in multivariate analysis. The role of age-adjusted International Prognostic Index (IPI) and CD3-positivity was not conclusive.

CASE (Continued)

Based on St Jude staging—it was a stage 3 disease, and according to ALCL99 risk stratification, a high-risk disease. He was started on ALCL99 Protocol.

6. What are the different chemotherapeutic options and basic principles of management of ALCL? What is the role of targeted agents as frontline therapy in this patient?

There are different treatment protocols used by European (BFM and Italian) and North American [the Pediatric Oncology Group (POG), the Children's Cancer Group (CCG) and the Children's Oncology Group (COG) groups. These two approaches have considerable differences.
1. European group—short, intensive B-NHL analogous therapy, higher doses of alkylating agents requiring admission, while avoiding anthracyclines
2. North American—long, less intensive, leukemia-based therapy on outpatient basis. It has high cumulative dose of anthracyclines with little or no alkylators.

Pediatric ALCL is a relatively chemosensitive tumor with high response rate and despite the difference in both the strategies the event-free survival (EFS) and OS remained between 65–70% and 70–90%, respectively across time. However, the survival in ALCL is slightly inferior to that of the mature B-NHL, i.e., BL and diffuse large B cell lymphoma (DLBCL). The EFS of ALK-negative ALCL is poor and ranges from 15 to 45%. NHL BFM 90 was the first trial to prospectively test short pulse B-NHL-type treatment strategy for ALCL, based on the retrospective analysis of previous NHL BFM studies. This resulted in a significant reduction in the dose as well as duration of chemotherapy to 2–5 months (as compared to 8–9 months previously), while maintaining a comparable EFS and OS.[7] The high risk of short-term side effects associated with high-dose methotrexate like oral and GI mucositis which leads to fulminant sepsis and even death in some cases, lead to the trial for testing lower concentrations of methotrexate administered in shorter pulses in NHL-BFM95. The trial found that 1 g/m^2 methotrexate infused over 4 hours was noninferior and less toxic than 5 g/m^2 over 24 hours infusion.[8] The low cumulative drug doses and short duration of therapy with comparable EFS and OS with BFM-NHL backbone makes it a standard of therapy for ALCL. The most commonly used protocol to treat ALCL worldwide is based on ALCL99 backbone, which itself is derived from BFM-NHL protocol. The treatment consists of a prephase followed by six alternating cycles of high-dose intensive chemotherapy over a short period of time. The trial recruited 352 children under 22 years of age regardless of ALK status. The total duration of therapy is around 4–5 months. This study proved that intrathecal chemotherapy can be safely omitted and higher dose with shorter infusion duration (3 g/m^2 over 3 hours) methotrexate has less toxicity and same EFS. Addition of vinblastine delayed but did not reduce the risk of relapse. The treatment resulted in excellent 10-year PFS and OS rates of 70 and 90%, respectively. The acute toxicities were high with grade 4 neutropenia reported in 60%, mucositis in 15%. There were very rare late relapses that too in a specific group of patients with poor biology/pathology. There was no report of SMN.[9]

Low stage ALCL needs special mention as the completely resected disease, has 2-year EFS of 100% versus incompletely resected disease with EFS of 30%.[10]

The EFS and OS of ALCL are almost static with different chemotherapeutic agents since 1980s. Moreover, the relapse rate is 30%, regardless of the treatment used. Progressive disease has a very poor prognosis with only 25–40% survival even with aggressive salvage chemotherapy including hematopoietic stem cell transplant (HSCT). So, there is need to develop new targeted therapies.

The different targeted agents are:
- *Drugs targeting CD30: Brentuximab Vedotin (BV)*

Study	Inclusion criteria	N	Treatment description	Results	Comments
Lowe et al. 2021[11]	Newly diagnosed nonlocalized ALK+ pediatric (<22 years) ALCL	68	• Phase II trial • (ANHL12P1) • ALCL99 backbone + BV, to test the toxicity and efficacy of BV • 5 days prophase with 6 cycles chemotherapy every 21 days. BV on day 1 of each cycle (@180 mg/kg)	• 2-year EFS and OS = 79% and 97%, respectively • Mean time of relapse = 7.5 months • No significant neurological toxicity • MDD positive has significant poor EFS (52%) than MDD negative (89%)	• Addition of brentuximab prevented relapse/progression during therapy in all cases, which is remarkable because these cases have worse outcome • MDD is an important prognostic marker

(ALCL: anaplastic large cell lymphoma; ALK: anaplastic lymphoma kinase; EFS: event-free survival; MDD: minimal disseminated disease; OS: overall survival)

- *ALK inhibitors: Crizotinib and ceritinib:* The result of crizotinib arm of ANHL12P1 trial is awaited. There are no studies till date establishing the role of crizotinib as frontline therapy in ALCL. Ceritinib has unacceptable gastrointestinal (GI) toxicity, which limits its use in pediatric ALCL.

Despite the exciting result with BV in ANHL12P1 trial, there are no guidelines to use targeted therapy in frontline; however, studies are ongoing to incorporate these agents as first-line therapy in high-risk ALCL.

CASE (Continued)

The patient came after 10 months of completing treatment with similar complaints of fever on and off with exertional breathlessness for past 20 days. He has also lost appetite for around 1 month. Chest X-ray showed left upper zone opacification. The infection workup including TB was negative. PET-CT was done which showed a local uptake. Fine needle aspiration cytology (FNAC) of the mass showed relapsed ALK+, CD3+ ALCL **(Figs. 6A to F)**.

7. What are the predictors of relapse?

The three most important independent predictors of relapse/refractory disease are: biological, pathological, and clinical factors. Biological factors are the most important among these, which include circulating tumor cells in PB or BM at diagnosis (MDD) and at the end of first cycle of chemotherapy (MRD) and anti-ALK antibody. There is a high rate of concordance between PB and BM so any of them can be used for the same.[12]

- *MDD:* MDD positivity at diagnosis is associated with high risk of relapse. The 5-year PFS was 41% in MDD+ versus 100% in MDD− cases in a study, MDD positivity also correlated with high-risk disease by conventional stratification and mediastinal involvement.[13]

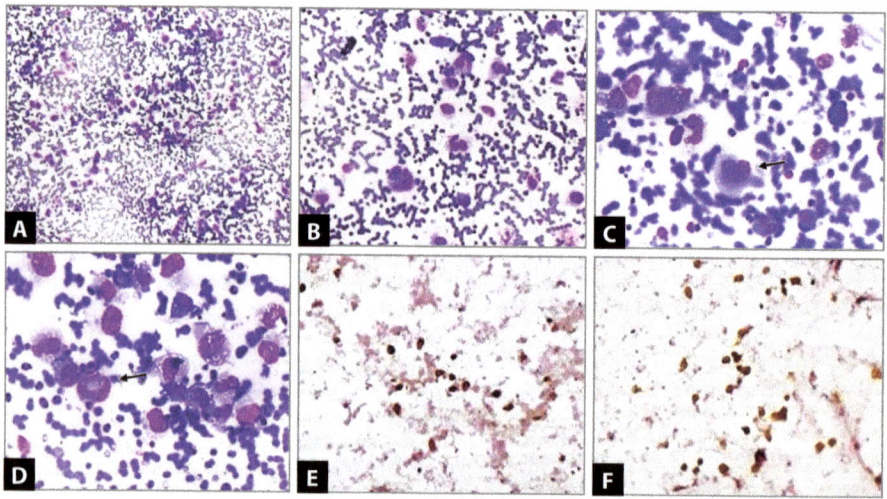

Figs. 6A to F: Fine needle aspiration cytology (FNAC) showing atypical large lymphoid cells with moderate amount of cytoplasm and large pleomorphic nuclei (A and B). Few hallmark cells (black arrows) with kidney- and doughnut-shaped nuclei were present (C and D). Tumor cells are immunopositive for anaplastic lymphoma kinase (ALK) (E) and CD30 (F).
Courtsey: Dr Saumyaranjan Mallik, Additional Professor, Pathology, AIIMS.

- *MRD:* Early MRD positivity is associated with high risk of relapse and inferior survival.[14] The combination of MDD and early MRD assessment helps in identifying patients with highest risk of relapse and very poor survival. 3-year PFS was significantly correlated with the MDD/MRD status: 81.1% in MDD−, 69.6% in MDD+/MRD−, and 15.2% in MDD+/MRD+ patients.[15]
- *Low circulating titers of anti-ALK antibodies:* <1:750 associated with high risk of relapse[14] as antibody titer is inversely proportional to MDD positivity.[16]
- *Histology:* Noncommon variant remains a poor prognostic factor.
- *Clinical high-risk feature:* Visceral, mediastinal, and skin involvement at baseline[17]

Few studies have shown significant correlation between mediastinal or visceral involvement, noncommon histology and MDD positivity.[12,14,15]

A new risk stratification based on biological features has been proposed based on MDD and antibody titers.[18]

8. What is the common time of relapse and what are the poor prognostic factors for relapsed/refractory ALCL?

The rate of relapse in ALCL is 25–35%. The median time of relapse between end of first-line chemotherapy and relapse is 2.6 months (0–69 months).

The poor prognostic factors are:
- *Time to relapse:* Relapse occurring within 12 months of diagnosis is the most consistent poor prognostic factor for subsequent relapse.[19,20]
- *Progressive disease on first-line therapy:* 5-year OS in patients with progressive disease was 25% as compared with 66% in those with later relapses.[19]
- *BM and CNS involvement:* In a study by BFM group, 5-year OS in patients with BM/CNS involvement was 27% versus 62% in those without BM/CNS involvement.[19]
- *CD3 positivity:* CD3 positivity at relapse was found to be a poor prognostic factor in a particular subgroup of relapsed population, i.e., those who had undergone autologous HSCT.[19] However, in ALCL-Relapse trial, higher relapse rate for CD3 positive tumors was seen only among patients who progressed during frontline therapy. No such association was observed in other risk subgroups.[21]

9. What are the treatment options in relapse/refractory ALCL?

There is no uniform consensus guideline for the treatment of relapsed ALCL. The different treatment options are:
- Single-agent Vinblastine
- Stem cell transplant
- Future treatment options—ALK inhibitors, agents targeting CD30, immunotherapy.

10. What is the role of Vinblastine in newly diagnosed and relapsed cases of ALCL?

Newly diagnosed ALCL: Vinblastine was investigated as a part of subtrial ALCL99-VBL. High-risk patients were randomized to receive either no vinblastine or weekly vinblastine for 1 year as maintenance therapy along with the protocol they were already receiving. The 1-year EFS in vinblastine arm was significantly better (91 vs. 74%). However, this effect was not sustained as the 2-year EFS was comparable in both the arms (73 vs. 70%). Thus, addition of Vinblastine as frontline therapy in ALCL, although delays relapse but does not prevent it.[9] Single-agent Vinblastine can replace multiagent chemotherapy in MDD negative ALCL, the studies for which are underway.

Relapsed ALCL: Single-agent Vinblastine given for a prolonged duration has high efficacy in relapsed ALCL. A study conducted by French Society of Pediatric Oncology found Vinblastine monotherapy led to complete remission (CR) in 83% of relapsed patients, which was sustained for 7 years in 36% cases.[22] Another trial, the EICNHL-ALCL-RELAPSE trial, recruited patients with low-risk relapse—CD3 negative and relapsed >12 months from initial diagnosis. Single-agent Vinblastine was given for 24 months. It achieved a 3-year EFS and OS of 85 and 90%, respectively.[21]

11. What is the role of HSCT in relapsed/refractory ALCL?

There is limited data on the role of HSCT in relapsed/refractory ALCL due to the rarity of the disease. Most of the studies are retrospective containing patients treated with different regimes. BFM group has reported the largest retrospective cohort which included 74 children with first relapse. The baseline disease was treated uniformly with BFM-based protocol. The survival was poor in CD3+, early relapse, and those with disseminated disease (CNS and BM). The survival was worse in those who had progression during first-line therapy (25% ± 11%) and who relapsed after treatment completion but within 12 months of diagnosis (50% ± 8%) versus those who relapsed after 12 months of diagnosis (67% ± 11%). EFS was better in CD3 negative relapse (72% ± 9%) versus CD3+ relapse (18% ± 12%). The study also concluded that autologous SCT is a feasible option in first relapse of CD3– ALCL, while allogenic SCT in progressive disease and CD3+ ALCL relapse.[19] Various other retrospective studies have suggested that allogenic SCT may be superior to autologous but with high treatment-related mortality (TRM).[23,24]

The largest and the only prospective trial on first relapsed ALCL was the ALCL-Relapse trial. The type of treatment was based on risk stratification **(Table 1)**.[21]

TABLE 1: Treatment based on risk stratification.

Risk stratification	Treatment received	Results	Conclusion
Very high risk (VHR): Progression/relapse during frontline therapy	Allogenic HSCT: Conditioning regime: TBI + Thiotepa + Etoposide (TBI replaced by busulfan in patients <24 months of age)	• EFS: 41% ± 12% • OS: 59% ± 12%	• Allogenic SCT is very effective in relapsed/refractory ALCL with a high survival of 75% • There is no role of autologous SCT in relapsed/refractory ALCL • Vinblastine monotherapy is effective only in late relapses
High risk (HR): CD3+ relapsed ALCL irrespective of timing of relapse	• Allogenic HSCT and Autologous HSCT if matched donor was not available • Conditioning regime: BEAM	• EFS: 62% ± 10% • OS: 73% ± 9%	
Intermediate risk (IR): CD3– ALCL relapsing within 12 months of starting therapy or prior exposure to Vinblastine	• Autologous HSCT • Conditioning regime: BEAM • Amendment in protocol: Switched to Vinblastine monotherapy due to high relapse rate	• EFS: 44% ± 9% • OS: 78% ± 7%	

Contd...

Contd...

Risk stratification	Treatment received	Results	Conclusion
Low risk (LR): CD3−ALCL relapsing after 12 months of starting therapy	Single-agent Vinblastine	• EFS: 81% ± 9% • OS: 90% ± 6%	• Time to relapse was the most important risk factor for subsequent relapses

(ALCL: anaplastic large cell lymphoma; EFS: event-free survival; HSCT: hematopoietic stem cell transplantation; OS: overall survival; TBI: total body irradiation)

CASE (Continued)

Our index case presented after 12 months of diagnosis (late relapse) and was CD3-negative, so he was started on single agent Vinblastine.

12. What are the upcoming treatment options?

Anaplastic lymphoma kinase inhibitors: Crizotinib was approved for pediatric (age >12 months) relapsed/refractory ALK+ ALCL in January 2021 **(Table 2)**.

TABLE 2: Studies with inclusion criteria, treatment description, results, and comments.

Study	Inclusion criteria	N	Treatment description	Results	Comments
Mosse et al. 2017[25]	Relapse/refractory ALK+ pediatric ALCL Age >12 months to <22 years	26	Single-agent oral Crizotinib twice daily @165 mg/m² (ALCL165) and 280 mg/m² (ALCL280) until disease progression/toxicity	ORR = 88% CR rate: • ALCL165 = 83% • ALCL280 = 80%	Recommended dose 280 mg/m² twice daily
Fischer et al 2021[26]	• Locally advanced/ metastatic ALK+ malignancy • Age >12 months to <18 years	83 (ALCL = 8)	• Phase 1 study • Single-agent oral Ceritinib once daily started @300 mg/m², dose was gradually increased to establish the maximum tolerated dose • Median follow-up duration = 34 months	• Recommended dose: Ceritinib 500 mg/m² once daily with food • Shows promising antitumor activity in ALK-rearranged malignancy • ORR = 75% (6/8)	
Bossi et al. 2020[27]	• Relapsed/ refractory ALK+ ALCL • Median age: 31 years	12	• Single-arm phase II trial • Single-agent oral Crizotinib	• ORR = 83% • 2-year EFS and OS = 65% • RT-PCR for NPM-ALK became negative within 1 month of therapy in 75%	Durable antitumor activity of Crizotinib as monotherapy in R/R ALCL

(ALCL: anaplastic large cell lymphoma; ALK: anaplastic lymphoma kinase; CR: complete remission; EFS: event-free survival; ORR: objective response rate; OS: overall survival; RR: relapsed or refractory; RT-PCR: reverse transcriptase polymerase chain reaction)

Agents targeting CD30 (brentuximab vedotin):

Study	Inclusion criteria	N	Study description	Results	Comments
Locatelli et al. 2018[28]	Relapsed/refractory pediatric ALCL/HL	36 (ALCL = 17)	Open-label, dose escalation, phase I/II study	• ORR = 53% for ALCL • Most common Grade III toxicity—neutropenia	Good response with manageable toxicity

(ALCL: anaplastic large cell lymphoma; HL: Hodgkin lymphoma; ORR: objective response rate)

Immunotherapy

Checkpoint inhibitors: *Nivolumab (PD1 inhibitor):* ALK rearrangement induces increased expression of PD-L1 on tumor cells which allows them to escape immune mechanism. There are two case reports, where Nivolumab has shown good response, where conventional chemotherapy, ALK inhibitors and CD30 inhibitors, have failed.[29,30]

REFERENCES

1. Lowe EJ, Gross TG. Anaplastic large cell lymphoma in children and adolescents. Pediatr Hematol Oncol. 2013;30(6):509-19.
2. Tole S, Wheaton L, Alexander S. Pediatric Anaplastic Large Cell Lymphoma—A Review. Oncol Hematol Rev (US). 2018;14(1):21.
3. Swerdlow SH, Campo E, Pileri SA, Harris NL, Stein H, Siebert R, et al. The 2016 revision of the World Health Organization classification of lymphoid neoplasms. Blood. 2016;127(20):2375-90.
4. Brugières L, le Deley MC, Rosolen A, Williams D, Horibe K, Wrobel G, et al. Impact of the methotrexate administration dose on the need for intrathecal treatment in children and adolescents with anaplastic large-cell lymphoma: results of a randomized trial of the EICNHL Group. J Clin Oncol. 2009;27(6):897-903.
5. Parrilla Castellar ER, Jaffe ES, Said JW, Swerdlow SH, Ketterling RP, Knudson RA, et al. ALK-negative anaplastic large cell lymphoma is a genetically heterogeneous disease with widely disparate clinical outcomes. Blood. 2014;124(9):1473-80.
6. Tsuyama N, Sakamoto K, Sakata S, Dobashi A, Takeuchi K. Anaplastic large cell lymphoma: pathology, genetics, and clinical aspects. J Clin Exp Hematop. 2017;57(3):120-42.
7. Seidemann K, Tiemann M, Schrappe M, Yakisan E, Simonitsch I, Janka-Schaub G, et al. (2001). Short-pulse B-non-Hodgkin lymphoma-type chemotherapy is efficacious treatment for pediatric anaplastic large cell lymphoma: a report of the Berlin-Frankfurt-Münster Group Trial NHL-BFM 90.
8. Woessmann W, Seidemann K, Mann G, Zimmermann M, Burkhardt B, Oschlies I, et al. The impact of the methotrexate administration schedule and dose in the treatment of children and adolescents with B-cell neoplasms: a report of the BFM Group Study NHL-BFM95. Blood. 2005;105(3):948-58.
9. le Deley MC, Rosolen A, Williams DM, Horibe K, Wrobel G, Attarbaschi A, et al. Vinblastine in children and adolescents with high-risk anaplastic large-cell lymphoma: results of the randomized ALCL99-vinblastine trial. J Clin Oncol. 2010;28(25):3987-93.
10. Attarbaschi A, Mann G, Rosolen A, Williams D, Uyttebroeck A, Marky I, et al. (2011). Limited stage I disease is not necessarily indicative of an excellent prognosis in childhood anaplastic large cell lymphoma.
11. Lowe EJ, Reilly AF, Lim MS, Gross TG, Saguilig L, Barkauskas DA, et al. Brentuximab vedotin in combination with chemotherapy for pediatric patients with ALK+ ALCL: results of COG trial ANHL12P1. Blood. 2021;137(26):3595-603.

12. Damm-Welk C, Busch K, Burkhardt B, Schieferstein J, Viehmann S, Oschlies I, et al. Prognostic significance of circulating tumor cells in bone marrow or peripheral blood as detected by qualitative and quantitative PCR in pediatric NPM-ALK–positive anaplastic large-cell lymphoma. Blood. 2007;110(2):670-7.
13. Mussolin L, Pillon M, d'Amore ES, Santoro N, Lombardi A, Fagioli F, et al. Prevalence and clinical implications of bone marrow involvement in pediatric anaplastic large cell lymphoma. Leukemia. 2005;19(9):1643-7.
14. Damm-Welk C, Mussolin L, Zimmermann M, Pillon M, Klapper W, Oschlies I, et al. Early assessment of minimal residual disease identifies patients at very high relapse risk in NPM-ALK-positive anaplastic large-cell lymphoma. Blood. 2014;123(3):334-7.
15. Rigaud C, Abbas R, Grand D, Minard-Colin V, Aladjidi N, Buchbinder N, et al. Should treatment of ALK-positive anaplastic large cell lymphoma be stratified according to minimal residual disease? Pediatr Blood Cancer. 2021;68(6):e28982.
16. Damm-Welk C, Kutscher N, Zimmermann M, Attarbaschi A, Schieferstein J, Knörr F, et al. Quantification of minimal disseminated disease by quantitative polymerase chain reaction and digital polymerase chain reaction for NPM-ALK as a prognostic factor in children with anaplastic large cell lymphoma. Haematologica. 2020;105(8):2141-9.
17. le Deley MC, Brugières L, Williams D, Reiter A. Prognostic Factors in Childhood Anaplastic Large Cell Lymphoma (ALCL): Results of the European Intergroup Study. Blood. 2006;108(11):2050-50.
18. Mussolin L, Damm-Welk C, Pillon M, Zimmermann M, Franceschetto G, Pulford K, et al. Use of minimal disseminated disease and immunity to NPM-ALK antigen to stratify ALK-positive ALCL patients with different prognosis. Leukemia. 2013;27(2):416-22.
19. Woessmann W, Zimmermann M, Lenhard M, Burkhardt B, Rossig C, Kremens B, et al. Relapsed or refractory anaplastic large-cell lymphoma in children and adolescents after Berlin-Frankfurt-Muenster (BFM)-type first-line therapy: a BFM-group study. J Clin Oncol. 2011;29(22):3065-71.
20. Brugières L, Quartier P, le Deley MC, Pacquement H, Perel Y, Bergeron C, et al. Relapses of childhood anaplastic large-cell lymphoma: treatment results in a series of 41 children—a report from the French Society of Pediatric Oncology. Ann Oncol. 2000;11(1):53-8.
21. Knörr F, Brugières L, Pillon M, Zimmermann M, Ruf S, Attarbaschi A, et al. Stem cell transplantation and vinblastine monotherapy for relapsed pediatric anaplastic large cell lymphoma: results of the international, prospective ALCL-relapse trial. J Clin Oncol. 2020;38(34):3999-4009.
22. Brugières L, Pacquement H, le Deley MC, Leverger G, Lutz P, Paillard C, et al. Single-drug vinblastine as salvage treatment for refractory or relapsed anaplastic large-cell lymphoma: a report from the French Society of Pediatric Oncology. J Clin Oncol. 2009;27(30):5056-61.
23. Fukano R, Mori T, Kobayashi R, Mitsui T, Fujita N, Iwasaki F, et al. Haematopoietic stem cell transplantation for relapsed or refractory anaplastic large cell lymphoma: a study of children and adolescents in Japan. Br J Haematol. 2015;168(4):557-63.
24. Strullu M, Thomas C, le Deley MC, Chevance A, Kanold J, Bertrand Y, et al. Hematopoietic stem cell transplantation in relapsed ALK+ anaplastic large cell lymphoma in children and adolescents: a study on behalf of the SFCE and SFGM-TC. Bone Marrow Transplant. 2015;50(6):795-801.
25. Mossé YP, Voss SD, Lim MS, Rolland D, Minard CG, Fox E, et al. Targeting ALK With Crizotinib in Pediatric Anaplastic Large Cell Lymphoma and Inflammatory Myofibroblastic Tumor: A Children's Oncology Group Study. J Clin Oncol. 2017;35(28):3215-21.
26. Fischer M, Moreno L, Ziegler DS, Marshall LV, Zwaan CM, Irwin MS, et al. Ceritinib in paediatric patients with anaplastic lymphoma kinase-positive malignancies: an open-label, multicentre, phase 1, dose-escalation and dose-expansion study. Lancet Oncol. 2021;22(12):1764-76.

27. Bossi E, Aroldi A, Brioschi FA, Steidl C, Baretta S, Renso R, et al. Phase two study of crizotinib in patients with anaplastic lymphoma kinase (ALK)-positive anaplastic large cell lymphoma relapsed/refractory to chemotherapy. Ame J Hematol. 2020;95:E319-21.
28. Locatelli F, Mauz-Koerholz C, Neville K, Llort A, Beishuizen A, Daw S, et al. Brentuximab vedotin for paediatric relapsed or refractory Hodgkin's lymphoma and anaplastic large-cell lymphoma: a multicentre, open-label, phase 1/2 study. Lancet Haematol. 2018;5(10):e450-61.
29. Rigaud C, Abbou S, Minard-Colin V, Geoerger B, Scoazec JY, Vassal G, et al. Efficacy of nivolumab in a patient with systemic refractory ALK+ anaplastic large cell lymphoma. Pediatr Blood Cancer. 2018;65(4).
30. Hebart H, Lang P, Woessmann W. Nivolumab for refractory anaplastic large Cell lymphoma: a case report. Ann Intern Med. 2016;165(8):607-8.

EXPERT OPINION

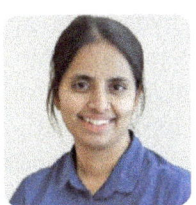

Bhavna Padhye MBBS FRACP MClinTRes PhD
Staff Specialist Pediatric Oncologist
Senior Clinical Lecturer University of Sydney
The Children's Hospital at Westmead Australia, Australia

1. Why do you think ALCL has a myriad of presentations and is often called the great mimicker?

Anaplastic large cell lymphoma, a form of NHL, accounts for 10-15% of all childhood lymphomas. ALCL is a T or null cell lymphoma characterized by the expression of CD30. In children >90% of cases are ALK positive, t (2:5) (p23; q35) involving the *ALK* gene on chromosome 2 and the *NPM* gene on chromosome 5. A minority of ALCL cases have alternative ALK translocation partners.

Pediatric ALCL is characterized by advanced disease, variety of symptoms and extranodal involvement at presentation. Three major presentations are: primary systemic ALCL, ALK+, primary systemic ALCL, ALK- and cutaneous ALCL. A form of ALCL associated with breast implants is described, with an excellent outcome. Cutaneous ALCL, presents with localized or solitary and often ulcerated skin tumors. Most patients with systemic ALCL present as advanced stages (stages III-IV) with peripheral, intra-abdominal or mediastinal lymphadenopathy, systemic symptoms, and extranodal spread including skin, liver, lung, soft tissue, and bone. BM involvement is detected by morphology in less than 15% of cases. As the majority of ALCL in children possess the genetic translocation, a PCR for NPM-ALK provides an ideal platform to assess minimal disease. Minimal disease in BM or peripheral blood found by PCR at diagnosis identified a group of patients with a high incidence of relapse. CNS involvement is rare.

2. Which protocol do you follow for ALCL in your center and why?

Frontline Therapy

Children's Oncology Group (COG) trial *ANHL0131* tested the substitution of vinblastine (APV) for vincristine in children with ALCL when given with APO (doxorubicin, prednisone, and vincristine) chemotherapy (52 weeks of therapy). Results showed similar EFS and no benefit to the patients receiving the additional vinblastine (3 year EFS of 74% for APO vs. 79% for APV, p = 0.68).

The *ALCL99* trial used chemotherapy based on BFM-NHL-90. The first randomization compared methotrexate 1 g/m^2 administered over 24 hours with intrathecal chemotherapy throughout therapy versus methotrexate 3 g/m^2 administered over 3 hours with intrathecal chemotherapy only in prophase of therapy. While the 2-year EFS (73.6 vs. 74.5%) did not differ between the two arms, the toxicity from the methotrexate administered over 3 hours was significantly less and the two CNS relapses both occurred on the arm with 1 g/m^2 and intrathecal chemotherapy. Therefore, it is now considered standard of care when using the ALCL99 regimen to use 3 g/m^2 of methotrexate over 3 hours and intrathecal chemotherapy only in the prophase. The second randomization was for patients with clinically "high-risk features", involvement of skin, mediastinum, liver, lung, and/or spleen. Patients were randomized to standard chemotherapy ± vinblastine weekly as maintenance for a total duration of 1 year of therapy. While vinblastine delayed relapses, there was no difference in the 2-year EFS (73 vs. 70%). Thus, the ALCL99 trial demonstrated a failure rate of approximately 30%, all but initial intrathecal chemotherapy can safely be omitted when using 3 g/m^2 of methotrexate administered over 3 hours, and the addition of vinblastine maintenance did not improve EFS.

ANHL12P1 determined the toxicity and efficacy of *BV* (CD30-directed antibody conjugated to monomethyl auristatin E) with chemotherapy (ALCL99) in children with *newly diagnosed* nonlocalized ALK+ and CD30+ ALCL. The 2-year EFS was 79.1% (95% CI, 67.2-87.1) and OS was 97.0% (95% CI, 88.1-99.2). The addition of BV prevented relapses during therapy, and the OS and EFS estimates compared favorably with results obtained using conventional chemotherapy.

This is our standard of care currently.

3. Your thoughts on the use of crizotinib in ALCL and its duration of use?
- Do you use single agent vinblastin for ALCL? your thoughts on it?
- In refractory/relapsed ALCL what chemotherapy do you use for salvage?

Relapsed/Refractory ALCL

Crizotinib is an inhibitor of receptor tyrosine kinases including ALK and hepatocyte growth factor receptor (HGFR, c-Met). A phase I/II Study ADVL0912 (NCT00939770) included 26 patients aged 1–21 years with *relapsed or refractory ALCL (R/R ALCL)* after at least one systemic treatment who received oral crizotinib at 280 mg/m^2 (n = 20 patients) or 165 mg/m^2 (n = 6) twice daily until disease progression or unacceptable toxicity. Objective response was observed in 23 patients (88%, 95% CI 71–96%), with CR in 21 (81%). Among responders, 39% maintained response for at least 6 months and 22% maintained response for at least 12 months. Crizotinib is approved by Food and Drug Administration (FDA) for treatment of pediatric patients 1 year of age and older and young adults with relapsed or refractory systemic ALK + ALCL.

ANHL12P1 is assessing role of crizotinib in combination with ALCL99 chemotherapy in newly diagnosed patients with ALCL.

Brugieres et al. reported the use of single-agent vinblastine in 36 patients included prospectively in the French database for pediatric ALCL who were treated with vinblastine for resistant primary disease, a first relapse, or subsequent relapses. 5-year OS was 65% (95% CI, 48–79%), and 5-year EFS was 30% (95% CI, 17–47%).

4. Autologous versus allogeneic HSCT for consolidation in R/R ALCL—your thoughts.

The largest reported retrospective cohort of R/R ALCL included 74 children with first relapse of ALCL who were uniformly treated with frontline BFM-type NHL therapy and were considered for reinduction chemotherapy with auto-HSCT at relapse. This study identified time to relapse and CD3 expression as potential prognostic factors, the optimal use of allo-HSCT versus auto-HSCT remained uncertain except in patients who relapse during initial therapy. Knorr et al. conducted the European Intergroup for Childhood Non-Hodgkin Lymphoma (EICNHL) International ALCL-Relapse study.[13] The study stratified patients in risk groups based on time to relapse and CD3 positivity. Those with recurrence during upfront treatment (very high risk) or a CD3-positive relapse (high risk) were recommended allogeneic SCT after reinduction chemotherapy. Patients with a CD3-negative relapse within 1 year after the diagnosis or prior exposure to vinblastine (intermediate risk) received autologous SCT after carmustine-etoposide-cytarabine-melphalan. Patients with a CD3-negative relapse >1 year after initial diagnosis (low risk) received vinblastine monotherapy. Allogeneic SCT offered a chance for cure in patients with high-risk ALCL relapse. For early relapsed ALCL auto-HSCT was not effective. Vinblastine monotherapy achieved cure in patients with late relapse; however, it was not effective for early relapses.

Depending on the agents used in upfront therapy BV, crizotinib (or other ALK inhibitors), and vinblastine are all efficacious agents to bridge to allo-HSCT or as protracted maintenance therapy in specific subgroups.

CHAPTER 9

Diffuse Large B Cell Lymphoma

Debabrata Mohapatra, Jagdish P Meena

CASE VIGNETTE

Miss R 12-year-old female, presented with left-sided neck swelling for 8 months prior to presentation. There was no history of weight loss, night sweat, or fever. There was no history of Koch's contact.

On examination, there was no pallor, icterus, or petechiae. She had left cervical and supraclavicular lymphadenopathy 3 × 3 cm, nontender, firm, noninflamed, and nonmatted. There was no hepatosplenomegaly or any other swelling over the body.

1. What are your clinical differentials?

Given below is a list of differential diagnosis of chronic cervical lymphadenopathy **(Table 1)**.[1]

TABLE 1: Differential diagnosis of chronic cervical lymphadenopathy.

Etiology	Causes (chronic)
Infective	Tuberculosis, CMV, EBV, and HIV
Immunologic	Sarcoidosis, systemic lupus erythematosus, common variable immune deficiency, and chronic granulomatous disease
Metabolic	Gaucher's disease, Niemann–Pick disease, and Tangier disease
Neoplastic	Non-Hodgkin lymphoma, Hodgkin lymphoma, nasopharyngeal carcinoma, rhabdomyosarcoma, and Langerhans cell histiocytosis

(CMV: cytomegalovirus; EBV: Epstein–Barr virus; HIV: human immunodeficiency virus)

Criteria that are more consistent with malignancy are size >2–2.5 cm, firm/hard consistency, supraclavicular/axillary localization, posterior edge of the sternocleidomastoid muscle, absence of tenderness, low mobility, progressive course, and B symptoms.

Criteria that are less consistent with malignancy: under 1.5 cm in size, soft consistency, tender, erythema, fluctuation, mobility, and regressive course.[1]

If there is a suspicion of malignancy in pediatric patients, the type of malignancy differs with age. Under 6 years of age, acute leukemia, neuroblastoma, rhabdomyosarcoma, and non-Hodgkin lymphoma (NHL) are common causes, while between ages 7 and 13 years, NHL and Hodgkin's lymphoma (HL) are roughly equal. After 13, Hodgkin's disease is the leading malignant cause of neck nodes till the rest of the adolescence.[2]

In the index child, NHL and HL were the initial differential diagnoses.

2. How will you approach the case to reach a diagnosis?

Initial investigations and approach to lymphadenopathy are given in the algorithm below **(Flowchart 1)**.[3]

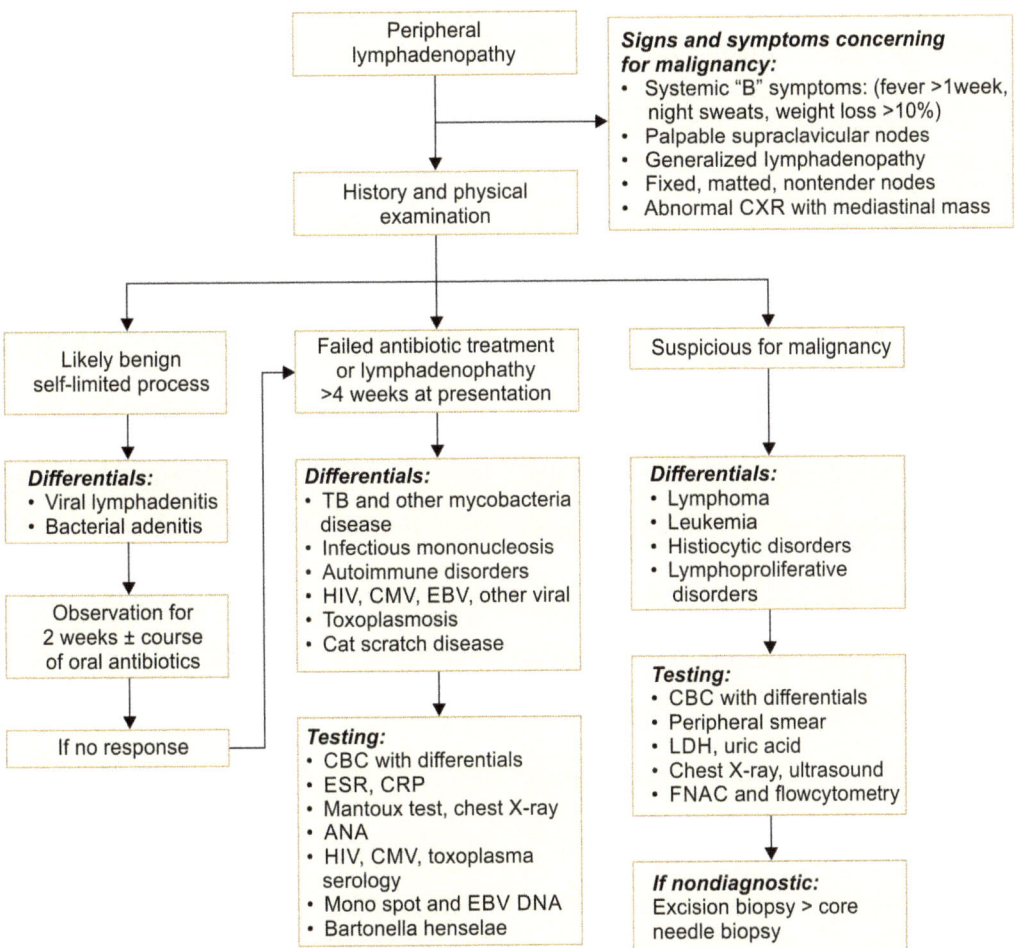

Flowchart 1: Initial investigations and approach to lymphadenopathy.

(ANA: antinuclear antibody; CBC: complete blood count; CRP: C reactive protein; CMV: cytomegalovirus; EBV: Epstein–Barr virus; ESR: erythrocyte sedimentation rate; FNAC: fine needle aspiration cytology; HIV: human immunodeficiency virus; LDH: lactate dehydrogenase)

Although excision biopsy remains the gold standard for the diagnosis of malignant lymph nodes, core needle biopsy is many times the only doable procedure in resource constraint settings due to logistic reasons. It can be used for immunohistochemistry and molecular diagnosis, with evidence suggesting that when performed by an experienced pathologist and by imaging guidance, it has comparable diagnostic efficacy as excision biopsy.[4]

In the index case, hemogram and biochemistry were within normal limits, with serum lactate dehydrogenase (LDH) of 368 U/L and Mantoux test was nonreactive. The patient underwent a core needle biopsy.

3. What morphological findings and immunohistochemistry will help you reach the specific diagnosis?

Pediatric lymphomas can be classified into HL and NHL. HL can be further divided into classic HL (CHL) and nodular lymphocyte-predominant HL (NLPHL) based on pathology.

Non-Hodgkin lymphoma is a heterogeneous group of lymphoid malignancies originating from B-, T- or NK cells. Common NHLs in children include:
- Burkitt lymphoma (BL)
- Lymphoblastic lymphoma (LBL)
- Diffuse large B-cell lymphoma (DLBCL)
- Anaplastic large cell lymphoma (ALCL).

The immunohistochemistry and molecular characterization of pediatric NHL is given in the **Table 2**.[5]

TABLE 2: Immunohistochemistry and molecular characterization of pediatric non-Hodgkin lymphoma.

	BL (50–60%)	LBCL (10–15%)		LL (20–25%)		ALCL (10–12%)
		DLBCL	PMBL	B-LL	T-LL	
Immunohistochemistry						
MIB1	~100%	40–90%	30–90%	Not informative	Not informative	Not informative
IHC panels typically positive	CD10 CD19 CD20 CD79a sIg Bcl-6	CD10 CD19 CD20 CD79a	CD30 CD10 CD19 CD20 CD79a MUM1 MAL	TdT CD19 CD20 CD79a	TdT cCD3 CD4 CD8 CD7	CD30 ALK
IHC panels sometimes positive		sIg Bcl-6 MUM1	Bcl-6	CD10 CD20	CD10 CD5	cCD3 CD4 CD8 CD7 CD5
Cytogenetic	t(8;14) t(2;8) t(8;22)	R8q24 (~30%)	Few data	Few data	Translocations involving 14q11-13; few other data	t(2;5) >90% or variants involving 2p23
Molecular biology	MYC/IGH IGK/MYC MYC/IGL	Translocations involving MYC, BCL-2, BCL-6	Nuclear factor-kB pathway dysregulation	IGH/TCR rearrangements	NOTCH/FBXW, PTEN IGH/TCR rearrangements	NPM/ALK >90% or variants

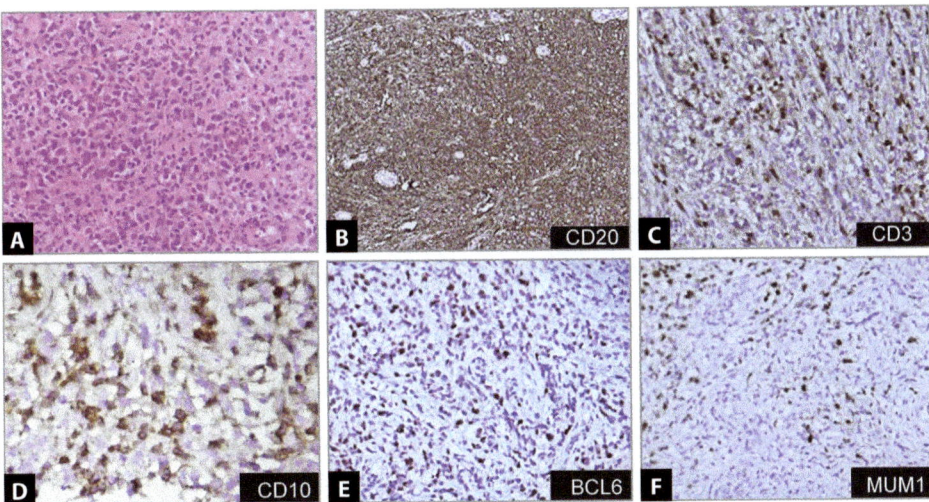

Figs. 1A to F: Microphotograph shows sheets of large atypical lymphoid cells(A). The cells are immuno-positive for CD20 (B), CD10 (D) while negative for CD3 (C), BCL6 (E) and MUM1 (F).
Courtesy: Dr Saumyaranjan Mallik, Additional Professor, Pathology, AIIMS.

Biopsy of the index case was suggestive of large atypical cells which were immune-positive for CD20 (Strong), CD10, Epstein–Barr virus (EBV) latent membrane protein (LMP), CD79a, and LCA. They were negative for CD3, CD30, ALK, and CD15. The final diagnosis of DLBCL-not otherwise specified (NOS) was made **(Figs. 1A to F)**.

4. What is the role of genetic testing in DLBCL?

Recurrent translocations involving BCL-6, BCL-2, and MYC are commonly found in DLBCL patients, though the prevalence of MYC amplification is less common than BL. The absence of these translocations doesn't rule out DLBCL due to the heterogeneous nature of the disease and in that case, it is labeled as DLBCL-NOS. These recurrent translocations impart worse prognosis to DLBCL as compared to the NOS subtype.

Diffuse large B-cell lymphomas that contain any two of these translocations (MYC/BCL2, MYC/BCL6, MYC/BCL2/BCL6) are labeled as double-hit lymphomas (DHLs) and are associated with a very poor prognosis in adults. These entities are relatively rare in the pediatric population.[6]

5. What are the differences between DLBCL and more common but closely mimicking BL?

Unlike in adults, DLBCL is less common in pediatrics as compared to BL. The clinic-pathological differences between these two mimicking diseases are highlighted in the **Table 3**.[7]

TABLE 3: Clinic-pathological differences between diffuse large B-cell lymphoma and Burkitt lymphoma.

Lymphoma type	Burkitt lymphoma	Diffuse large B-cell lymphoma
Clinical	<ul><li>Children > adults</li><li>Extranodal (abdominal) > nodal</li><li>Bulky, rapidly growing masses</li><li>Commonly go into tumor lysis syndrome (TLS)</li></ul>	<ul><li>Adults > children</li><li>Nodal or extranodal</li><li>Sometimes large mass lesions, often localized</li><li>TLS less common</li></ul>
Histological	<ul><li>Medium sized cells</li><li>Cytoplasmic vacuolation</li><li>Starry-sky pattern common</li></ul>	<ul><li>Large oval cells</li><li>Irregular nuclei, scant cytoplasm</li><li>Sometimes starry sky</li></ul>
Immunohistochemistry	<ul><li>Ki67~100%</li><li>CD20+, CD10+, Bcl-6+, sIg+</li><li>Bcl-2–, CD5–, TdT–,</li></ul>	<ul><li>Ki67~90–95%</li><li>CD20+, CD10–/+, Bcl-6+/–, Bcl-2+/–, sIg+/–</li></ul>
Molecular	<ul><li>t(8;14), t(2;8), or t(8;22) (myc and IgH or IgL)</li><li>No bcl-2 or bcl-6 translocation</li></ul>	bcl-2 and bcl-6 abnormalities common, myc abnormal in a minority

6. What are the differences between pediatric DLBCL and the adult counterpart?

Though DLBCL can occur both in adults as well as pediatrics, there are biologic as well as prognostic difference between these two. Pediatric DLBCL appears to behave as more uniform manner with a better prognosis as compared to the adults. The differences between the two are given in the **Table 4**.[8]

TABLE 4: Differences between pediatric diffuse large B-cell lymphoma (DLBCL) and adult DLBCL.

Age group	Pediatric DLBCL	Adult DLBCL
Origin	Mostly germinal center origin and named as germinal center B-cell–like, GCB type	Mostly post germinal center origin and named as activated B-cell–like, ABC type
Transformation	Most pediatric DLBCL are de novo and behave more uniformly	A subset of adult DLBCL result from transformation of indolent follicular lymphoma
Immunohistochemistry	70% are CD10+ and bcl-6+	30% are CD10+
Molecular	Lack of t(14;18) and NF-kB alteration in pediatrics	t(14;18) and NF-kB alteration are found
Prognosis	Good and uniform prognosis	Worse and variable prognosis depending on GCB vs. ABC origin

7. What additional investigations will you do to stage the disease?

Most of the trials in NHL have used Murphy/St Jude's staging system. The details of the staging system is given **Table 5**.[9]

TABLE 5: Details of the staging system.

Stage	Criteria for extent of disease
I	A single tumor (extranodal) or single anatomic area (nodal) with the exclusion of the mediastinum and abdomen
II	• A single tumor (extranodal) with regional node involvement • Two or more nodal areas on the same side of the diaphragm • Two single (extranodal) tumors with or without regional node on the same side of the diaphragm • A primary gastrointestinal tract tumor with or without mesenteric nodes, grossly and completely excised
III	• Two single tumors (extranodal) on opposite sides of the diaphragm • Two or more nodal areas above and below the diaphragm • All of the primary intrathoracic tumors (mediastinal, pleural, thymic) • All extensive primary intra-abdominal disease • All paraspinal or epidural tumors, regardless of the other tumor site(s)
IV	Any of the above with initial central nervous system (CNS) and/or bone marrow involvement (<25% malignant cells)

Considering the extent of extranodal diseases in NHLs, a revised International Pediatric NHL Staging System (IPNHLSS) was proposed and remains to be validated.[10]

Positron emission tomography-computed tomography (PET-CT) is increasingly used in staging and response assessment of malignant lymphomas. [18F]Fluorodeoxyglucose (FDG)-PET-CT is more accurate than CT for staging in HL and NHL with increased sensitivity, particularly for extranodal disease. Upstaging occurs more commonly than downstaging, with management alterations in some patients, particularly patients with the limited disease in CT.[11] The good interobserver agreement has been reported in NHL when the five-point Deauville scores are used to stage the disease as follows objectively:

1. No uptake
2. Uptake ≤ mediastinum
3. Uptake > mediastinum but ≤ liver
4. Uptake moderately higher than liver
5. Uptake markedly higher than liver and/or new lesions.

Although most pediatric NHL protocols still use bone marrow biopsy (BMB) to detect marrow infiltration by lymphoma and label it as the gold standard, some new evidence suggests contrary. The guidelines issued by the European Society for Medical Oncology (ESMO) in 2018 indicated that FDG-PET/CT is sufficient for body mass index (BMI) assessment in adults. The pediatric evidence for the same were poor till a recent meta analysis by Zhizhuo-Li et al.,[12] in 2021 concluded that as compared to BMB, FDG-PET/CT was a better diagnostic method to evaluate marrow involvement in pediatric Hodgkin and NHL patients with extremely high diagnostic accuracy.

Lactate dehydrogenase has long been known as an adverse prognostic indicator of lymphomas and can predict tumor load and indirectly survival.[13]

We use PET/CT, BMB, cerebrospinal fluid (CSF), and baseline LDH for all NHL patients at diagnosis. The index patient had LDH 368 U/L, baseline PET/CT s/o multiple enlarged nodes at left cervical level IB, II, III, IV, and supraclavicular location. Baseline BMB and CSF were negative. The final staging of the case was stage II.

8. How will you risk stratify this patient for deciding the treatment intensity?

Risk stratification in NHL is a composite analysis of multiple parameters and slightly varies based on the protocol used in treatment. Below is the summary of risk stratification and treatment recommendations as per the two commonly used protocols for BL/leukemia and DLBCL **(Table 6)**.

TABLE 6: Summary of risk stratification and treatment recommendations.

Trial	Stratum	Disease manifestations	Treatment
FAB/LMB-96	A	Completely resected stage I and abdominal stage II	Two cycles of chemotherapy
	B	Multiple extra-abdominal sites Nonresected stage I and II, III (normal LDH)	Prephase + four cycles of chemotherapy (reduced-intensity arm)
		Stage III (elevated LDH), marrow <25% blasts, no stage IV CNS disease	Prephase + four cycles of chemotherapy (reduced-intensity arm) + six doses of rituximab
	C	Mature B-cell ALL (>25% blasts in marrow) and/or stage IV CNS disease	Prephase + six cycles of chemotherapy (full-intensity arm) and only two maintenance cycles + six doses of rituximab
NHL-BFM-95	R1	Completely resected stage I and abdominal stage II	Two cycles of chemotherapy
	R2	Nonresected stage I/II and stage III with LDH <500 IU/L	Prephase + four cycles of chemotherapy (24-hour methotrexate infusion)
	R3	Stage III with LDH 500–999 IU/L, stage IV, B-cell ALL (>25% blasts), and LDH <1,000 IU/L No CNS disease	Prephase + five cycles of chemotherapy (24 h methotrexate infusion)
	R4	Stage III, IV, B-cell ALL with LDH >1,000 IU/L any CNS disease	Prephase + 6 cycles of chemotherapy (24 hours methotrexate infusion)

(ALL: acute lymphoblastic leukemia; BFM: Berlin-Frankfurt-Munich; CNS: central nervous system; FAB: French–American–British; LDH: lactate dehydrogenase; LMB-96: lymphomes malins B-96; NHL: non-Hodgkin lymphoma)

The index case was a nonresected stage II disease with LDH <500 IU/L, so final risk stratification as R2 in Berlin-Frankfurt-Munich (BFM) protocol and stratum B in lymphomes malins B (LMB) protocol.

9. How will you treat this patient?

Most of the NHL protocols start the patient on a less intensive prephase chemotherapy before starting the multidrug intense regimen to prevent infectious and metabolic complications associated with the high tumor load at the beginning. In a study[14] on 100 DLBCL patients there was a significant improvement in performance status of the patients who received prephase and also febrile neutropenia was lower (16%) in the prephase cohort as compared with the nonprephase cohort (34%; $p = 0.03$). In view of significant undernutrition and bulky disease in our patients, we always initiate therapy with prophase, i.e., dexamethasone 5 mg/m^2/day OD on days 1–2 followed by 10 mg/m^2/day in two divided doses on days 3–5, cyclophosphamide 200 mg/m^2/day on day 1–2 along with triple intrathecal therapy.

Most of the pediatric DLBCL are treated as per one of the two commonly used protocols producing almost similar outcomes.

The LMB-96 protocol treated both DLBL and other high-grade mature B-cell lymphomas on the same regimen resulting in a 4-year event-free survival (EFS) of 92% was reported for children with DLBCL [excluding those with primary mediastinal large B-cell lymphoma (PMLBL)].[15] To further improve outcomes, an international B-NHL protocol for children with high-grade mature B-cell lymphomas, which featured a rituximab randomization for those with high-risk disease (stage III with LDH 2X upper limit of normal, stage IV) was tested by the LMB group. The first interim analysis indicated a survival advantage for rituximab group as a result of which the randomization was stopped.[16] Rituximab has been accepted as the standard of care for high-risk mature B-NHLs.

A similar observation was made in the BFM mature B-cell study in which children with DLBCL were treated with a contemporary regimen designed for those with BL.[17]

The outcomes as per the study groups are outlined in **Table 7**.[18]

TABLE 7: Risk groupwise survival in B-NHL in both the major NHL study groups.

Protocol	Risk group	5 years EFS
B-NHL (FAB-LMB-96)	A	98%
	B	92%
	C	84%
B-NHL (BFM)	R1	94%
	R2	94%
	R3	85%
	R4	81%

(BFM: Berlin-Frankfurt-Munich; FAB: French–American–British; LMB-96: lymphomes malins B-96; NHL: non-Hodgkin lymphoma)

As per unit protocol, the patient was started on BFM NHL-95 protocol. She received a prephase and was planned for four cycles of high-dose methotrexate-based chemotherapy cycles.

10. How will you assess the response in this patient?

The response evaluation is conventionally established by CT or MRI of involved sites in conjunction with a morphologic evaluation of BM and CSF if involved at diagnosis. The standard NHL response criteria were defined by Sandlund et al., in 2015 **(Table 8)**.[19]

The lack of universal availability of FDG-PET is accounted for in this system; however, in centers where FDG-PET is available, it is recommended to be used and designated accordingly. Pathologic evaluation of a residual FDG-PET-negative mass provides the most direct evidence

TABLE 8: Response assessment criteria in NHL.

Response	Definitions
CR	The disappearance of all diseases (three designations) • Resected residual mass that is pathologically (morphologically) negative for the disease • BM and CSF morphologically free of disease • CT or MRI reveals no residual disease or new lesions
CRb	• Residual mass has no morphologic evidence of disease from limited or core biopsy, with no new lesions by imaging examination • BM and CSF morphologically free of disease • No new and/or progressive disease elsewhere
CRu	• Residual mass is negative by FDG-PET; no new lesions by imaging examination • BM and CSF morphologically free of disease • No new and/or progressive disease elsewhere
PR	• *50% decrease in SPD on CT or MRI*; FDG-PET may be positive (Deauville score of 4–5 with reduced uptake compared with baseline) with no new and/or PD • Morphologic evidence of disease may be present in BM or CSF if present at diagnosis; however, there should be 50% reduction in percentage of lymphoma cells
MR	• *Decrease in SPD > 25% but < 50% on CT or MRI*; no new and/or PD • Morphologic evidence of disease may be present in BM or CSF if present at diagnosis; however, there should be 25–50% reduction in percentage of lymphoma cells
NR	• For those who do not meet CR, PR, MR, or PD criteria
PD	• For those with >25% increase in SPD on CT or MRI, Deauville score 4 or 5 on FDG-PET with an increase in lesional uptake from baseline • OR development of new morphologic evidence of disease in BM or CSF

(BM: bone marrow; CR: complete response; CRb: complete response biopsy negative; CRu: complete response unconfirmed; CSF: cerebrospinal fluid; CT: computed tomography; FDG: [18F]fluorodeoxyglucose; MR: minor response; MRI: magnetic resonance imaging; NHL: non-Hodgkin lymphoma; NR: no response; PD: progressive disease; PET: positron emission tomography; PR: partial response; SPD: sum of product of greatest perpendicular diameters)

of whether a true CR has been achieved. The need for a CR unconfirmed designation may become unnecessary if sufficient evidence becomes available that FDG-PET-negative masses reflect a true CR in children and adolescents with NHL.

After starting on BFM-95 protocol risk group-R2, the patient went into partial response after AA and BB cycles. Following one more cycle of CC, she still remained in partial response, labeling it as refractory NHL.

11. What is the evidence for minimal disseminated disease (MDD) monitoring in B-NHL?

Similar to minimal residual disease (MRD) monitoring in children with acute lymphoblastic leukemia, MDD as detected by polymerase chain reaction (PCR) or flow cytometry is now reported as an evidence for sub-microscopic involvement of marrows that are morphologically free of disease. MDD testing (by either flow cytometric or molecular method), which can detect one in 10,000 to one in 100,000 cells, is increasingly being done. MDD technology has been developed for the major pediatric NHL subtypes. It includes flow cytometric determination of PCR products of immunoglobulin gene rearrangements for mature B-cell lymphomas (e.g., BL and DLBCL). Though the inclusion of these data is not a part of the current standard B-NHL response evaluation systems in the literature, this information can now be included in the description of response evaluation as supportive data, in centers where facility for the same is available. Like the role of MDD in deciding refractoriness in some pediatric NHLs like ALCL, DLBCL patients with MDD positivity are at an increased chance of relapse compared to those who are MDD negative and may deserve therapy intensification in coming future as newer evidences emerge.[20]

12. What are the treatment options for relapsed/refractory NHL at this stage?

There is a paucity of evidence about the best conditioning regimen for refractory or relapsed NHL in pediatric patients.

There is limited data on salvage regimens for pediatric relapsed/refractory B-NHL in small series of patients with variable histology and disease status. The various available options reported are given in **Table 9**.[21]

TABLE 9: Salvage chemotherapy options for relapsed pediatric NHL.

Author	Group	Age (years)	Histology	N (ref/rel)	Salvage regimen	CR	ORR
Gentet et al., 1990[22]	SFOP	<18	B-NHL	12 (NA)	CYVE	33%	66%
Griffin et al., 2009[23]	COG	<21	B-NHL/BAL	20 (NA)	R-ICE	NA	60%
Jourdain et al., 2015[24]	SFOP	<18	BL/BAL, DLBCL, PMBCL	31 (0/31)	CYVE	48%	61%
Jourdain et al., 2015	SFOP	<18	BL/BAL, DLBCL, PMBCL	5 (0/5)	ICE	40%	60%
Osumi et al., 2016[25]	JPLSG	<17	B-NHL	22 (NA)	R-ICE	NA	72%
Rigaud et al., 2019[26] SFOP		<18	BL/BAL, DLBCL, PMBCL	18 (0/18)	R-CYVE	56%	72%
Rigaud et al., 2019[26]	SFOP	<18	BL/BAL, DLBCL, PMBCL	7 (0/7)	R-ICE	43%	57%

(BAL: B mature acute lymphoblastic leukemia; BL: Burkitt lymphoma; B-NHL: B-cell non-Hodgkin lymphoma; CCSG: Children Cancer Study Group; COG: Children's Oncology Group; CR: complete response; CYVE: high-dose cytarabine and etoposide; DECAL: dexamethasone, etoposide, cisplatin, cytarabine, and l-asparaginase; DLBCL: diffuse large B-cell lymphoma; ICE: ifosfamide, carboplatin, etoposide; JPLSG: Japanese Pediatric Leukemia/Lymphoma Study Group; N: number of patients; NA: not available (not reported/not analyzed); ORR: overall response rate; PMBCL: primary mediastinal B-cell lymphoma; R: Rituximab; rel: relapse; ref: refractory; SFOP: Société Française d'Oncologie Pédiatrique)

The overall response rate (ORR) ranges from 50 to 72%, with CR rates of 33–56%. In a SFOP phase II study, high-dose cytarabine and etoposide (CYVE) has proven effective and safe, with an ORR of 66%.[22] In the study by Jourdain et al.,[24] CYVE was the most frequent option in patients who relapsed from LMB favorable treatment groups A or B resulting in the ORR of 61%.

The ICE (ifosfamide, carboplatin, and etoposide) regimen was first shown to be effective and safe in pediatric patients with NHL Kung et al.[27] The ICE regimen has the advantages of no further anthracycline exposure and acceptable extra hematological toxicity. Rituximab, in combination with ICE (R-ICE), produced an ORR of 60% in a single-arm COG study [23] and 72% in the Japanese pediatric leukemia-lymphoma group,[25] confirming the efficacy of the R-ICE regimen.

In patients who relapsed from the LMB 2001 study, rituximab was combined with the CYVE regimen in groups A and B, showing an ORR of 72%, and with the ICE regimen in group C patients with an ORR of 57%.[26] Rituximab is added to all salvage regimens, irrespective of previous exposure to the drug, and the R-ICE regimen remains the most used treatment in pediatric patients with r/r B-NHL.

The index patient was started on the R-ICE protocol, and after two cycles, she achieved a complete metabolic response. After CMR, she was planned for consolidation with an autologous stem cell transplant (ASCT).

13. What stem cell source and conditioning regimen will you use for ASCT in relapsed/refractory DLBCL?

Autologous stem cell transplant is more commonly used than allogeneic stem cell transplant in r/r B-NHL. Burkhardt et al.,[28] in a study conducted on 693 relapsed/refractory NHLs in children and adolescents, found that there was no clear advantage of allogeneic versus autologous hematopoietic stem cell transplantation (HSCT); likely because the graft-versus-lymphoma effect was balanced by higher transplant-related mortality (TRM) for allogeneic HSCT. Remission status pre-HSCT was highly associated with the outcome. An OS probability progressively declines parallel to the depth of response, from 60% for patients transplanted in CR to 11% for those transplanted with progressive disease.

In a Children's Oncology Group Study A5962[29], relapsed lymphoma patients achieving CR or PR after 2–4 courses of reinduction underwent peripheral blood stem cell (PBSC) mobilization and apheresis with a target collection dose of 5×10^6 CD34$^+$/kg. Eligible subjects received autologous PBSCT after CBV (cyclophosphamide, BCNU, and etoposide) conditioning regimen (7,200 mg/m^2, 450–300 mg/m^2, 2,400 mg/m^2). The 3-year OS for all patients was 51%, 64% for transplanted patients. The initial duration of remission had a significant effect on OS, with those relapsing after 12 months having better outcomes (3-year OS 70 vs. 34%) ($p = 0.003$).

A study published in 2015 American Society for Blood and Marrow Transplantation (ASBMT) evaluated the impact of a conditioning regimen on outcomes for adult patients with lymphoma undergoing high-dose therapy with ASCT.[30] Among patients with DLBCL, CBV resulted in worse outcomes than BEAM, i.e., BCNU, etoposide, cytarabine, and melphalan (3-year OS 43 vs. 58%). Though no direct comparison of conditioning regimens is available in pediatric patients, BEAM appears to be less toxic and provides better OS than other chemotherapy or total body irradiation (TBI)-containing regimens.

In the index case; after stem cell mobilization using granulocyte-colony stimulating factor (G-CSF) and one dose of injection plerixafor, PBSC harvest was done and her stem cells were cryopreserved. She was started with ursodeoxycholic acid (UDCA), fluconazole, acyclovir, and prednisolone eye drops. She received BEAM (BCNU on day-7, etoposide, and cytarabine on days 6, 5, 4, 3, and melphalan on day 2) as conditioning and the cryopreserved stem cells were infused. Both neutrophil and platelet engraftment occurred on day + 18.

14. What is the survival rate after ASCT in this setting, and are there any alternative methods to salvage this child if the facility of ASCT is not available?

In the largest, most extensive pediatric NHL relapse study by Burkhardt et al.,[28] that analyzed treatment and outcome of 639 relapsed NHLs in children and adolescents, survival was in the range of 50% for patients who underwent HSCT, while survival for r/r NHL without HSCT was below 10%. Only a few low-risk individual patients were alive without HSCT, particularly with very late relapses.

15. What are the advances in the management of DLBCL?

With promising results, numerous novel therapies are being tested in adults with r/r B-NHL, mostly in DLBCL. The small number of children with r/r B-NHL limits the conduction of such trials in exclusive pediatric age groups. Some of the trials of newer agents are mentioned in the Table 10.[21]

TABLE 10: Trials of newer agents.

	Agent	Target	Age years	Disease	Phase	Reference
Next-generation monoclonal antibodies	Obinutuzumab (increased FcR affinity)	CD20	CAYA (3–31 y)	B-NHL	Phase II	Barth et al., 2018
Checkpoint blockade inhibitors (anti-PD1)	Pembrolizumab	PD1	Adults	PMBCL	Phase I	Zinzani et al., 2017
				PMBCL	Phase II	Armand et al., 2019
B-cell signaling inhibitors-Bruton TK (BTK) inhibitors	Ibrutinib	BTK	CAYA (1–30 y)	B-NHL	Phase III	Burke et al., 2019
Bi-specific T-cell engagers (BiTE)	Blinatumomab	CD19/CD3	Adults	DLBCL	Phase II	Viardot et al., 2016
	FBTA05 (increased ADCC)	CD20/CD3	CA < 18	B-NHL	Compassionate	Schuster et al., 2015
Chimeric antigen receptor T (CAR) T-cells	CD19 CAR-T (tisagenlecleucel)	CD19	CA < 18	B-NHL	Phase II	–
	CD22 CAR-T	CD22	CAYA (3–30 y)	BAL, B-NHL	Phase I	–
	CD19/CD22 CAR-T	CD19/CD22	CAYA (3–30 y)	BAL, B-NHL	Phase I	–

(ADCC: antibody-dependent cell-mediated cytotoxicity; ALL: acute lymphoblastic leukemia; BAL: B mature acute lymphoblastic leukemia; BL: Burkitt lymphoma; B-NHL: B non-Hodgkin lymphoma; CA: children/adolescents; CAYA: children, adolescents, young adults; DLBCL: diffuse large B cell lymphoma; PMBCL: primary mediastinal large B cell lymphoma)

16. How will you follow this patient after ASCT?

Mounier et al.[31] extensively described the late effects in NHL survivors. These were cardiovascular in 20%, neuropsychiatric effects in 17%, musculoskeletal disorders in 11%, and pulmonary diseases in 8%. Second cancer was reported in 8% of patients. This mandates long-term follow-up in these patients by echocardiography, pulmonary function testing, and screening for second cancer.

REFERENCES

1. Lang S, Kansy B. Cervical lymph node diseases in children. GMS Curr Top Otorhinolaryngol Head Neck Surg. 2014;13:Doc08.
2. Brown RL, Azizkhan RG. Pediatric head and neck lesions. Pediatr Clin North Am. 1998;45(4):889-905.
3. Grant CN, Aldrink J, Lautz TB, Tracy ET, Rhee DS, Baertschiger RM, et al. Lymphadenopathy in children: a streamlined approach for the surgeon—a report from the APSA Cancer Committee. J Pediatr Surg. 2021;56(2):274-81.
4. Chatani S, Hasegawa T, Kato S, Murata S, Sato Y, Yamaura H, et al. Image-guided core needle biopsy in the diagnosis of malignant lymphoma: comparison with surgical excision biopsy. Eur J Radiol. 2020;127:108990.
5. Minard-Colin V, Brugières L, Reiter A, Cairo MS, Gross TG, Woessmann W, et al. Non-Hodgkin lymphoma in children and adolescents: Progress through effective collaboration, current knowledge, and challenges ahead. J Clin Oncol Off J Am Soc Clin Oncol. 2015;33(27):2963-74.
6. Sandlund JT, Martin MG. Non-Hodgkin lymphoma across the pediatric and adolescent and young adult age spectrum. Hematology. 2016;2016(1):589-97.
7. Ferry JA. Burkitt's lymphoma: clinicopathologic features and differential diagnosis. The Oncologist. 2006;11(4):375-83.
8. Oschlies I, Klapper W, Zimmermann M, Krams M, Wacker HH, Burkhardt B, et al. Diffuse large B-cell lymphoma in pediatric patients belongs predominantly to the germinal-center type B-cell lymphomas: a clinicopathologic analysis of cases included in the German BFM (Berlin-Frankfurt-Münster) Multicenter Trial. Blood. 2006;107(10):4047-52.
9. Murphy SB, Fairclough DL, Hutchison RE, Berard CW. Non-Hodgkin's lymphomas of childhood: an analysis of the histology, staging, and response to treatment of 338 cases at a single institution. J Clin Oncol Off J Am Soc Clin Oncol. 1989;7(2):186-93.
10. Rosolen A, Perkins SL, Pinkerton CR, Guillerman RP, Sandlund JT, Patte C, et al. Revised International Pediatric Non-Hodgkin Lymphoma Staging System. J Clin Oncol. 2015;33(18):2112-8.
11. Barrington SF, Mikhaeel NG, Kostakoglu L, Meignan M, Hutchings M, Müeller SP, et al. Role of imaging in the staging and response assessment of lymphoma: consensus of the International Conference on Malignant Lymphomas Imaging Working Group. J Clin Oncol Off J Am Soc Clin Oncol. 2014;32(27):3048-58.
12. Li Z, Li C, Chen B, Shi L, Gao F, Wang P, et al. FDG-PET/CT versus bone marrow biopsy in bone marrow involvement in newly diagnosed paediatric lymphoma: a systematic review and meta-analysis. J Orthop Surg. 2021;16(1):482.
13. Endrizzi L, Fiorentino MV, Salvagno L, Segati R, Pappagallo GL, Fosser V. Serum lactate dehydrogenase (LDH) as a prognostic index for non-Hodgkin's lymphoma. Eur J Cancer Clin Oncol. 1982;18(10):945-9.

14. Lakshmaiah KC, Asati V, Babu K G, D L, Jacob LA, M C SB, et al. Role of prephase treatment prior to definitive chemotherapy in patients with diffuse large B-cell lymphoma. Eur J Haematol. 2018;100(6):644-8.
15. Cairo MS, Sposto R, Gerrard M, Auperin A, Goldman SC, Harrison L, et al. Advanced stage, increased lactate dehydrogenase, and primary site, but not adolescent age (≥ 15 years), are associated with an increased risk of treatment failure in children and adolescents with mature B-cell non-Hodgkin's lymphoma: Results of the FAB LMB-96 Study. J Clin Oncol. 2012;30(4):387-93.
16. Minard-Colin V, Auperin A, Pillon M, Burke A, Anderson JR, Barkauskas DA, et al. Results of the randomized Intergroup trial Inter-B-NHL Ritux 2010 for children and adolescents with high-risk B-cell non-Hodgkin lymphoma (B-NHL) and mature acute leukemia (B-AL): Evaluation of rituximab (R) efficacy in addition to standard LMB chemotherapy (CT) regimen. J Clin Oncol. 2016;34 (15suppl):10507.
17. Reiter A, Schrappe M, Tiemann M, Ludwig WD, Yakisan E, Zimmermann M, et al. Improved treatment results in childhood B-cell neoplasms with tailored intensification of therapy: a report of the Berlin-Frankfurt-Münster Group Trial NHL-BFM 90. Blood. 1999;94(10):3294-306.
18. Thacker N, Bakhshi S, Chinnaswamy G, Vora T, Prasad M, Bansal D, et al. Management of Non-Hodgkin Lymphoma: ICMR Consensus Document. Indian J Pediatr. 2017;84(5):382-92.
19. Sandlund JT, Guillerman RP, Perkins SL, Pinkerton CR, Rosolen A, Patte C, et al. International Pediatric Non-Hodgkin Lymphoma Response Criteria. J Clin Oncol Off J Am Soc Clin Oncol. 2015;33(18):2106-11.
20. Mussolin L, Damm-Welk C, Pillon M, Woessmann W. Minimal disease monitoring in pediatric non-Hodgkin's lymphoma: current clinical application and future challenges. Cancers. 2021;13(8):1907.
21. Moleti ML, Testi AM, Foà R. Treatment of relapsed/refractory paediatric aggressive B-cell non-Hodgkin lymphoma. Br J Haematol. 2020;189(5):826-43.
22. Gentet JC, Patte C, Quintana E, Bergeron C, Rubie H, Pein F, et al. Phase II study of cytarabine and etoposide in children with refractory or relapsed non-Hodgkin's lymphoma: a study of the French Society of Pediatric Oncology. J Clin Oncol Off J Am Soc Clin Oncol. 1990;8(4):661-5.
23. Griffin TC, Weitzman S, Weinstein H, Chang M, Cairo M, Hutchison R, et al. A study of rituximab and ifosfamide, carboplatin, and etoposide chemotherapy in children with recurrent/refractory B-cell (CD20+) non-Hodgkin lymphoma and mature B-cell acute lymphoblastic leukemia: a report from the Children's Oncology Group. Pediatr Blood Cancer. 2009;52(2):177-81.
24. Jourdain A, Auperin A, Minard-Colin V, Aladjidi N, Zsiros J, Coze C, et al. Outcome of and prognostic factors for relapse in children and adolescents with mature B-cell lymphoma and leukemia treated in three consecutive prospective "Lymphomes Malins B" protocols. A Société Française des Cancers de l'Enfant study. Haematologica. 2015;100(6):810-7.
25. Osumi T, Mori T, Fujita N, Saito AM, Nakazawa A, Tsurusawa M, et al. Relapsed/refractory pediatric B-cell non-Hodgkin lymphoma treated with rituximab combination therapy: a report from the Japanese Pediatric Leukemia/Lymphoma Study Group. Pediatr Blood Cancer. 2016;63(10):1794-9.
26. Rigaud C, Auperin A, Jourdain A, Haouy S, Couec ML, Aladjidi N, et al. Outcome of relapse in children and adolescents with B-cell non-Hodgkin lymphoma and mature acute leukemia: A report from the French LMB study. Pediatr Blood Cancer. 2019;66(9):e27873.
27. Kung FH, Harris MB, Krischer JP. Ifosfamide/carboplatin/etoposide (ICE), an effective salvaging therapy for recurrent malignant non-Hodgkin lymphoma of childhood: a Pediatric Oncology Group phase II study. Med Pediatr Oncol. 1999;32(3):225-6.

28. Burkhardt B, Taj M, Garnier N, Minard-Colin V, Hazar V, Mellgren K, et al. Treatment and outcome analysis of 639 relapsed non-Hodgkin lymphomas in children and adolescents and resulting treatment recommendations. Cancers (Basel). 2021;13(9):20752021.
29. Harris R, Termuhlen A, Smith L, Lynch J, Henry M, Perkins S, et al. Autologous Peripheral Blood Stem Cell Transplantation in Children with Refractory or Relapsed Lymphoma: Results of Children's Oncology Group Study A5962. Biol Blood Marrow Transplant J Am Soc Blood Marrow Transplant. 2011;17:249-58.
30. Chen YB, Lane AA, Logan B, Zhu X, Akpek G, Aljurf M, et al. Impact of conditioning regimen on outcomes for patients with lymphoma undergoing high-dose therapy with autologous hematopoietic cell transplantation. Biol Blood Marrow Transplant J Am Soc Blood Marrow Transplant. 2015;21(6):1046-53.
31. Mounier N, Anthony S, Busson R, Thieblemont C, Nerich V, Ribrag V, et al. Long term toxicity and fatigue after treatment for non-Hodgkin lymphoma (NHL): An analysis of twelve collaborative lymphoma study association (LYSA) trials, the Simonal Study. J Clin Oncol. 2016;34(15_suppl):7518–18.

EXPERT OPINION

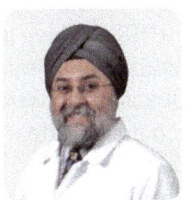

Vikramjit S Kanwar MBA MRCP(UK) FAAP
Professor Emeritus Pediatrics, Albany Medical College, NY
Chief of Pediatric Oncology, Homi Bhabha Cancer Hospital, Lahartara
Varanasi, Uttar Pradesh 221005

Non-Hodgkin lymphoma accounts for almost half of all pediatric lymphomas seen at our institution, with mature B-cell NHL comprising the majority of those cases. BL represents 40–50% of overall NHL, and DLBCL 10–20%, similar to our numbers from our institution. PMBCL is rare, biologically distinct, requiring a different therapeutic approach, and will not be discussed further.

Diffuse large B-cell lymphoma in pediatric patients differs biologically from that in adult patients, with relatively high proliferation rates and an increased frequency of the favorable germinal cell (GC) phenotype. In addition, t(14;18) translocation is virtually absent. Thus, many of the topics discussed by adult hematologists have little relevance in pediatric patients, e.g., poor outcomes are seen in the 10% of adult patients with DLBCL who display "double hit" and "triple hit" tumor abnormalities (impacting c-MYC, Bcl-2, and Bcl-6 in various combinations), but these abnormalities are almost never seen in childhood. Therefore, the molecular analysis does not play a role in pediatric DLBCL. Similarly, while MDD assessment is occasionally used for treatment optimization in adult NHL, it has no value in pediatric DLBCL. The excellent outcomes achieved in pediatric DLBCL with standard therapy means that while novel agents are in the adult pipeline, there is little incentive to bring these into the market for children, where they would be of value for a small number of chemorefractory patients.

Definitive diagnosis of DLBCL is by tissue biopsy, and fine needle aspiration (FNAC) is actively discouraged. Histology shows a diffuse infiltrate of medium to large-sized cells that efface the lymph node architecture. There is often overlap in the morphologic and immunophenotypic appearance within pediatric mature B-NHL (BL and DLBCL) with no defining cytogenetic abnormalities for DLBCL, and c-MYC translocation present in 5–10% of pediatric DLBCL cases. The immunophenotypic signature can also be identical, with an expression of mature B-cell antigens CD19 and CD20, GC-associated antigens CD10 and Bcl-6, and absence of terminal deoxynucleotidyl transferase (tdt). While all mature B-NHL expresses the proliferation antigen Ki-67 at high rates, in BL, it is often >99%. A distinguishing marker is Bcl-2, expressed in 40% of DLBCL but rarely found in BL. Staging of DLBCL with PET combined with CT is now routine, comprehensively evaluating nodal disease and more accurately detecting BM involvement than BMB.

Treatment protocols for DLBCL in childhood in high-income countries (HIC) are virtually identical to those for pediatric BL. They are based on the French Society of Pediatric Oncology

LMB-89/96 trials, which yielded a 3-year EFS of 92%. Significant myelosuppression led to a high rate of febrile neutropenia, mucositis, and blood product transfusion, making it harder to implement in our setting. Accordingly, our frontline protocol remains MCP-842 (multicenter protocol), with LMB-89/96 reserved for CNS-positive or poorly responsive diseases. MCP-842 excludes high-dose methotrexate and consists of alternating cycles of regimens A and B, the former including cyclophosphamide, doxorubicin, vincristine, and cytarabine, and the latter etoposide, methotrexate, vincristine, and ifosfamide with mesna. Patients with St Jude stages I–II receive six cycles, and stages III–IV eight cycles.

Tata Memorial Hospital Mumbai retrospectively reviewed 15 children with DLBCL treated from 2013–2018, the majority with advanced stage III-IV disease: after two cycles of chemotherapy, most achieved complete metabolic and morphologic response (CMR), with the remainder achieving CMR by end of treatment with a 3-year EFS of $77.1 \pm 11.7\%$. Our institution has treated nine children since 2018 with similar outcomes (unpublished observation). The InPOG-NHL-16-01 study audited pediatric DLBCL patients in India (n = 26), mostly treated with LMB and BFM protocols, and reported a 3-year EFS of $88.1 \pm 6.4\%$; the small numbers and overlapping confidence intervals makes it hard to draw definitive conclusions as to which NHL protocol provides optimal outcomes in India. Adverse prognostic factors still remain advanced stage, serum LDH level >2,000 U/L, and BM/CNS disease (fortunately rare in DLBCL, with isolated CNS relapse rare).

With strong CD20 expression in mature B-NHL, rituximab was a logical choice for targeted therapy. LMB-89/96 served as the backbone for the multinational intergroup Phase III study COG ANHL1131, where the randomized addition of rituximab for advanced-stage BL and DLBCL showed survival benefit. However, rituximab is associated with hypogammaglobulinemia and infection risk, and in the Indian setting has negatively impacted survival. As a result, we only rarely use rituximab in advanced disease, and for those with inadequate response after two cycles of chemotherapy and, along with colleagues in US and Europe, we do not use it for low- and standard-risk patients with DLBCL.

Very few children/adolescents with DLBCL experience relapsed/refractory disease, those who do have dismal outcomes with no current standard of care. Salvage may be attempted with ifosfamide, carboplatin, etoposide and rituximab (R-ICE) which provides a complete/partial response in 60–70% of cases, despite which only 50–60% of patients proceed to an HSCT, with the available data not showing a clear advantage for autologous versus allogeneic HSCT. The prognosis was poor for those with primary or secondary chemorefractory disease who do not benefit from HSCT and such patients should be offered palliation. A large series (n = 104) of relapsed/refractory B-NHL patients from the FAB/LMB96 protocol reported an overall survival rate of 23% at 2 years, and higher survival from retrospective registry data probably overestimate real-world outcomes. Novel therapies for chemoresistant relapsed DLBCL being tested in adults include ibrutinib, obinutuzumab (anti-CD20), inotuzumab (anti-CD22 antibody conjugate), and anti-CD19 CAR-T cells, but experience in children is limited or absent.

In summary, pediatric DLBCL comprises 10–20% of all childhood NHL, is distinct from the corresponding entity in adults, fortunately has better outcomes when treated at pediatric oncology centers, and has excellent long-term survival with current protocols and adequate supportive care. The role of chemotherapy regimens which lack high-dose methotrexate should be confirmed in the Indian setting by prospective trials with larger numbers of patients.

CHAPTER 10

Burkitt Lymphoma

Meena H, Aditya Kumar Gupta

CASE VIGNETTE

A 6-year old child presented with history of abdominal distension, nodal swellings, and weight loss of 1.5 month duration. A contrast-enhanced computed tomography (CT) of the abdomen revealed a hypodense soft tissue mass extending from the posterior mediastinum, encircling the esophagus and extending into the abdominal cavity. There was a 17 × 7.5 mm focus in the pancreatic neck. Biopsy from the mesenteric tissue showed immature lymphoid cells in a starry-sky pattern **(Fig. 1A)**, positive for CD 20, CD10, and B-cell lymphoma 6 (BCL-6) **(Fig. 1B)**. MIB-1 labeling index was 100% **(Fig. 1B)**. He was diagnosed with a Burkitt's lymphoma (BL). Bone marrow aspirate and biopsy were not involved. Initial lactate dehydrogenase (LDH) was 1,846 IU/L. Positron emission tomography (PET) CT showed metabolically active disease involving lymph nodes on both sides of the diaphragm, involvement of gastrointestinal tract (GIT), omentum, mesentery, and bilateral pleural effusion **(Fig. 2)**.

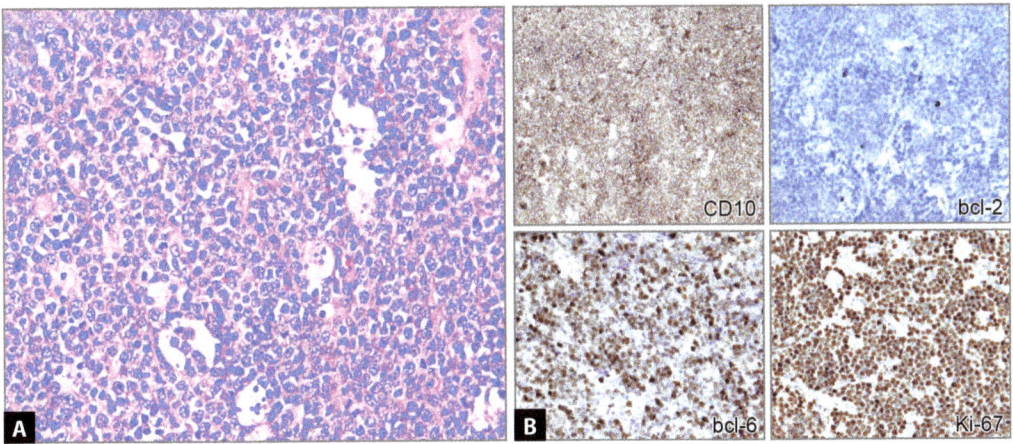

Figs. 1A and B: Histopathology and immunohistochemistry of tissue from abdominal biopsy.

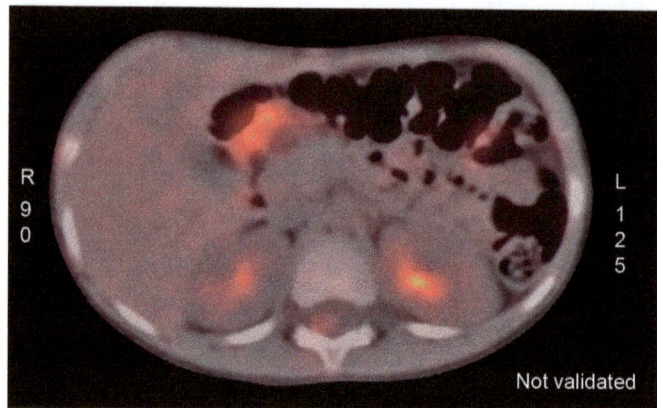

Fig. 2: Baseline positron emission tomography-computed tomography (PET-CT).

1. What are the various approaches to his risk stratification?

The major determinants for risk stratification are rooted in the original Murphy staging, the improvised form of which is the International Pediatric Non-Hodgkin Lymphoma Staging System (INHLSS).[1] The French–American–British/Lymphomes Malins B (FAB/LMB) approach has risk-stratified pediatric B cell non-Hodgkin lymphoma (B-NHL) into three groups and built the treatment platform upon that. It predominantly differs from Berlin-Frankfurt-Münster (BFM) stratification in the inclusion of LDH in the latter **(Table 1)**. Our child belongs to group B as per LMB-FAB and R4 as per BFM-NHL-95.

TABLE 1: Comparison of FAB/LMB and BFM risk stratifications.

Risk stratification	BFM-NHL	FAB-LMB
Low risk	R1: Stage I or II, completely resected	Group A: • Resected Stage I • Abdominal completely resected Stage II
↓	R2: Stage I or II, not resected Stage III with LDH <500 U/L	Group B: • All patients not in group A or C
↓	R3: Stage III with LDH ≥500 to <1,000 U/L	
High risk	R4: Stage III or IV with LDH ≥1,000 U/L and/or CNS-positive	Group C: • Bone marrow disease (≥25% L3 blasts) and/or CNS-positive

(BFM: Berlin-Frankfurt-Münster; CNS: central nervous system; FAB/LMB: French–American–British/Lymphomes Malins B; LDH: lactate dehydrogenase; NHL: non-Hodgkin lymphoma)

2. What is its oncogenic role of *MYC* gene?

MYC has the function of a proto-oncogene in the human body and is the gene involved in production of transcription factor MYC (or c-Myc). Approximately one-tenth of the human genes are regulated by MYC by its actions on deoxyribonucleic acid (DNA) and protein metabolism pathways. Elevated expression of MYC due to mutations can result in increased activation of cyclin-dependent kinases and CCND2 and this results in downregulation of cell cycle inhibitors, contributing to oncogenesis. MYC plays a very important role in the formation and maintenance of germinal centers.[2]

The most important genomic feature of Burkitt is the presence of MYC translocation. The typical t(8;14) (q24;q32) rearrangement (MYC-IGH) occurs in 80%, with less frequent rearrangements to the light chain loci IGL t(2;8) or IGK t(8;22). Rarely, MYC translocation may be absent in morphologically evident BL, usually resulting from cryptic rearrangements.[3]

3. What is the latest understanding of signaling pathways implicated in Burkitt pathogenesis?

Mutations in TCF3 and/or ID3 can lead to decreased transactivation of ID3 by disruption of the negative feedback of TCF3 **(Fig. 3)**. TCF3 is important for survival of BL cell lines as it is a transcription factor in normal germinal center responses. The PI(3) kinase activity in BL is regulated via multiple mechanisms.[4] Transactivation of MIR17HG by MYC and its amplification in some cases contributes to increased PTEN and PI(3) kinase signaling mediated by MicroRNA-19 (miR-19). The PI(3) kinase activity is also promoted by TCF3, by upregulation of B-cell receptor (BCR) expression by transactivation of immunoglobulin loci. CCND3 which regulates G1-S phase transition is another target of TCF3 and this is a regulator of the germinal center reaction.[5] Cyclin D3 and its partner CDK6 are required for the proliferation of BL cells, even in cell line models with wild type CCND3, probably reflecting the

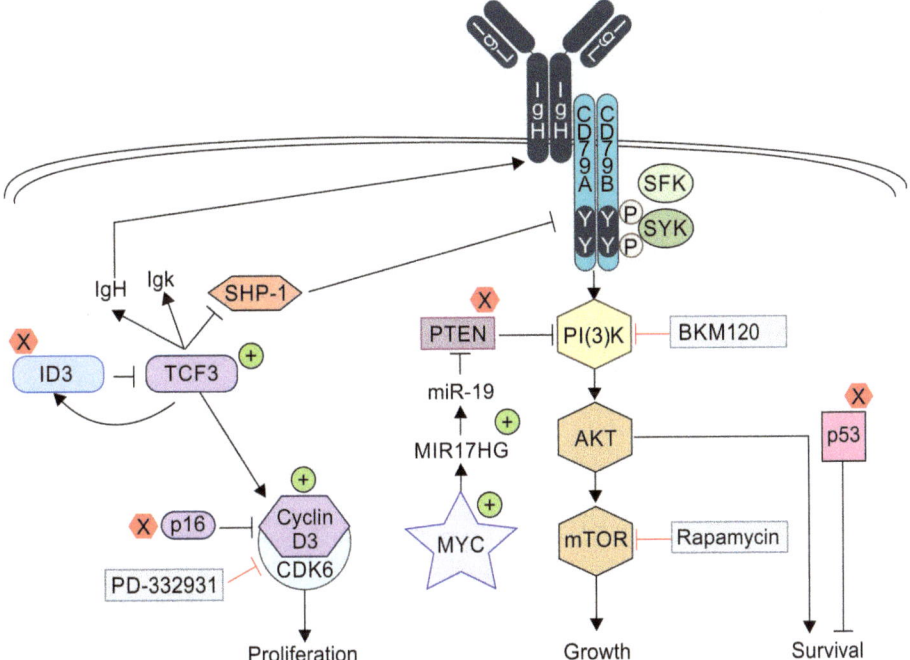

Fig. 3: Pathways in the pathogenesis of Burkitt lymphoma.
Source: Modified from Lenz G, Salles G (Eds). Aggressive Lymphomas in "Hematologic Malignancies".

role of cyclin D3 in normal germinal center B cells.[6] Mutations in CCND3 result in highly stable isoforms of cyclin D3, that drive cell proliferation, and this is a mechanism on which the BL proliferation is dependent. Inactivating mutations and deletions targeting p16 can deregulate the G1-S restriction resulting in increased proliferation.[7]

4. What is the role of Epstein-Barr virus (EBV) in pathogenesis of BL?

In endemic BL, EBV is present in majority of the malignant cells. In the sporadic BL, the presence of EBV is less common. The resting human B cells can be stimulated to proliferate by EBV leading to transformation into lymphoblastoid cell lines (LCLs)[8] **(Fig. 4)**. These LCLs express

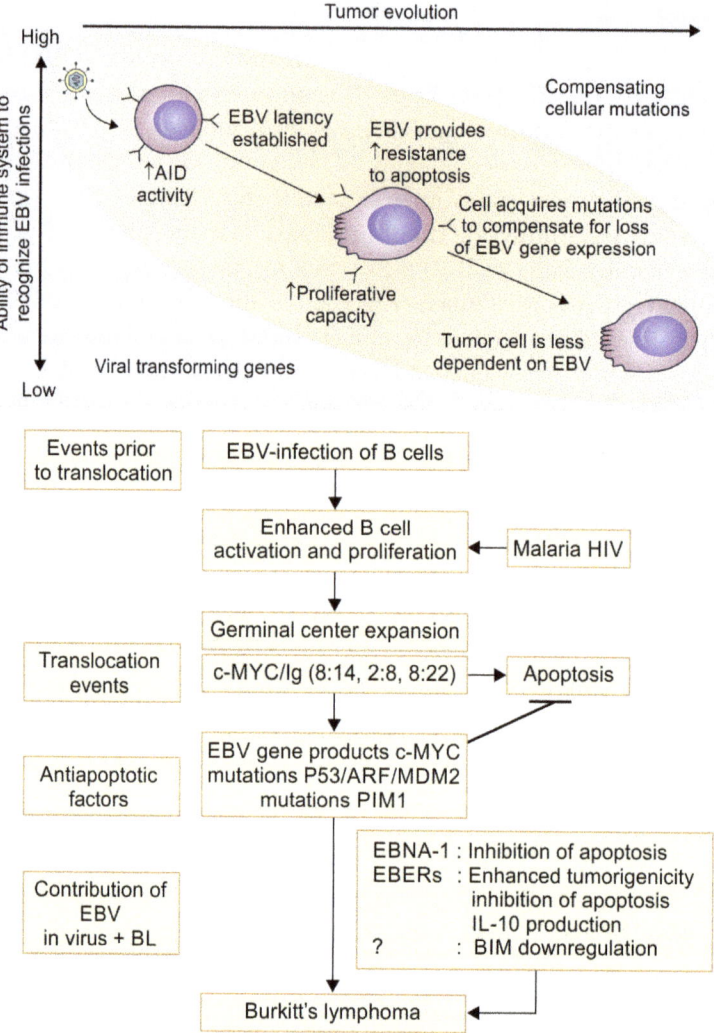

Fig. 4: Burkitt lymphoma evolve and escape dependency on Epstein-Barr virus (EBV).
(EBV: Epstein-Barr virus; HIV: human immunodeficiency virus)
Source: Modified from Hutcheson RL, Chakravorty A, Sugden B. Burkitt Lymphomas Evolve to Escape Dependencies on Epstein-Barr Virus. Front Cell Infect Microbiol. 2021;10:606412.[9]

on their surface a variety of EBV proteins, which serve as key regulators of metabolic pathways such as PI3K and NF-kB. The BL cell express a restricted pattern of viral products mainly EBNA1. In the absence of functional T cells, the EBV-induced LCLs can proliferate without restriction. A hit and run model in which EBV inhibits the apoptosis of the premalignant tumor cells (at which point the majority of its latency proteins are no longer necessary), allowing for a second hit to transform it into a malignancy is likely with EBV in BL.

5. What is MIB-1 index?

MIB-1 is a monoclonal antibody directed against the nuclear protein Ki-67, which is expressed in all phases of the cell cycle except G0. For this reason it is used as a cellular marker for proliferation; the presence of nuclear staining indicates an active cycling cell. Numerous studies indicate that a high proliferation rate is associated with a more aggressive disease course, and hence a poorer prognosis.

6. Where do double/triple hit lymphomas stand in the spectrum of high-grade B-NHL?

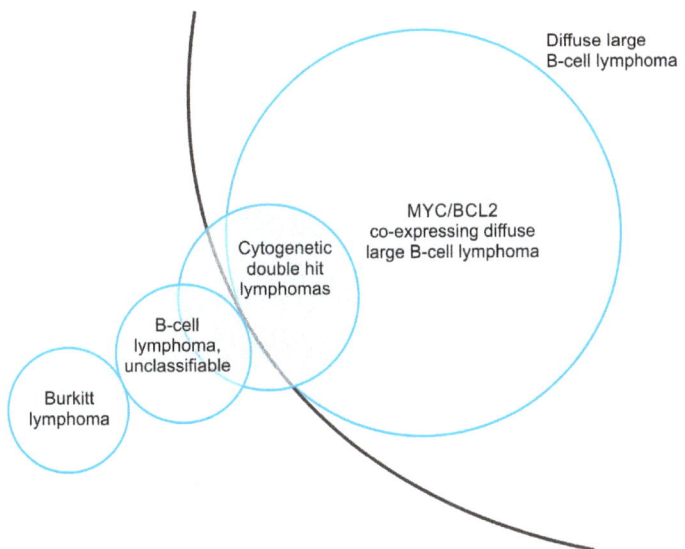

Fig. 5: Double-hit, triple-hit, and double expressor lymphomas: where do they stand?

The term "double-hit lymphoma" implies B-cell lymphomas with a number of activating oncogenes, one of them being *MYC*. *MYC/BCL2* double-hit are the most common, while *MYC/BCL6* double hit lymphoma and *MYC/BCL2/BCL6* "triple hit" lymphomas are the least common **(Fig. 5)**. The term "double-expressor" on the other hand refers to protein expression of MYC/BCL2 and/or BCL6.

7. In this child we have used PET-CT as the primary imaging modality. Is it justified? What is available evidence?

PET, when combined with CT, offers the advantage of combining functional information with anatomic imaging. There is a growing body of literature evaluating the utility of PET/CT in both pediatric and adult BL patients. Carrillo-Cruz et al. have shown that PET/CT has a 100% negative predictive value in predicting treatment response as well 100% positive predictive values in predicting recurrence.[10] Similarly, Wei et al. showed significant reduction in SUVmax on interim and post-therapy PET/CT was a good prognostic factor for BL patients.[11] In the pediatric population, PET/CT has demonstrated better ability to detect both nodal and extranodal sites of disease and greater impact on initial staging compared to CT.[12] With regard to treatment response and prognosis, despite preliminary evidences no shared data are available in the literature as yet.

8. Which protocol will you use to treat the index child? On what factors does the choice of a protocol depend?

As per FAB/LMB, our child will receive group B backbone consists of a low-dose COP reduction (cyclophosphamide 300 mg/m², vincristine, and prednisone), followed by two induction cycles [COPAD plus methotrexate (MTX) 3 g/m²] and two consolidation cycles (cytarabine 500 mg/m² plus MTX 3 g/m²), each with intrathecal chemotherapy given throughout. This group B intermediate-risk therapy was established by Patte and colleagues in 2007, ultimately demonstrating equivalent event-free survival (EFS) rates of 91% despite reduced total doses of cyclophosphamide and deletion of maintenance cycles.[13] The details of chemotherapy under BFM-95 has been given in **Table 2**.

TABLE 2: Comparison of FAB/LMB versus BFM-95 for the index child.

Protocol	FAB/LMB	BFM
Stratification	Group B	R4
Definition	Not resected, I, II, III, IV, CNS-negative	LDH >1,000 and/or CNS-positive
Number of courses	4	6
Methotrexate	1 g/m² × 4 4 hours infusion	5 g/m² × 4 24 hours infusion
Doxorubicin g/m²	120	100
Cyclophosphamide g/m²	3.3	2.4
Ifosfamide g/m²	–	8
Etoposide mg/m²	–	1,400

(BFM-95: Berlin-Frankfurt-Münster-95; CNS: central nervous system; FAB/LMB: French–American–British/Lymphomes Malins B; LDH: lactate dehydrogenase)

9. The treating team decided to treat the child as per BFM-95 protocol. The child was started on prephase. What is the role of prephase?

In comparison with standard dose of chemotherapy, prephase limits the risk of tumor lysis syndrome (TLS) by decreasing the release of cytokines, a situation that can be lethal given the aggressiveness and chemosensitivity of the tumor. Moreover, this procedure allows finalizing the staging process. The NHL-B2 trial[14] was the first to utilize prephase therapy with an aim to prevent the "first-cycle effect" [described as deepest absolute neutrophil count (ANC) nadir, longest duration of neutropenia, and highest rate of therapy-associated deaths]. However, there are no large studies in pediatric setting establishing the superiority of prephase by a head-to-head comparison.

10. What is variation in dose and duration of MTX administration across various protocols?

In BFM-NHL-86, stage III patients were treated with 0.5 g MTX and had a relatively poor prognosis: 43% EFS at 6 years, hence the dose of methotrexate was elevated to 5 g/m^2 and the EFS rate at 6 years improved to 81%.

The BFM-NHL-95 trial showed that a shorter infusion time of high-dose (HD) MTX to 4 hours (from 24 hours) decreased the incidence of severe mucositis.[15] In the higher risk groups however, viz., R3 and R4, a shorter infusion time was associated with more failures in contrast to the low- and intermediate-risk groups where it did not affect outcomes. Thus in the subsequent study, i.e., BFM-NHL 04: 1 g/m^2 IV over 4 hours in risk groups R1 and R2, and 5 g/m^2 IV over 24 hours in risk groups R3 and R4 was used. In LMB protocol group C, the dose of MTX is 8 g/m^2 over 4 hours. Further evidence has shown higher dose and longer duration is beneficial in the central nervous system (CNS)-positive setting.

11. If this child were CNS-positive, how would you approach as per different protocols? Which trial provided the evidence for omission of radiotherapy in such cases?

CNS$^+$ disease is diagnosed based if one or more of the following are there: any L3 cerebrospinal fluid (CSF) blasts, cranial nerve palsy that cannot be explained by extradural lesion, isolated intracerebral mass or clinical spinal cord compression. In LMB96 and LMB2001 studies, patients with cranial or spinal tumor and parameningeal extension beyond meninges were also considered as CNS$^+$ irrespective of clinical symptoms.

Patients with CNS$^+$ were assigned to high-risk group C in all the three LMB protocols.

1. In LMB89, cranial irradiation (CRT, 24 Gy) was delivered to patients with CSF$^+$ or nerve palsy.[16]
2. In LMB96, CRT was omitted and replaced by an additional dose of 8 g/m^2 MTX. The pEFS at 4 years for CNS-positive patients in these studies was comparable, 71% (FAB96) and 77% (LMB89), respectively. Further, half of the patients were randomized to receive the reduced-intensity chemotherapy arm (cytarabine 2 g vs. 3 g/m^2 dose × 4 days and etoposide 100 mg vs. 200 mg/m^2 dose × 4 days during the consolidation phase, and shortened maintenance).[13]
3. In LM2001, treatment of CNS$^+$ patients was similar to LMB96 with HD MTX administrated over 24 hours instead of 4 hours.[17] In NHL-BFM-90 and NHL-BFM-95[15] studies, CNS-positive B-NHL patients received intraventricularly administered triple-drug therapy to achieve a better distribution within the CSF and MTX was fractionated during 4 days. The outcome for CNS-positive B-NHL patients in these studies was comparable to that in studies LMB89 and LMB96, in which MTX and cytarabine were administered via lumbar puncture.

CASE (Continued)

Postprephase, our child received R-AA and R-BB cycles. PET-CT after the first two cycles showed significant response to treatment but some residual disease at L3 vertebral level. He had two episodes of febrile neutropenia which did not require intensive care support.

12. What is the estimated incidence of toxic deaths in low- and middle-income countries (LMICs)? How will you prevent?

Toxic death in the first month of therapy may be up to 30% in higher-risk patients in LMIC.[16] Patients whose diagnosis is delayed present with more advanced disease and a higher risk of malnutrition, TLS, comorbid infections, and great risk for early toxic death. Renal failure at diagnosis is found to be a *predictor of toxic deaths in LMIC. Good supportive care in the first few weeks is of utmost importance.*

13. State the evidence for use of rituximab in pediatric BL.

In a study of 328 children on LMB96 backbone, at a median follow-up duration of ~40 months in both arms, patients receiving rituximab plus chemotherapy had a significantly improved 3-year EFS rate (93.9% vs. 82.3%, $p = 0.00096$).[18]

CASE (Continued)

The child went on to receive CC cycle. PET-CT after CC cycle showed suspicion of residual disease and reappearance of metabolic activity in known sites of involvement. Close follow up was advised. The child was continued on the same protocol and went to complete his course. PET-CT postcompletion of 6 cycles showed increase in the extent of involvement and metabolic activity **(Figs. 6A and B)**.

14. He was labeled to have refractory/relapsed (r/r) BL. What are the prognostic factors at relapse?

Cairo et al.[19] have shown that in the patients who were refractory or relapsed on the LB protocols and inferior overall survival (OS) was associated with LDH ≥2 upper normal limit at diagnosis ($p = 0.0006$), refractoriness or relapse within 6 m of diagnosis ($p = 0.038$) and involvement of bone marrow ($p = 0.0001$). Jourdain's[20] and in Rigaud's studies demonstrated that survival was significantly better for patients who underwent a hematopoietic stem cell transplantation (HSCT) in complete remission.[21]

15. What are the salvage chemotherapy options for this child? Compare their outcome.

In the French Paediatric Oncology Society (SFOP) study (phase II) the combination of HD cytarabine and etoposide (CYVE) has proven effective and safe in pediatric r/r B-NHL (66% overall response rate).[22] In the study by Jourdain et al., CYVE was the most frequent option in patients relapsed from LMB treatment groups A or B with an overall response rate (ORR) of approximately 61%.[20] With the DECAL (dexamethasone, etoposide, cisplatin, cytarabine, L-asparaginase) regime a ORR of 50% has been reported.[23]

The ICE regimen is now the preferred option in r/r pediatric B-NHL, with the advantages of no further anthracycline exposure and acceptable extrahematological toxicity. Rituximab in combination with ICE (R-ICE) has been proven to be safe and effective with response rates up to 60%.[24] The Japanese Pediatric Leukemia Lymphoma Group has also shown an ORR of 72% in 20 r/r B-NHL patients with the R-ICE regimen.[25] The patients from the LMB2001 study who relapsed, R-CYVE was used for group A and B with ORR of 72% and R-ICE for group C with ORR of 57%.[17]

16. **The child received four cycles of R-ICE and PET-CT done showed complete metabolic response (Fig. 6C). Is hematopoietic stem cell transplant mandatory at this point?**

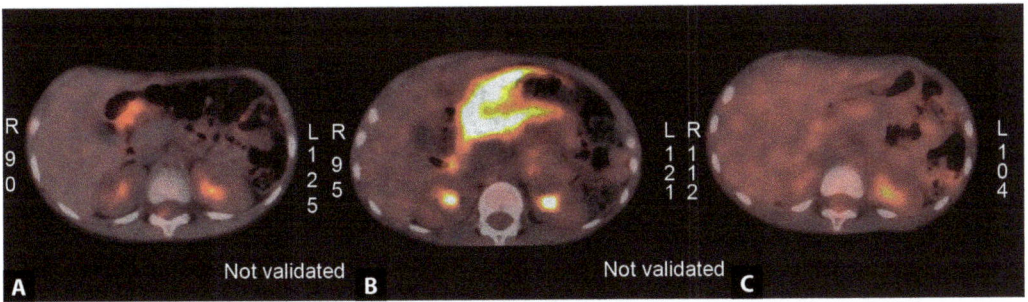

Figs. 6A to C: (A) Positron emission tomography-computed tomography (PET-CT) at baseline; (B) At relapse; and (C) Postsalvage chemotherapy.

The role of HSCT for consolidation in r/r BL is supported by data. With HSCT the survival was approximately 50% compared to 10% without HSCT.[26] Only a few low-risk late relapses have been documented to be alive without HSCT. In general, all pediatric patients with r/r BL are candidates for HSCT.

In a study of 646 patients with r/r NHL, the survival rate was 55% for autografted and 48% for allografted patients.[26] There is no advantage of allogeneic HSCT over autologous HSCT as the benefit of survival due to the graft-versus-lymphoma (GVL) effect is mitigated by the transplantation-related mortality (TRM) of allogeneic HSCT. Death from BL progression was similar in allogeneic and autologous HSCT (34 and 31% respectively).

The conditioning regimens for autologous HSCT in literature are based on busulfan, BEAM, total body irradiation (TBI), or individualized regimens. For allogeneic HSCT, the most frequently used conditioning regimens were TBI-based, Burkitt-specific combination of rituximab, fludarabine, thiotepa, carboplatin, mitoxantrone and paclitaxel, busulfan, treosulfan, or individualized regimens.

17. **What are the newer transplant strategies in the pipeline for BL?**

One strategy is to obtain the maximum response prior to allogeneic transplant with a myeloablative conditioning (MAC) autologous HSCT, followed by a reduced-intensity conditioning (RIC) allogeneic HSCT (tandem MAC, auto-HSCT-RIC allo-HSCT). This may decrease the morbidity and mortality associated with a conventional MAC allogeneic transplant while maintaining its GVL effect. Radioimmunotherapy may further increase the efficacy of the HSCT strategies. Excellent results (91% EFS) have been achieved by addition of yttrium-90 ibritumomab tiuxetan—that has already proven effective and safe in children with r/r B-NHL.[27]

18. Is there any potential role of minimal detectable disease (MDD) assessment in BL/leukemia?

The long distance polymerase chain reaction (LD-PCR)-based assay for the MYC-IGH fusion has been used by the Associazione Italiana di Ematologia e Oncologia Pediatrica (AIEOP) group.[28] Approximately, 70% of BL have a detectable MYC-IGH fusion by the LD-PCR and that 30% of patients with available BM were MDD-positive. The progression-free survival (PFS) for MDD-positive patients is inferior compared to MDD-negative ones. According to another study,[29] MDD correlated with BM and peripheral blood (PB) samples, suggesting the possibility of monitoring MDD by blood testing in the future.

19. Describe the novel therapy under trials for BL.

Antibody-drug conjugates have been combined with chemotherapy in rr-NHL, and multiple antibody-drug conjugates are in development. Additionally, bispecific T-cell-engaging antibody constructs and autologous chimeric antigen receptor (CAR) T-cells have been successful. Programmed death-ligand 1 (PD-L1) and PD-L2 on tumor cells can be targeted with checkpoint inhibitors to augment responses. Lastly, trials of small molecule inhibitors targeting cell signaling pathways in NHL subtypes are underway **(Fig. 7)**.

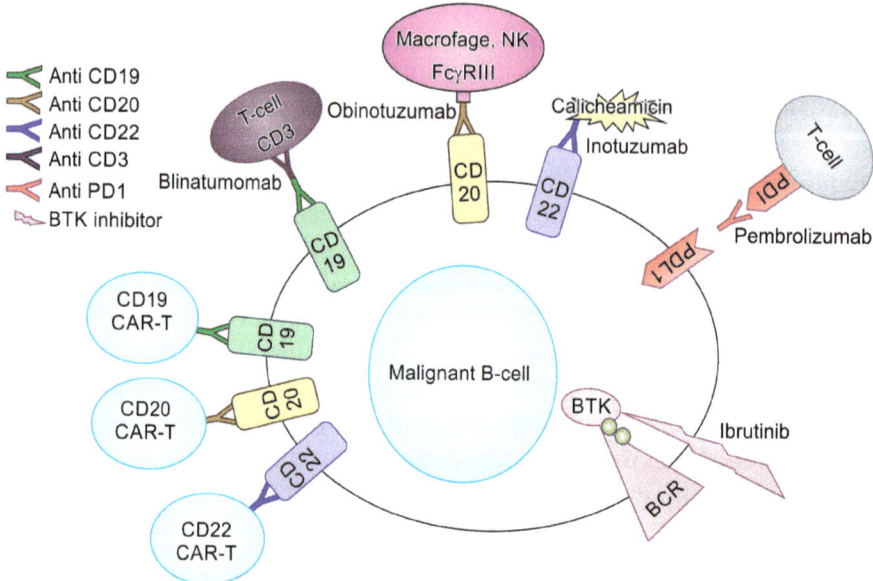

Fig. 7: Select target therapy in Burkitt lymphoma.
Source: Modified from Moleti et al.[22]
(BCR: B-cell receptor; BTK: Bruton's tyrosine kinase; PD1: programmed death 1; PDL1: programmed death ligand 1)

REFERENCES

1. Rosolen A, Perkins SL, Pinkerton CR, Guillerman RP, Sandlund JT, Patte C, et al. Revised International Pediatric Non-Hodgkin Lymphoma Staging System. J Clin Oncol. 2015;33(18):2112-8.
2. Schmitz R, Ceribelli M, Pittaluga S, Wright G, Staudt LM. Oncogenic mechanisms in Burkitt lymphoma. Cold Spring Harb Perspect Med. 2014;4(2):a014282.
3. Dunleavy K, Little RF, Wilson WH. Update on Burkitt Lymphoma. Hematol Oncol Clin North Am. 2016;30(6):1333-43.
4. Rohde M, Bonn BR, Zimmermann M, Lange J, Möricke A, Klapper W, et al. Relevance of ID3-TCF3-CCND3 pathway mutations in pediatric aggressive B-cell lymphoma treated according to the non-Hodgkin Lymphoma Berlin-Frankfurt-Münster protocols. Haematologica. 2017;102(6):1091-8.
5. Schmitz R, Young RM, Ceribelli M, Jhavar S, Xiao W, Zhang M, et al. Burkitt lymphoma pathogenesis and therapeutic targets from structural and functional genomics. Nature. 2012;490(7418):116-20.
6. Cato MH, Chintalapati SK, Yau IW, Omori SA, Rickert RC. Cyclin D3 is selectively required for proliferative expansion of germinal center B cells. Mol Cell Biol. 2011;31(1):127-37.
7. Sánchez-Beato M, Sánchez-Aguilera A, Piris MA. Cell cycle deregulation in B-cell lymphomas. Blood. 2003;101(4):1220-35.
8. Shannon-Lowe C, Rickinson A. The Global Landscape of EBV-Associated Tumors. Front Oncol. 2019;9:713.
9. Hutcheson RL, Chakravorty A, Sugden B. Burkitt Lymphomas Evolve to Escape Dependencies on Epstein-Barr Virus. Front Cell Infect Microbiol. 2021;10:606412.
10. Carrillo-Cruz E, Marín-Oyaga VA, Solé Rodríguez M, Borrego-Dorado I, de la Cruz Vicente F, Quiroga Cantero E, et al. Role of 18F-FDG-PET/CT in the management of Burkitt lymphoma. Eur J Haematol. 2015;94(1):23-30.
11. Wei WX, Huang JJ, Li WY, Zhang X, Xia Y, Jiang WQ, et al. Prognostic values of interim and post-therapy 18F-FDG PET/CT scanning in adult patients with Burkitt's lymphoma. Chin J Cancer. 2015;34(12):608-13.
12. Paes FM, Kalkanis DG, Sideras PA, Serafini AN. FDG PET/CT of extranodal involvement in non-Hodgkin lymphoma and Hodgkin disease. Radiographics. 2010;30(1):269-91.
13. Patte C, Auperin A, Gerrard M, Michon J, Pinkerton R, Sposto R, et al.; FAB/LMB96 International Study Committee. Results of the randomized international FAB/LMB96 trial for intermediate risk B-cell non-Hodgkin lymphoma in children and adolescents: it is possible to reduce treatment for the early responding patients. Blood. 2007;109(7):2773-80.
14. Pfreundschuh M, Trümper L, Kloess M, Schmits R, Feller AC, Rübe C, et al.; German High-Grade Non-Hodgkin's Lymphoma Study Group. Two-weekly or 3-weekly CHOP chemotherapy with or without etoposide for the treatment of elderly patients with aggressive lymphomas: results of the NHL-B2 trial of the DSHNHL. Blood. 2004;104(3):634-41.
15. Woessmann W, Seidemann K, Mann G, Zimmermann M, Burkhardt B, Oschlies I, et al.; BFM Group. The impact of the methotrexate administration schedule and dose in the treatment of children and adolescents with B-cell neoplasms: a report of the BFM Group Study NHL-BFM95. Blood. 2005;105(3):948-58.
16. Patte C, Auperin A, Michon J, Behrendt H, Leverger G, Frappaz D, et al.; SociétéFrançaise d'Oncologie Pédiatrique. The Société Française d'Oncologie Pédiatrique LMB89 protocol: highly effective multiagent chemotherapy tailored to the tumor burden and initial response in 561 unselected children with B-cell lymphomas and L3 leukemia. Blood. 2001;97(11):3370-9.
17. Dourthe ME, Phulpin A, Auperin A, Bosq J, Couec ML, Dartigues P, et al. Rituximab in addition to LMB-based chemotherapy regimen in children and adolescents with primary mediastinal large B-cell lymphoma: results of the French LMB2001 prospective study. Haematologica. 2022;107(9):2173-82.

18. Goldman S, Smith L, Anderson JR, Perkins S, Harrison L, Geyer MB, et al. Rituximab and FAB/LMB 96 chemotherapy in children with Stage III/IV B-cell non-Hodgkin lymphoma: a Children's Oncology Group report. Leukemia. 2013;27(5):1174-7.
19. Cairo M, Auperin A, Perkins SL, Pinkerton R, Harrison L, Goldman S et al. Overall survival of children and adolescents with mature B cell non-Hodgkin lymphoma who had refractory or relapsed disease during or after treatment with FAB/LMB 96: A report from the FAB/LMB 96 study group. Br J Haematol. 2018;182(6):859-69.
20. Short NJ, Kantarjian HM, Ko H, Khoury JD, Ravandi F, Thomas DA, et al. Outcomes of adults with relapsed or refractory Burkitt and high-grade B-cell leukemia/lymphoma. Am J Hematol. 2017;92(6):E114-E117.
21. Rigaud C, Auperin A, Jourdain A, Haouy S, Couec ML, Aladjidi N, et al. Outcome of relapse in children and adolescents with B-cell non-Hodgkin lymphoma and mature acute leukemia: A report from the French LMB study. Pediatr Blood Cancer. 2019;66(9):e27873.
22. Moleti ML, Testi AM, Foà, R. Treatment of relapsed/refractory paediatric aggressive B-cell non-Hodgkin lymphoma. Br J Haematol. 2020;189(5):826-43.
23. Kobrinsky NL, Sposto R, Shah NR, Anderson JR, DeLaat C, Morse M, et al. Outcomes of treatment of children and adolescents with recurrent non-Hodgkin's lymphoma and Hodgkin's disease with dexamethasone, etoposide, cisplatin, cytarabine, and L-asparaginase, maintenance chemotherapy, and transplantation: Children's Cancer Group Study CCG-5912. J Clin Oncol. 2001;19(9):2390-6.
24. Griffin TC, Weitzman S, Weinstein H, Chang M, Cairo M, Hutchison R, et al.; Children's Oncology Group. A study of rituximab and ifosfamide, carboplatin, and etoposide chemotherapy in children with recurrent/refractory B-cell (CD20+) non-Hodgkin lymphoma and mature B-cell acute lymphoblastic leukemia: a report from the Children's Oncology Group. Pediatr Blood Cancer. 2009;52(2):177-81.
25. Osumi T, Mori T, Fujita N, Saito AM, Nakazawa A, Tsurusawa M, et al. Relapsed/refractory pediatric B-cell non-Hodgkin lymphoma treated with rituximab combination therapy: A report from the Japanese Pediatric Leukemia/Lymphoma Study Group. Pediatr Blood Cancer. 2016;63(10):1794-9.
26. Burkhardt B, Taj M, Garnier N, Minard-Colin V, Hazar V, Mellgren K, et al. Treatment and Outcome Analysis of 639 Relapsed Non-Hodgkin Lymphomas in Children and Adolescents and Resulting Treatment Recommendations. Cancers (Basel). 2021;13(9):2075.
27. Cooney-Qualter E, Krailo M, Angiolillo A, Fawwaz RA, Wiseman G, Harrison L, et al.; Children's Oncology Group. A phase I study of 90yttrium-ibritumomab-tiuxetan in children and adolescents with relapsed/refractory CD20-positive non-Hodgkin's lymphoma: a Children's Oncology Group study. Clin Cancer Res. 2007;13(18 Pt 2):5652s-5660s.
28. Mussolin L, Damm-Welk C, Pillon M, Woessmann W. Minimal Disease Monitoring in Pediatric Non-Hodgkin's Lymphoma: Current Clinical Application and Future Challenges. Cancers (Basel). 2021;13(8):1907.
29. Busch K, Borkhardt A, Wossmann W, Reiter A, Harbott J. Combined polymerase chain reaction methods to detect c-myc/IgH rearrangement in childhood Burkitt's lymphoma for minimal residual disease analysis. Haematologica. 2004;89(7):818-25.

EXPERT OPINION

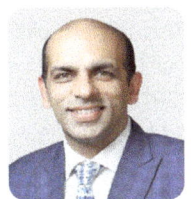

Manas Kalra MD DNB FNB (Pediatric Hematology Oncology)
Fellowship Pediatric Oncology, BMT (Sydney)
Senior Consultant, Sir Ganga Ram Hospital, New Delhi.
email: manaskalra27@gmail.com

1. Do you regularly use PET-CTs in the management of BL?

I do use PET-CT scan for all patients with BL. PET-CT has found a unique role in evaluation and treatment decisions of lymphomas. PET scan allows for accurate staging and picks ^{18}F-fluorodeoxyglucose (FDG) avid sites that are not always apparent on a CT scan. It has increasingly replaced the need of bone marrow biopsy which in children invariably needs sedation and carries its risks. However, as the grouping and therapy allocation in B-NHL still depends on the extent of bone marrow involvement, we continue to do a bone marrow aspirate and biopsy for all children with NHL. The change in metabolic activity helps assess response which is more accurate than merely a change in size of the lymph nodal mass. PET-CT is standard of care for response assessment in FDG avid lymphomas. However, the decision to change therapy for a suspected progressive disease or a refractory neoplastic mass should always be confirmed by a biopsy. A negative PET scan is reassuring and carries a good predictive value. For patients with group B disease, a negative PET-CT after CYM-1 block obviates the need to escalate further treatment.

2. Which protocol do you use for Burkitt lymphoma at your center and why?

We use a modified Inter-B-NHL ritux 2010 protocol. We have modified the MTX and cytarabine doses in the high-risk patients (Group C) to diminish the toxic morbidity and mortality. In a sick patient, we use COP cytoreductive phase twice and sometimes omit MTX from the first Rituximab, Cyclophosphamide, Oncovin (Vincristine), Prednisone, Adriamycin (Doxorubicin), Methotrexate (R-COPADAM) block in children with massive disease burden, active sepsis or significant renal dysfunction. The chance of getting multidrug resistant (MDR) gram-negative sepsis is maximum after the first R-COPADAM when the gut is loaded with malignant cells. The disease melts with chemotherapy and the resultant mucositis allows the transmigration of MDR bacteria in the blood stream leading to septicemia. In my experience, children with bone marrow involvement are not able to handle this septic episode as they suffer from severe neutropenia after initiation of chemotherapy and prompt initiation of antimicrobials is a must. Also, we administer only one dose of rituximab on day 1 in each cycle as opposed to the two doses recommended in the original protocol.

3. What are your views on role of rituximab in BL and use of intravenous immunoglobulin (IVIg) postrituximab?

We have been using rituximab for all our patients with Burkitt's or diffuse large B-cell lymphoma (DLBCL) since 2014. This was initiated in view of the encouraging results both by the BFM group (Meinhardt et al. JCO. 2010) and the COG group (Goldman et al. Leukemia. 2013) that was later confirmed by FAB-LMB group (Minard Colin et al. NEJM. 2020). However, we have modified the protocol and give only one dose of rituximab per cycle of chemotherapy and a maximum of six doses for both Group B and Group C patients. The main reason for toxicity is due to MTX usage in combination with other multiagent chemotherapy. Rituximab appears to be tolerated well. We do need to supplement patients with IVIg from time to time. We check the immunoglobulin G (IgG) levels every other cycle or during an episode of infection and administer IVIg at a dose of 400 mg/kg. We have a lower threshold for IVIg infusion in children admitted with MDR sepsis and a borderline IgG level.

4. How do you treat double hit and triple hit lymphomas at your center?

According to the 2017 WHO classification of lymphomas, DLBCL is classified as double hit (MYC translocation and BCL2/BCL6 rearrangement) or triple hit (MYC translocation and BCL2 and BCL6 rearrangement) lymphoma. These are aggressive cancers with poor response to conventional therapy, higher CNS involvement and higher chances of relapse. They are treated with intense protocols such as dose-adjusted EPOCH-R or R-Hyper-CVAD/MA or R-CODOX-M/IVAC. Unlike adults, all pediatric B-cell lymphomas are aggressive and broadly classified as DLBCL, Burkitt's or lymphoblastic lymphomas. DLBCL and Burkitt lymphoma are treated with similar protocols. The distinction between double hit or triple hit lymphomas is not a common practice in pediatric B-NHLs. The therapy does not alter based on these findings. Even if a distinction is made, there are no unique innovative strategies to manage them. Collation of pediatric data to better understand the biology of tumors carrying above mutations may help devise novel therapies.

5. What is your approach to relapsed and refractory BL?

Relapsed BL carries a dismal outcome. In case a patient is naïve to agents such as rituximab, ifosfamide, MTX, or etoposide, a trial of induction chemotherapy followed by a stem cell transplant may be done. Often that is not the case. Most patients in this era are treated with multiagent chemotherapy along with rituximab. In such a situation, inducing remission can be a challenge. Even if a remission is achieved, the relapse-free period is short lived. An allogeneic transplant carries an advantage of graft versus lymphoma effect, but comes with a risk of graft-versus-host disease, infection, or graft rejection. Alternatively, an autologous transplant can be performed in absence of a suitable allogeneic donor. Most patients are suitable for palliative care only.

CHAPTER 11

Relapsed/Refractory Hodgkin Lymphoma

Piali Mandal, Rachna Seth

CASE VIGNETTE

N, a 10-year female, was diagnosed with Hodgkin lymphoma (HL) 8 years ago. She had presented with fever, weight loss, and neck swelling. Lymph node biopsy was suggestive of classical HL [atypical mononuclear cells were immunopositive for CD30 and Epstein–Barr virus latent membrane protein 1 (EBV-LMP1), while negative for CD3, CD20, and CD15]. contrast-enhanced computed tomography (CECT) neck, chest, abdomen, pelvis was done along with bilateral bone marrow biopsy, as a part of staging work up though currently positron emission tomography computed tomography (PET-CT) has replaced bone marrow examination for staging in HL. After baseline work up she was staged as IV B, nonbulky, based on involvement of multiple nodal sites above and below diaphragm (cervical, supraclavicular, liver 7 cm below right costal margin, spleen 6 cm below costal margin), lung involvement and presence of B symptoms (weight loss and fever). From treatment perspective, she was risk stratified as advanced stage HL and was treated with 8 cycles of BEACOPP (Bleomycin, Etoposide, Doxorubicin, Cyclophosphamide, Vincristine, Procarbazine, Prednisolone) without radiotherapy (RT) and was in remission at the end of therapy. She continued to be under follow up for disease recurrence and treatment related late effects at the survivor clinic. One year into survivorship, she developed cardiac dysfunction in the form of low left ventricular ejection fraction (LVEF) (45%). She was started on cardioprotection comprising enalapril and carvedilol on which her cardiac function improved.

Seven years later she started having pain abdomen without any altered bowel habits or abdominal discomfort, along with off and on fever. On examination, she had severe thinness, pallor, and splenomegaly. With the suspicion of relapse/chronic infection like tuberculosis, an abdominal ultrasound followed by PET/CT was performed.

Her PET/CT **(Figs. 1A to D)** revealed metabolically active lymph nodes on both sides of diaphragm, left supraclavicular nodes, enlarged spleen with multiple hypodense splenic lesions, peritoneal and left paracolic gutter nodules, paravertebral soft tissue, L2 vertebral lesion with corresponding sclerotic changes on CT, and pelvic ascites. These findings were suggestive of lymphomatous involvement. Biopsy was performed on the abdominal nodes. Awaiting the biopsy report, she developed acute abdomen requiring emergency visit and underwent exploratory laparotomy with Graham's patch repair of duodenal perforation, gastrostomy, reverse duodenostomy along with placement of feeding jejunostomy.

Retroperitoneal lymphnode histology and the surgical sample were suggestive of HL. Immunohistochemistry (IHC) was positive for (CD30, CD15, and CD20) and negative for [CD3, anaplastic lymphoma kinase (ALK), epithelial membrane antigen (EMA), and EBV-LMP1]. Perforation edge showed transmural ischemic necrosis and serositis. Blood vessels had shown fibrin thrombi.

With all the above investigations, diagnosis of relapsed of HL was made. This was a late relapse (relapsing >1 year from completion of treatment), stage IV with B symptoms, and thus risk stratified as "high-risk relapse". For her initial disease she had received, 8 cycles of first-line chemotherapy without RT. The treatment planned included salvage chemotherapy followed by high-dose chemotherapy (HDCT) and autologous bone marrow transplant (BMT). She was started on gemcitabine and vinorelbine (GV)-based protocol. Due to poor performance status, malnutrition and underlying cardiac dysfunction she received 75% dose for the first cycle. After two cycles she had partial response (PR) on PET/CT and thus was continued on two more cycles of GV. After four cycles of GV, she showed progressive disease (PD), requiring change of salvage regime to ifosfamide, carboplatin, and etoposide (ICE) with a plan to transplant when she goes into complete remission (CR).

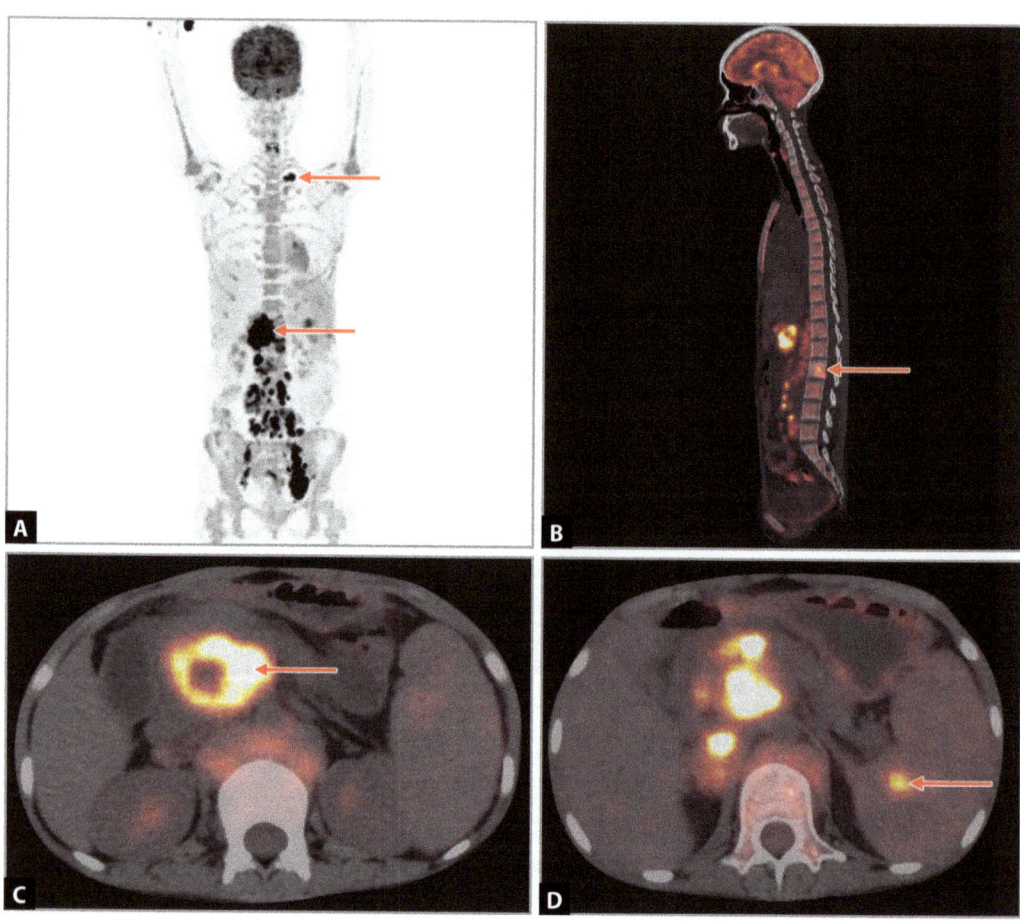

Figs. 1A to D: Maximum intensity projection (MIP) and fused positron emission tomography-computed tomography (PET-CT) images. (A) MIP image is showing multiple FDG lesions above and below the diaphragm; (B) Fused PET-CT images, arrow showing L2 vertebral lesion; (C) Arrow indicating abdominal lymph nodes; and (D) Arrow indicating splenic lesion.
Courtesy: Department of nuclear medicine, AIIMS, New Delhi.

1. How do you stage HL? What is the significance in newly diagnosed cases and in a relapsed setting?

Staging for any lymphoma is done for choosing appropriate treatment with maximum effect and at the same time minimizing the late effects and for prognostication. HL is staged on the basis of sites of nodal involvement, any extranodal disease, and presence of B symptoms. (Ann Arbor staging system, **Table 1 and Fig. 2**). At the time of relapse also the above parameters are taken into account, along with other attributes (primary progressive/refractory disease, time to relapse, and chemoresistance) described later. Proper staging and risk stratification at relapse is of paramount importance for deciding treatment strategy—conventional chemotherapy or HDCT followed by stem cell rescue.

TABLE 1: Ann Arbor staging classification.

Stage	Definition
Stage I	Involvement of a single lymph node region (I) or of a single extralymphatic organ or site (IE)
Stage II	Involvement of two or more lymph node regions on the same side of the diaphragm (II) or localized involvement of an extralymphatic organ or site and one or more lymph node regions on the same side of the diaphragm (IIE)
Stage III	Involvement of lymph node regions on both sides of the diaphragm (III), which may be accompanied by involvement of the spleen (IIIS) or by localized involvement of an extralymphatic organ or site (IIIE) or both (IIISE)
Stage IV	Diffuse or disseminated involvement of one or more extralymphatic organs or tissues with or without associated lymph node involvement

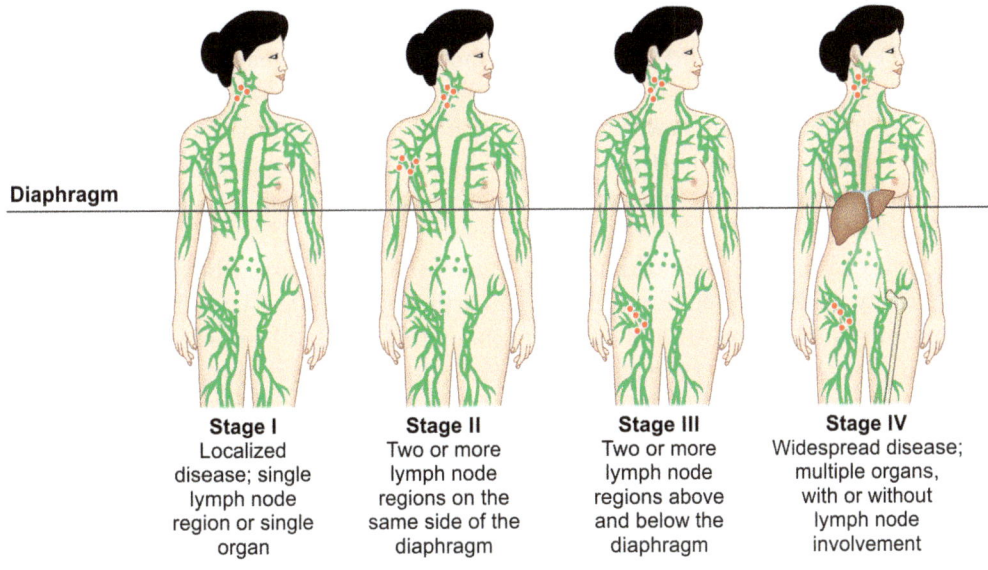

Fig. 2: Ann Arbor staging classification.

2. How do we risk stratify newly diagnosed HL? What is the optimum management of newly diagnosed advanced HL and could this child be managed on any other protocol?

Treatment of HL is the one of the success story in pediatric cancer treatment. With modern treatment estimate 5-year survival exceeds 90%. Some Indian studies have also documented an overall survival (OS) of 85–90%. Recently published reports from Indian Pediatric Oncology Group (InPOG) have also shown OS of 95% and 90% for early and advanced phase HL.[1,2] However, India is still struggling with issues of lack of awareness, poor social support, lack of facilities for early diagnosis, and delay in referral to cancer treatment centers leading to presentation in advanced stage. Availability of chemotherapy drugs, access to RT, and treatment abandonment are also contributory to the not so uniform outcomes across India.

Focus in the current era is to manage cases based on a risk based, response adapted strategy that has optimized not only treatment outcomes but also reduced the occurrence of late effects. For the purpose of treatment allocation and prognostication, at diagnosis patients are risk stratified based on stage, presence of B symptoms, number of nodal regions, peripheral nodal and mediastinal bulk, and extranodal extension of the disease. Risk group allocation varies substantially across different study groups. Advance stage, B symptoms and bulk is usually taken as high risk.

Currently first-line treatment of HL is multiagent chemotherapy with sparingly used consolidative RT only to slow/partial responders or baseline bulky disease. Regimens which are commonly used in newly diagnosed HL are Adriamycin, bleomycin, vinblastine, dacarbazine (ABVD), Cyclophosphamide, vincristine, procarbazine, prednisolone (COPP), Cyclophosphamide, vincristine, prednisone, Dacarbazine (COPDAC), Vincristine, etoposide, prednisone, doxorubicin/ Vincristine, prednisone, procarbazine, doxorubicin (OEPA/OPPA), Bleomycin, etoposide, adriamycin, cyclophosphamide, vincristine, procarbazine, prednisone (BEACOPP). Various published literature have shown that RT can be safely omitted in rapid responders on early interim assessment. Recently published report from multicentric study (InPOG-HL) of children with newly diagnosed HL from India have also used risk stratified and response adapted model with RT only for initial bulky and slow responders/residual disease. Can we quote from literature/ongoing studies that consider RT only for those with baseline bulky disease?

Our index case was treated with BEACOPP almost a decade ago, which causes hematological toxicity, cardiopulmonary toxicity, secondary malignancy, and infertility as side effects. Currently our unit is using ABVD as first-line chemotherapy for all stages and across all risk groups. At our center, stages I and IIA are classified as low risk, and stages IIB to IV as high risk. Low-risk patients receive 2–4 cycles of ABVD and high-risk receives 6 cycles. Bulky sites receive RT after completion of chemotherapy cycles. Most of the time, the choice of first-line chemotherapeutic regimen is based on the discretion of the treating center's preference.

3. How was she followed up postcompletion of her treatment?

Relapse of the primary malignancy is a constant threat for any cancer survivor. Even with the most effective pediatric regimens, treatment failure rates are approximately 10% in low stage and 15-20% in advanced HL. The child was under clinical follow up at periodic intervals (6 monthly in initial 2 years then annually). There is no role of surveillance imaging in the follow up of HL survivors.

Survivors of pediatric HL are at risk of diverse sequelae, including organ dysfunction and secondary malignancies. This mandates constant follow up not only for disease relapse but also for growth, endocrine, cardiopulmonary, fertility, bone health, and second malignant neoplasms. She was followed at the after treatment completion clinic, for disease recurrence, late effects, integration with peers, etc. special emphasis on vaccination, and breast self-examination.

4. What are the prognostic markers for newly diagnosed HL?

Pretreatment prognostic factors can help tailoring treatment for patients with HL, to achieve high cure rates in advance stage disease and at the same time decreasing toxicity in early stage disease.

Various prognostic factors have been studied in adult patients with HL across different study groups. Several prognostic indices have been developed to guide treatment. The most widely accepted risk stratification tool, in adults, is *International Prognostic Score* (IPS), but these cannot be extrapolated to pediatric patients. The IPS incorporates seven clinical parameters (male sex, age ≥45 years, hemoglobin <105 g/L, WBC count ≥15 × 10^9/L, lymphocyte count <0.6 × 10/L or <8% of differential, albumin <40 g/L, stage IV) and each parameter is independently associated with a poorer outcome. As per IPS, on the basis of the number of factors present at diagnosis, 5-year freedom from progression (FFP) ranged from 42 to 84% in different subgroups of patients.[3]

Pediatric studies have identified male sex; hemoglobin <11.0 g/dL and WBC >13.5 × 103/mm^3; stages IIB, IIIB, or IV disease; bulky mediastinal disease; as significant predictors for inferior disease-free survival (DFS). A prognostic index, incorporating the five significant factors, assigning each a score of 1 showed that DFS was worst in those with score of 4-5. The 5-year DFS and OS for children with a score of 0-1 were 94 and 99%; score 2-85% and 96%; score 3-71% and 92%; and score 4 or 5-49% and 72%, respectively.[4]

Children's Oncology Group (COG) has developed prognostic score known as Childhood Hodgkin International Prognostic Score (CHIPS) for children and adolescents with intermediate risk HL. Fever, stage IV disease, large mediastinal mass, and albumin (<3.5) were assigned one point each and were independent predictors of event-free survival (EFS). 4-year EFS for patients with CHIPS = 0 was 93.1%, CHIPS = 2, 77.6% and CHIPS = 3, 69.2%.[5] These prognostic scores can improve the ability to tailor the treatment better. With development of functional imaging (FI), the early response to chemotherapy assessed by PET-CT has become an important prognostic tool.

5. How do we diagnose and risk stratify at relapse?

Despite high initial cure rates, management of relapsed refractory Hodgkin lymphoma (RR-HL) is a challenge, in part because of lack of randomized trials defining best salvage regimen as well as absence of head to head trial for comparison of conventional chemotherapy versus HDCT followed by autologous stem cell transplant (ASCT) for pediatric HL.

For diagnosis, all patients should undergo excisional or trucut biopsy to document relapse as fine needle aspiration cytology (FNAC) does not provide sufficient material and is not advisable. All patients should be restaged at the time of relapse, preferably with FI to help in better comparison at the time of response assessment.

Similar to the newly diagnosed cases, certain clinical features and FI holds prognostic implications for freedom from subsequent relapses in RR-HL. Risk stratification at relapse helps in fine tuning the treatment strategy as to who can be treated with only standard-dose chemotherapy (SDCT) and/or RT, without ASCT. Though various study groups have reported prognostic factors at relapse, but there are no standard criteria for defining risk groups nor is there standard treatment regimen, which may be attributed to low accrual rates in the studies, due to rarity of relapses. Nonetheless, primary progressive/refractory disease, time to relapse, and chemoresistance are certain prognostic factors which are consistent across various studies.

Primary progressive/refractory disease (relapse or progression <3 months from completion of therapy), carries a very poor prognosis with EFS of 40–50% and has worse outcomes than early (3–12 months) or late relapse (>12 months) regardless of retrieval strategy (conventional chemotherapy or HDCT with stem cell rescue). Similarly, patients with early relapse fair worse than late relapse. *ST-HD-86 trial*, revealed the time to progression/relapse as the strongest prognostic factor. Patients with progression had an inferior DFS of 41% and OS of 51% whereas patients with late relapse did well with a DFS of 86% and OS of 90%, although none of them received stem cell transplantation (SCT) in second remission.[6] In a retrospective study from France, including, 70 patients with RR-HL, also reported time to progression/relapse and response to therapy as an important prognostic factor. Patients treated on *UK HD3* relapse treatment strategy, also showed that duration of first remission was strongly associated with OS.[7]

Response to reinduction chemotherapy is also highly predictive of outcome. A retrospective study from St. Jude Children's Research Hospital showed that patients with complete response (CR) or PR following initial salvage chemotherapy had a 5-year OS of 97.2% compared to 17.9%, for nonresponders.[8] In a study from Saudi Arabia[9], 15 patients who had CR/CRu before HDC ASCT were alive as compared to only 49% with no CR/CRu, $P = 0.0001$.

Few other less consistent factors are stage of the disease at relapse, presence of B symptoms and extranodal disease, bulk, mediastinal mass, relapse at original and distant new sites, anemia, and raised erythrocyte sedimentation rate (ESR). But these studies did not utilized PET/CT as response assessment criteria. PET negativity after salvage therapy is now the most consistent prognostic factor in relapse setting also it is in the first-line treatment. Reasons for inconsistent risk stratification among different study groups are mostly prognostic factors are studied in retrospective fashion and in prospective studies, the n is small to provide power to the study. The initial treatment of newly diagnosed HL, choice of salvage therapy is varied, along with evolution of treatment to novel agents in the upfront treatment and more and more use of FI, every study with RR-HL uses own set of risk stratification.

The ability to attain a *complete remission prior to AHSCT* is highly prognostic. Study from Memorial Sloan Kettering showed that patients transplanted with negative ^{18}F-fluorodeoxyglucose positron emission tomography (FDG-PET), pre-high-dose therapy/autologous stem cell transplant (pre-HDT/ASCT) post 1 or 2 second-line chemotherapy regimens, had an EFS of >80%, versus 28.6% for patients with a positive scan (p <0.001).[10] Another study from Memorial Sloan Kettering Cancer Center (MSKCC) demonstrated, 4-year EFS rates of 33% versus 77% for patients transplanted with positive versus negative FI.[11] CR on FI correlate better with higher EFS compared to chemosensitivity to CT criteria but positive by FI prior to AHSCT. Retrospective study from Egypt[12], including 43 patients, also showed an OS (89.4 vs. 60%) and EFS (78.3 vs. 40%) advantage for patients with negative PET scan as compared to those with positive PET scan before AHSCT. Earlier studies reporting prognostic factors did not use PET-CT as response, which is now commonly used as a modality for reassessment. PET negativity after salvage therapy is now the most consistent prognostic factor in relapse setting, as it is in the first-line treatment. Lately, EURONET pediatric Hodgkin Lymphoma group has come up with recommendations for risk stratification and treatment of RR-HL. They propose using three most important presalvage prognostic factors to allocate patients into low risk and standard risk groups.[13] An ongoing study on pediatric RR-HL by InPOG has also proposed a risk based response adapted approach for pediatric RR-HL. **Table 2** depicts the presalvage prognostic factors and risk stratification as per the two groups.

TABLE 2: Risk stratification according to study groups.

	EURONET	InPOG	AIIMS
Presalvage prognostic factors	• Time to relapse • Prior treatment • Stage at relapse	• Primary refractory disease • Early relapse (<12 months) • B symptoms at relapse • Relapse in an irradiated site • Extranodal disease at relapse • Stage IV disease at relapse	• InPOG criteria is being followed at our center • Primary refractory disease • Early relapse (<12 months) • B symptoms at relapse • Relapse in an irradiated site • Extranodal disease at relapse • Stage IV disease at relapse

Relapse risk category	Low-risk group:
	• Early relapse after a maximum four cycles of first-line chemotherapy
	• Late relapse after a maximum of six cycles of first-line chemotherapy
	• And all of the following:
	  – Stage at relapse is I-III
	  – No prior RT or relapse only outside prior RT field
		High-risk:
		• If any of the above risk factor is present
		Low-risk:
		• None of the above should be present
			As per InPOG-RR-HL protocol

Contd...

Contd...

Euronet	InPOG	AIIMS
– No excessive RT fields required in salvage *Standard risk group:* • Primary progressive HL • Early relapse after >4 cycles of first-line chemotherapy • Stage IV relapse • Relapse in a prior RT field • Relapse requiring RT in salvage that is considered as having unacceptable toxicity *On the basis of response to salvage therapy, EURONET further risk stratify patients into three groups:* • Low risk • Standard risk • High risk High risk are those who fail to achieve a CMR after two lines of SDCT on PET4		

(CMR: complete metabolic response; HL: Hodgkin lymphoma; InPOG: Indian Pediatric Oncology Group; RT: radiotherapy; SDCT: standard-dose chemotherapy)

6. What is the treatment strategy and salvage regimen for RR-HL and do the cumulative doses have bearing on treatment of RR-HL?

Treatment of RR-HL is based on the risk stratification and response to salvage regimen. HDCT followed by AHSCT is the standard of care for adults with high-risk relapsed HL. This is supported by two RCT done in adult patients, showing superiority in terms of high 3-year EFS, though OS did not differ.[14,15] These results are being extrapolated for pediatric patients with relapsed HL, but growing body of evidence suggest that only chemotherapy with/without RT, is a feasible option for low-risk pediatric relapses.

After initial risk stratification based on the above mentioned prognostic factors, salvage chemotherapy should be given, following which response assessment is done. Salvage regimen is chosen keeping in mind the cumulative doses from the previous treatment as well as status of RT. Second next step in deciding the individual retrieval plan is based on the response to salvage regimen. Achieving complete metabolic response (CMR) or adequate response with SDCT on FDG-PET, is the most important prognostic marker for long-term disease control. Response assessment previously used conventional imaging but FI with FDG-PET response is more accurate as it may distinguish residual sclerotic tissue from viable tumor. Thus the goal of salvage SDCT should be to achieve a negative FDG-PET pre-HDCT. Patients with residual FDG-PET positivity after first salvage SDCT, who achieved a FDG-PET negativity after second line, noncross resistant salvage, had a similar post-transplant outcome to those in CMR after first line. The poor prognostic impact of failure to achieve a CMR with first-line SDCT can therefore be overcome by switching to alternative salvage regimens if a CMR is achieved with second-line SDCT. **Flowchart 1** showing the treatment plan suggested by InPOG. **Flowchart 2** depicts the treatment plan followed at our institute.

To summarize the treatment for low- or standard/intermediate-risk relapse group is SDCT followed by consolidative RT. After two cycles of salvage depending on CMR or PR at post two cycle reassessment by FI, they can either continue to receive two more cycles of same chemotherapy or can switch to second-line chemotherapy. Low risk and good responders can thus be salvaged with SDCT followed by consolidative RT. All high risk and poor responders to salvage should be transplanted as soon as they achieve CMR. Some might need to be transplanted in PR, though outcome may be dismal.

Summary of treatment strategy by various groups (EURONET recommendations and InPOG):
- *Low-risk group/intermediate group (variably named) treatment summary:* The intention in this group is to select patients that may avoid the toxicity of HDCT/ASCT and in whom SDCT plus RT is an effective option without excessive RT toxicity. Usual strategy is induction treatment with two cycles of first-line salvage SDCT, followed by response assessment. If PET2 is CMR (D1–3 or qPET <1.3), consolidation treatment is 1–2 further cycles of SDCT followed by consolidation involved-field radiotherapy (IFRT). In cases of no CMR/PR

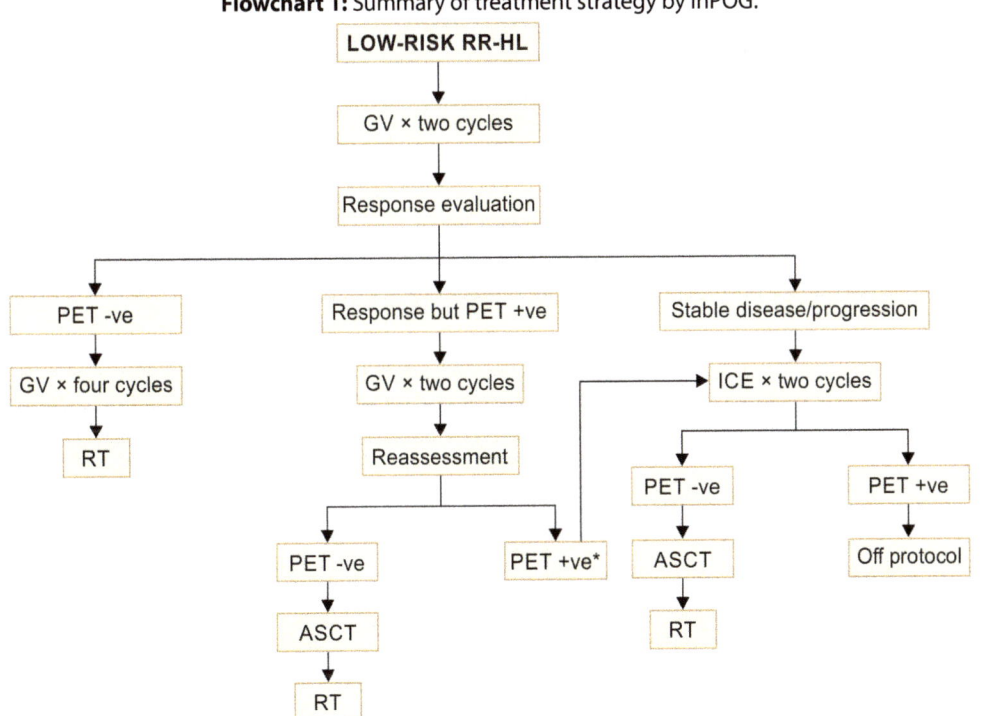

Flowchart 1: Summary of treatment strategy by InPOG.

Contd...

Contd...

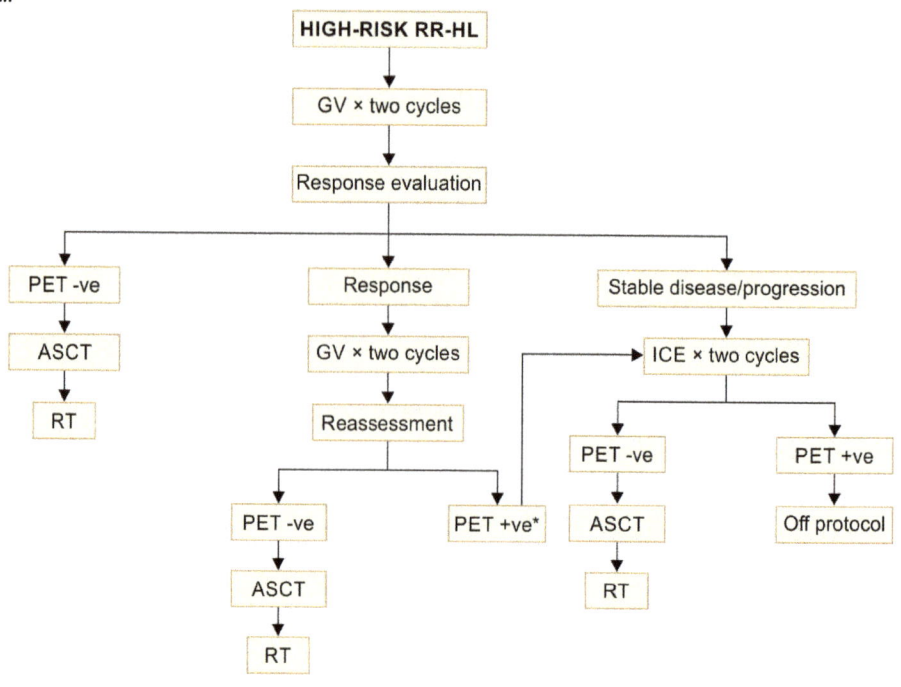

*Second-line salvage to be used if PET positive even after four cycles of first salvage.
(ASCT: autologous stem cell transplant; CMR: complete metabolic response; GV: gemcitabine and vinorelbine; ICE: Ifosfamide, carboplatin, etoposide; InPOG: Indian Pediatric Oncology Group; PD: progressive disease; PET: positron emission tomography; PR: partial response; SD: stable disease; RR-HL: relapsed refractory Hodgkin lymphoma; RT: radiotherapy)

Flowchart 2: Summary of treatment strategy followed at our institute.

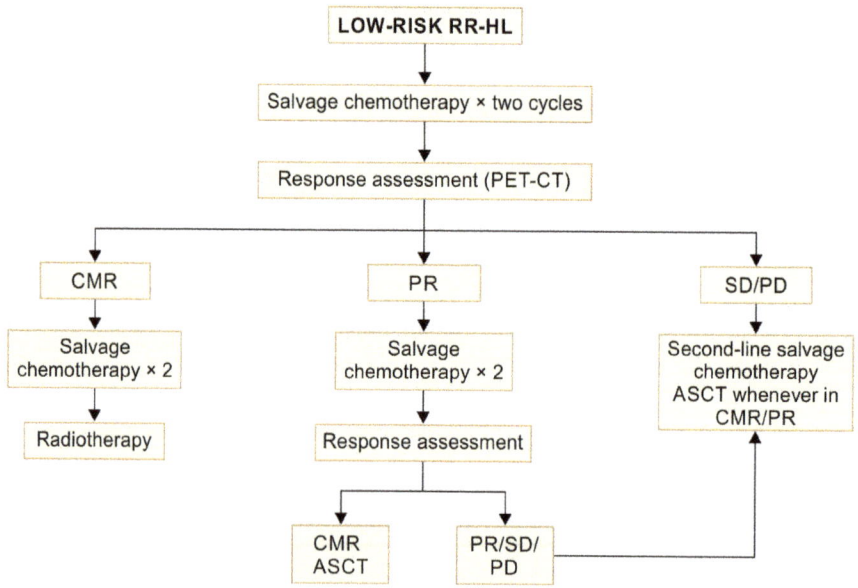

Contd...

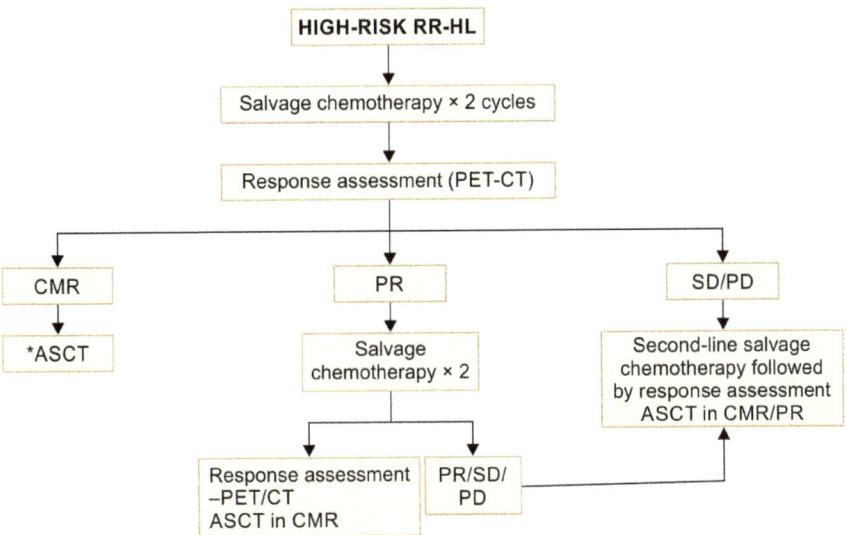

*1 or 2 chemotherapy cycles can be given, while arranging transplant.
(ASCT: autologous stem cell transplant; CMR: complete metabolic response; GV: gemcitabine and vinorelbine; ICE: Ifosfamide, carboplatin, etoposide; PD: progressive disease; PET/CT: positron emission tomography/computed tomography; PR: partial response; SD: stable disease; RR-HL: relapsed refractory Hodgkin lymphoma; RT: radiotherapy)

(D4–5 or qPET >1.3) but not stable disease (SD) or PD, some may choose to continue with same salvage for two more cycles or else may switch to second salvage regimen. Selection of chemotherapy is guided by the factors mentioned later. If CMR is achieved in second interim assessment (PET4) they should proceed to consolidative HDCT/ASCT as soon as possible. But if PET4 or second reassessment also shows no CMR, they should be treated as high-risk patients.

- *Standard-risk group/high-risk (variably named) treatment summary:* The intention in this group is to select patients for whom SDCT plus consolidation HDCT/ASCT is indicated and deescalation to nontransplant salvage is not recommended. These patients should receive salvage chemotherapy followed by response assessment. If CMR on PET2 can proceed to consolidative treatment with HDCT/ASCT. If PET2, no CMR, patients can be switched to second-line salvage or can continue with two more cycles of same chemotherapy, depending upon centers protocol. Following this if PET4 is in CMR, they should pursue HDCT/ASCT. At any time, disease progression or fail to achieve CMR after two lines of salvage chemotherapy they should be treated as chemorefractory patients.
- *Prognosis of chemorefractory is dismal and options are:*
  - Use of novel agents, immunotherapy, or further lines of noncross resistant chemotherapy to achieve a CMR on FDG-PET before HDCT/ASCT and consider addition of further treatments after HDCT/ASCT
  - Proceed with HDCT/ASCT anyway in responding patients despite no CMR on pretransplant PET and consider addition of further treatments after HDCT/ASCT such as RT and/or maintenance brentuximab vedotin (BV)
  - Enrol patients in clinical trials where available
  - Consider nonstandard transplant strategies such as allogeneic transplantation.

7. What are the available conventional standard-dose salvage chemotherapy (SDCT) regimens?

There is no best salvage SDCT regimen because of lack of randomized trials comparing salvage regimens in children (or adults), which demonstrate the superiority of one regimen over another. Salvage response rates come from single arm or retrospective studies, which are difficult to compare because of inconsistency in the prior treatment regimens and prognostic factors between various studies. The choice of salvage regimen is guided by individual patient factors, previous chemotherapy received to use noncross-resistant drugs and avoid excess cumulative drug toxicities and individual patient factors as well as preference of the treating center for the regimen. Desirable qualities in salvage regimens include high efficacy and low toxicity, no impairment in the ability to mobilize and collect peripheral blood stem cells (PBSCs) and minimal late effects, including secondary myelodysplastic syndrome (MDS) and myeloid leukemia. The overall response rates (ORR = CR and PR >50%) of salvage regimens vary between 70 and 90%. For patients failing to achieve a CMR at PET2 a switch to second-line salvage SDCT is recommended and similar assessment of factors applies as for choice of first-line regimen, though based on previous chemotherapy used center may choose to continue with two more cycles of first-line chemotherapy in cases of less than CR (i.e., PR, but not SD or PD). Various categories of salvage regimens are listed in **Table 3**.

TABLE 3: Various salvage regimen and the ORR and CR rates needs alignment.

Salvage chemotherapy regimens (ORR %, CR %)	Targeted therapy	Immunotherapy
Gemcitabine-based: • *IGEV:* Ifosfamide, gemcitabine, vinorelbine, prednisolone (81%, 54%) • *BeGV:* Bendamustine, gemcitabine, vinorelbine (83%, 73%) • *GV:* Gemcitabine, vinorelbine (76%, 24%) • *GDP:* Gemcitabine, dexamethasone, cisplatin (70%, 17%) • *GVD:* Gemcitabine, vinorelbine, liposomal doxorubicin (70%, 19%)	**Brentuximab-based regimens** (can be used as second-line salvage) • BV single agent (47%, 33%) • *BV:* Bendamustine (93%, 74%) • *BV:* Nivolumab (90%, 62%) • *BV:* ESHAP (96%, 70%) • *BV:* ICE (94%, 69%) • *BV:* DHAP (100%, 92%) • *BV:* IGEV (100%, 71%)	Nivolumab
Ifosfamide/etoposide based: • *ICE:* Ifosfamide, carboplatin, etoposide (88%, 26%) • *IVE:* Ifosfamide, etoposide, epirubicin (84%, 60%) • *IEP-ABVD:* Ifosfamide, etoposide, prednisolone-adriamycin, bleomycin, vinblastine, dacarbazine (85%, NR)		Pembrolizumab
Cisplatin-based: • *DHAP:* Cytarabine, cisplatin, dexamethasone (88%, 21%) • *ESHAP:* Etoposide, methylprednisolone, high-dose cytarabine, cisplatin (73%, 40%) • *ASHAP:* Doxorubicin, methylprednisolone, high-dose cytarabine, cisplatin		

(BV: brentuximab vedotin; CR: complete response; ORR: overall response rate)

8. What is the role of targeted therapy and immunotherapy in HL?

Novel agents are increasingly being used in RR pediatric HL. They have been extensively studied in adults and pediatric data is scarce. So mostly it is extrapolated from the adult data and that is why they are usually used as a second-line salvage. Outside clinical trials use of novel agents BV is considered the first-line novel agent in RR-HL. This is an anti-CD30 antibody conjugated to auristatin [monomethyl auristatin E (MMAE)], an antitubulin agent, and is highly effective in RR-cHL. In phase II study in adults with single agent BV, ORR was 75% (CR 34%). Pediatric phase II trials with single agent BV, the CR rates were 33% in HL patients with manageable toxicity profile at 1.8 mg/kg.[16] BV in combination with either chemotherapy or immunotherapy drugs has shown more promising results and so single agent BV generally is no longer recommended as second-line salvage. Response rates of BV-based salvage regimens are given in **Table 3**.

Single agent bendamustine achieved CR rates of 33% in a phase II trial including patients receiving a median of four prior treatment including ASCT. This study confirmed the efficacy of bendamustine in heavily pretreated patients.[17] There appears to be synergy between BV and bendamustine in the BV-B combination. A phase 1/2 study evaluating this in RR-HL, has reported a CR rates of 74% and ORR of 93% including 85.7% among patients with primary refractory HL and 100% among patients with relapsed disease.[18] The majority of CRs are achieved after two cycles of BV-B and stem cell mobilization and collection was adequate in all patients who underwent this procedure ($n = 24$). This outpatient-based regimen has a manageable safety profile, very high CR rate, durable response and successful stem cell mobilization and collection and represents a promising approach for maximizing response prior to ASCT at an earlier stage in salvage. In a single center experience of the combination of BV + B used as second-line or greater salvage for RR-cHL in children and young people under 30 years, ORR was 83% (24/29), with CMR in 79% patients. Various other combinations of BV with chemotherapy and bendamustine with chemotherapy have been used. Multicentric phase 2 study of Benda with GV has shown promising results with ORR of 83% and CR of 73%.[19]

The immune checkpoint inhibitors nivolumab and pembrolizumab are an option in patients' refractory to two initial lines of salvage and are thus reserved for high-risk patients. These agents target the programmed death 1 (PD1) pathway, which is a checkpoint to limit T-cell-mediated immune responses. The two programmed death 1 ligands (PD-L1 and PD-L2), engage the PD1 receptor resulting in a reversible inhibition of T-cell activation and proliferation. Tumors, expressing PD1 ligands, can engage with the PD1 pathway to evade an immune response. This provides a potential therapeutic target in HL because Hodgkin and Reed–Sternberg (HRS) cells aberrantly overexpress PD-L1 and PD-L2, which can inhibit T-cell activation. Antibodies blocking PD1/PD-L1/PD-L2 engagement can facilitate and enhance T-cell activation and induction of T-cell-mediated antitumor response. CheckMate 205 phase 2 trial of Nivo showed an ORR of 69%.[20]

Pediatric study including 21 heavily pretreated patients receiving Nivo-based therapy showed an ORR of 86%. Nivo as a monotherapy resulted in ORR of 92%, combination therapy demonstrated similar effectiveness, i.e., ORR of 75%. Three-year OS and progression-free survival (PFS) were 95 and 29%, respectively.

Nivolumab + BV has shown 67% CMR and a high 2-year PFS rate as first salvage in adults with RR-cHL. CheckMate 744 (NCT02927769) is an ongoing phase 2 study for CAYA with RR-cHL, evaluating a risk-stratified, response-adapted approach using nivolumab + BV and, for patients without CMR, BV + bendamustine. After Nivo + BV induction ORR in primary refractory and pediatric age group was 79 and 81%, respectively.

9. What are the RT indications in relapse setting?

Radiotherapy is a highly effective modality for treatment of HL. With increasing use of radiation sparing protocols in pediatric HL treatment, >50% patients are RT naïve at relapse. RT is used as a consolidation postcompletion of salvage chemotherapy in low-risk patients. RT is also used as a consolidation post-ASCT in certain selected patients for better local control and DFS/PFS. In extensive nodal involvement and in previously irradiated sites, the RT dose and field may be way too much and thus toxicity may not be acceptable. For patients where the disease sites at relapse and first presentation are similar then the radiation fields can incorporate all sites of disease. If there is a change in disease distribution at relapse, then those relapsing within 12 months of first-line treatment should get RT at the unirradiated sites at first presentation and relapse as long as the RT fields and toxicity is considered acceptable by the treating team, but for patients who relapse >12 months after primary treatment, RT includes only FDG avid sites at relapse. RR-HL is more aggressive than de novo disease, and therefore, the recommended ISRT dose in salvage is a standard 3,000 cGy (150 cGy/day) or 3,060 cGy (180 cGy/day) to the ISRT volume. This higher dose of RT should be applied to all FDG-PET positive sites at relapse. In patients with early relapse previously unirradiated FDG-PET positive sites that were involved at first presentation but negative at relapse may also be considered for irradiation and these sites may have lower RT dose as applied in first line which is 1,980cGy (180cGY/day). *As per InPOG trial*, radiation is recommended to all sites of original disease and the site of relapse. The recommended doses are 35–40 Gy. If there is relapse at an irradiated site, careful discussion needs to be undertaken with the radiation oncology team bearing in mind the doses delivered at the previous at the time of initial treatment and plan the treatment.

Involved-field radiotherapy shall begin within 4 weeks of completion of the last cycle of chemotherapy subject to complete recovery of blood counts including an absolute neutrophil count (ANC) >1,000/µL and platelets >100,000/µL. For patients who undergo ASCT, this may be delayed to 6 weeks post-transplant.

10. What are the conditioning agents for RR-HL and is it advisable to transplant in PR?

There are no randomized trials to supporting one HDCT conditioning regimen over other. The choice of conditioning regimen is often based on institutional preference or familiarity of the treating team. Currently, in Europe, the consensus is chemotherapy-only conditioning, in both in adult and pediatric patients, as there is no evidence of superiority of total body irradiation (TBI), total lymphoid irradiation (TLI), or subtotal lymph node irradiation (STLI)-containing regimens. At the same time risk of MDS and secondary malignancy increases with use of radiation. Most popular regimens are the BEAM regimen (BCNU/carmustine, etoposide, cytarabine, and melphalan) or the alternative LEAM regimen with lomustine replacing

BCNU with almost equivalent toxicity and efficacy. The CBV regimen (cyclophosphamide, carmustine, and etoposide) is preferred in the United States of America. In a retrospective comparative analysis of patients with RR lymphoma undergoing ASCT with BEAM/LEAM/CLV (cyclophosphamide, lomustine, etoposide) as conditioning, showed no difference regarding engraftment, early toxicity, and transplant-related mortality (TRM).[21]

Bendamustine, a very active drug in HL may also be used in a conditioning regimen. Studies comparing BEAM and Benda-EAM (with bendamustine replacing BCNU) have recently shown similar 4 years PFS and OS but more of acute nonhematological toxicity with Benda-EAM. In view of unknown long-term toxicity, there is no clear evidence that Benda-EAM is superior to BEAM.

11. What are the indications for BV maintenance after HDCT/ASCT?

Post-ASCT consolidation with BV, in high-risk patients have shown improved PFS. Though this study was done in adults, results can be extrapolated to pediatric patients. Patients with two or more risk factors: (i) early relapse or primary progression, (ii) extranodal disease at relapse, (iii) B symptoms at relapse, (iv) no CMR to most recent SDCT, and (v) patients who needed two or more lines of SDCT pre-HDCT.

12. Role of allogeneic HSCT in RR-HL setting.

Allogeneic HSCT in RR-HL setting is reserved for those relapsing after autologous transplant/PET positive after two/more salvage therapy. There are no clear cut indications for allogeneic transplant in first salvage or in preference to autologous transplant. It is an option in high-risk patients who remain PET positive after two lines of salvage regimen, but this should be borne in mind that pretransplant PET positivity even in allogeneic transplant is associated with low PFS and OS. In a retrospective study of 70 patients undergoing reduced intensity conditioning (RIC) allogeneic transplant, resistant disease at allogeneic-ASCT-impacted survival. Nonrelapse mortality (NRM) in this was 17% at 1 year. In another large recent retrospective series of allogeneic-SCT outcomes, patients with pretransplant CR had a significantly lower rate of relapse compared to patients not in CR, 43% [95% confidence interval (CI) 25–56] versus 59% (95% CI 41–69), $p = 0.04$. The NRM was 13% at day 100 and 24% at 2 years for the whole cohort, which far exceeds that of autologous transplantation, and the overall 2-year PFS was 27%.[22] With novel targeted therapy achievement of CMR pretransplant has improved, which predicts good results with auto-ASCT and thus avoiding allogeneic-SCT. Use of post-HDCT/ASCT, consolidation strategies, and the outline is likely for less use of allogeneic-SCT.

13. Role of rituximab in classical HL and experience with R-DHAP [rituximab, dexamethasone, high-dose cytosine arabinoside (Ara-C), and cisplatin].

Rituximab is a commercially available chimeric antibody against CD20. Although the malignant HRS cells are predominantly of B cell origin, they infrequently express CD20. Apart from activity against CD20 positive HRS cells, rituximab acts on the benign B lymphocytes in the HL microenvironment which promotes HRS survival. So regardless of CD20 expression by HRS cells, by eliminating B cells, rituximab may deprive the malignant cells of survival signals and makes them more susceptible to chemotherapy.[23] Classical HL stem cells are small subpopulations, with memory B cell phenotype [immunoglobulin (Ig)-light chain, CD27, CD20, and stem cell marker aldehyde dehydrogenase], which are responsible for the generation and maintenance of the predominant HRS cell population. Thus, the expression of CD20 antigen by the putative HRS stem cells provides an additional rationale for the use of rituximab in patients with cHL. Rituximab as a single agent ORR of (22%) as well as with gemcitabine (ORR 46%), GIFOX (gemcitabine, ifosfamide, and oxaliplatin) (ORR 86%), and ABVD have been used in newly diagnosed classical HL as well as RR-HL. We have used R-DHAP in RR-HL with CD20 expression in HRS cells. After two cycles response assessment has shown CMR in one patient, who was chemoresistant and heavily pretreated with three lines of salvage chemotherapy and not affording novel agents. Patient has been autotransplanted successfully. In another high-risk patient response assessment is awaited. R-DHAP regimen is readily available and can be further explored in the setting of classical HL.

14. Why did our patient develop cardiac dysfunction and what is the evidence for giving cardioprotective agents?

Cardiac dysfunction is known complication of various anticancer drugs, especially anthracyclines, though cyclophosphamide, high-dose Ara-C, ifosfamide, cisplatin, pactitaxel, fluorouracil, and amsacrine, small molecules like tyrosine kinase inhibitors can also cause cardiotoxicity. There are no published Indian guidelines for the follow-up of patients for cardiotoxiciy, though COG long-term follow-up guidelines are available for reference. The regimen used in this case was BEACOPP, which contains doxorubicin and cyclophosphamide. *She received cumulative dose as 270 mg/m² of doxorubicin and 9,400 mg/m² of cyclophosphamide.*

The incidence of congestive heart failure is <5% with cumulative anthracycline exposure of <250 mg/m²; approaches 10% at doses between 250 mg/m² and 600 mg/m² and exceeds 30% for doses higher than 600 mg/m² for survivors of childhood cancer.[24]

However, there is a different level of risk for each patient scheduled for anthracycline therapy: patients <5 years old or >65 years old, with prior or concurrent chest irradiation, preexisting heart disease, or already known cardiovascular risk factors, have an increased risk for cardiotoxicity. As per COG, highest risk factors for cardiomyopathy are ≥300 mg/m² of anthracyclines, ≥30 Gy RT involving heart, anthracyclines + chest RT, younger age at treatment and pregnancy. Screening should began ≥2 years after treatment or ≥5 years after diagnosis (whichever is first). At our center we do a baseline cardiac evaluation at start of chemotherapy and also at end of chemotherapy when the child registers at the survivor clinic.

Cardiotoxicity can be acute (during or days to weeks of completion of chemotherapy), early (weeks or months of treatment and if often dose related) or late (years to develop and always dose related). Studies have shown β-blockers and angiotensin-converting enzyme (ACE) inhibitors as an effective agent for cardioprotection.

■ SUMMARY

To summarize, childhood RR-HL, is still a challenge to manage, but given a chance except primary progressive chemoresistant disease, early and late relapses have good outcome.

Management is risk adapted and response based. There is no standard salvage chemotherapy protocol, but the ultimate goal is to use no cross-resistant and least toxic drugs, to achieve remission and decrease late effects. Low risk can be salvaged without the need for HDCT/ASCT. High risk would still need HDCT/ASCT. RT is an effective modality for consolidation. With newer novel agents, there has been improved rate of CR prior to ASCT, leading to better PFS/EFS.

REFERENCES

1. Mahajan A, Singh M, Bakhshi S, Jain S, Radhakrishnan V, Verma N, et al. Treating early-stage Hodgkin lymphoma in resource-limited settings: InPOG-HL-15-01 experience. Pediatr Blood Cancer. 2021;68(10):e29219.
2. Jain S, Bakhshi S, Seth R, Verma N, Singh M, Mahajan A, et al. Risk based and response adapted radiation therapy for children and adolescents with newly diagnosed advanced stage Hodgkin lymphoma treated with ABVD chemotherapy: a report from the Indian pediatric oncology group study InPOG-HL-15-01. Leuk Lymphoma. 2022;63(5):1111-8.
3. Moccia AA, Donaldson J, Chhanabhai M, Hoskins PJ, Klasa RJ, Savage KJ, et al. International Prognostic Score in advanced-stage Hodgkin's lymphoma: altered utility in the modern era. J Clin Oncol. 2012;30(27):3383-8.
4. Smith RS, Chen Q, Hudson MM, Link MP, Kun L, Weinstein H, et al. Prognostic Factors for Children With Hodgkin's Disease Treated With Combined-Modality Therapy. J Clin Oncol. 2003;21(10): 2026-33.
5. Schwartz CL, Chen L, McCarten K, Wolden S, Constine LS, Hutchison RE, et al. Childhood Hodgkin International Prognostic Score (CHIPS) Predicts event-free survival in Hodgkin Lymphoma: A Report from the Children's Oncology Group. Pediatr Blood Cancer. 2017;64(4):10.1002/pbc.26278.
6. Schellong G, Dörffel W, Claviez A, Körholz D, Mann G, Scheel-Walter HG, et al. Salvage therapy of progressive and recurrent hodgkin's disease: results from a multicenter study of the pediatric DAL/GPOH-HD study group. 2005;23(25):6181-9.
7. Shankar A, Hayward J, Kirkwood A, McCarthy K, Hewitt M, Morland B, et al. Treatment outcome in children and adolescents with relapsed Hodgkin lymphoma—results of the UK HD3 relapse treatment strategy. Br J Haematol. 2014;165(4):534-44.
8. Metzger ML, Hudson MM, Krasin MJ, Wu J, Kaste SC, Kun LE, et al. Initial response to salvage therapy determines prognosis in relapsed pediatric Hodgkin lymphoma patients. Cancer. 2010;116(18): 4376-84.
9. Akhtar S, El Weshi A, Rahal M, Abdelsalam M, Al Husseini H, Maghfoor I. High-dose chemotherapy and autologous stem cell transplant in adolescent patients with relapsed or refractory Hodgkin's lymphoma. Bone Marrow Transplantation. 2010;45(3):476-82.
10. Moskowitz CH, Matasar MJ, Zelenetz AD, Nimer SD, Gerecitano J, Hamlin P, et al. Normalization of pre-ASCT, FDG-PET imaging with second-line, non-cross-resistant, chemotherapy programs improves event-free survival in patients with Hodgkin lymphoma. Blood. 2012;119(7):1665-70.
11. Moskowitz CH, Yahalom J, Zelenetz AD, Zhang Z, Filippa D, Teruya-Feldstein J, et al. High-dose chemo-radiotherapy for relapsed or refractory Hodgkin lymphoma and the significance of pre-transplant functional imaging. Br J Haematol. 2010;148(6):890-7.
12. Abdalla A, Hammad M, Hafez H, Zaghloul MS, Taha H, El-Hennawy G, et al. Outcome predictors of autologous hematopoietic stem cell transplantation in children with relapsed and refractory Hodgkin lymphoma: single-center experience in a lower middle-income country. Pediatr Transplant. 2019;23(6):e13531.
13. Daw S, Hasenclever D, Mascarin M, Fernández-Teijeiro A, Balwierz W, Beishuizen A, et al. Risk and response adapted treatment guidelines for managing first relapsed and refractory classical Hodgkin

lymphoma in children and young people. Recommendations from the EuroNet Pediatric Hodgkin Lymphoma Group. Hemasphere. 2020;4(1):e329.
14. Linch DC, Winfield D, Goldstone AH, Moir D, Hancock B, et al. Dose intensification with autologous bone-marrow transplantation in relapsed and resistant Hodgkin's disease: results of a BNLI randomized trial. Lancet. 1993;341(8852):1051-4.
15. Schmitz N, Pfistner B, Sextro M, Sieber M, Carella AM, Haenel M, et al. Aggressive conventional chemotherapy compared with high dose chemotherapy with autologous hematopoietic stem-cell transplantation for relapsed chemo-sensitive Hodgkin's disease: a randomized trial. Lancet. 2002;359(9323):2065-71.
16. Locatelli F, Mauz-Koerholz C, Neville K, Llort A, Beishuizen A, Daw S, et al. Brentuximab vedotin for paediatric relapsed or refractory Hodgkin's lymphoma and anaplastic large-cell lymphoma: a multicentre, open-label, phase 1/2 study. Lancet. Haematol. 2018;5(10):e450-e461.
17. Moskowitz AJ, Hamlin PA Jr, Perales MA, Gerecitano J, Horwitz SM, Matasar MJ, et al. Phase II study of bendamustine in relapsed and refractory Hodgkin lymphoma. J Clin Oncol. 2013;31(4):456-60.
18. LaCasce AS, Bociek RG, Sawas A, Caimi P, Agura E, Matous J, et al. Three-year outcomes with brentuximab vedotin plus bendamustine as first salvage therapy in relapsed or refractory Hodgkin lymphoma. Br J Haematol. 2020;189(3):e86-e90.
19. Santoro A, Mazza R, Pulsoni A, Re A, Bonfichi M, Zilioli VR, et al. Bendamustine in combination with gemcitabine and vinorelbine is an effective regimen as induction chemotherapy before autologous stem-cell transplantation for relapsed or refractory Hodgkin lymphoma: final results of a multicenter phase II study. J Clin Oncol. 2016;34(27):3293-9.34.
20. Armand P, Engert A, Younes A, Fanale M, Santoro A, Zinzani PL, et al. Nivolumab for relapsed/refractory classic Hodgkin lymphoma after failure of autologous hematopoietic cell transplantation: extended follow-up of the multicohort single-arm phase II checkMate 205 Trial. J Clin Oncol. 2018;36(14):1428-39.
21. Colita A, Colita A, Bumbea H, Croitoru A, Orban C, Lipan LE, et al. LEAM vs. BEAM vs. CLV conditioning regimen for autologous stem cell transplantation in malignant lymphomas. Retrospective comparison of toxicity and efficacy on 222 patients in the first 100 days after transplant, on behalf of the Romanian Society for Bone Marrow Transplantation. Front Oncol. 2019;9:892.
22. Spina F, Radice T, De Philippis C, Soldarini M, Di Chio MC, Dodero A, et al. Allogeneic transplantation for relapsed and refractory Hodgkin lymphoma: long-term outcomes and graft-versus-host disease-free/relapse-free survival. Leuk Lymphoma. 2019;60(1):101-109.
23. Oki Y, Younes A. Does rituximab have a place in treating classic Hodgkin lymphoma? Curr Hematol Malig Rep. 2010;5(3):135-9.
24. Purkayastha K, Seth R, Seth S, Lyon AR. Cancer therapy-induced cardiotoxicity: review and algorithmic approach toward evaluation. J Pract Cardiovasc Sci. 2017;3:82-93.

EXPERT OPINION

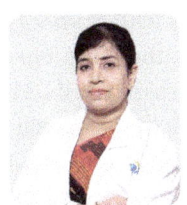

Amita Mahajan MBBS MD
Senior Consultant in Pediatric Oncology
Indraprastha Apollo Hospital, New Delhi

Management of Relapsed/Refractory Hodgkin Lymphoma in Children and Adolescents

Treatment outcomes of children with newly diagnosed HL currently exceed 90 and 80% for early-stage and advanced-stage disease, respectively. Excellent outcomes can be achieved even in low-middle income countries. Nevertheless, a proportion of patients have primary refractory disease and about 20–30% relapse. A significant proportion of them can be salvaged successfully and the current paradigm for the management of this cohort is risk stratified and response adapted.

For a definitive diagnosis of relapse, it is strongly recommended that a diagnostic biopsy be repeated, wherever feasible, especially in our setting where chronic infections such as tuberculosis may confound the diagnosis on imaging. FI with FDG-PET is essential for accurate staging and response evaluation.

There have been no randomized trials in children to define the optimal strategy for this cohort. Current recommendations are largely based on evidence from retrospective or nonrandomized studies but it is clearly evident that a proportion of patients can be cured without HDCT and ASCT. All patients receive salvage chemotherapy with the aim of achieving CMR (Deauville score 1–3) at reassessment. Response evaluation should ideally be done after two cycles of chemotherapy.

Many regimen for salvage chemotherapy have been evaluated in this setting with no clear superiority of any one specific regimen. Commonly used regimen are: GV with or without dexamethasone, ICE, IGEV (ifosfamide/gemcitabine/vinorelbine/prednisolone), ESHAP (etoposide, methylprednisolone, high-dose cytarabine, and cisplatin), and DHAP (cytarabine, cisplatin, dexamethasone). The regimen chosen depends on what agents have been used in frontline therapy and access to optimal supportive care. The efficacy of salvage chemotherapy must be balanced by toxicity and the impact on subsequent PBSC mobilization as many of these patients will go on to receive ASCT. Most centers in India use GV, ICE or IGEV.

Myeloablative chemotherapy with autologous ASCT has been considered the standard of care based on two randomized trials that compared SDCT with HDCT and ASCT in adults. These trials predated the FDG-PET era and though they did demonstrate improved PFS, there was no difference in the OS. There is however, increasing evidence that a proportion of patients can have equivalent outcomes with conventional chemotherapy with or without adjuvant radiation. In pediatric studies aimed at addressing this question, improved survival has been demonstrated only in patients with primary refractory or multiply relapsed disease. The treatment algorithm for this cohort, therefore, currently adopts risk stratification. Patients with primary refractory disease (progression within 3 months of completion of therapy), early relapse (<12 months from completion of therapy), stage IV, B symptoms, those with relapse in a previously irradiated site or extranodal disease and those who have a suboptimal response to salvage chemotherapy are considered to be high risk and warrant more aggressive therapy including ASCT. Patients without these high-risk features are deemed to have low-risk relapse and are likely to be cured with conventional chemotherapy with or without adjuvant radiation. ASCT has been preferred for patients with relapsed HL because of the historically high transplant-related morbidity and mortality associated with allogeneic transplantation. Patients can proceed to ASCT once they achieve metabolic remission. The projected PFS rate is 30–89% with improved outcomes for patients with metabolic remission prior to ASCT. Salvage rates for patients with primary refractory HL are suboptimal even with ASCT and radiation. The most commonly used conditioning regimen currently used prior to ASCT is BEAM chemotherapy with carmustine (BCNU), etoposide, cytarabine, and melphalan. Adverse prognostic features for outcome post-ASCT include primary refractory disease or poor response to salvage chemotherapy, extranodal disease or advanced stage at relapse, bulky mediastinal mass at time of transplant and a positive PET scan prior to transplant.

Patients who relapse post-ASCT are candidates for allogeneic BMT after achieving remission.

Patients with low-risk relapse who have achieved metabolic remission following salvage chemotherapy and patients with high-risk relapse both benefit from adjuvant radiation. The doses administered are higher than those used in frontline therapy, i.e., 35–40 Gy. The current recommendation from the EURONET group is that for patients with low-risk relapse, all sites that were FDG-PET positive sites should receive this higher dose of RT. In patients with high-risk relapse sites which were involved at first presentation but negative at relapse should also be considered for RT though lower doses (19.8 Gy) as employed in frontline treatment. Patients who have had a suboptimal response to salvage chemotherapy may benefit from radiation prior to ASCT.

Immunotherapy is being increasingly explored in this setting both to limit toxicity and to enhance response rates. Rituximab in combination with chemotherapy has been used for CD20+ HL, especially for nodular lymphocyte predominant HL. BV (anti-CD30) has been evaluated in this setting in combination with chemotherapy with response rates of 60–70%. It is currently recommended for second-line salvage therapy.

Immune checkpoint inhibitors (ICIs), pembrolizumab and nivolumab, are promising in this setting with impressive response rates and low toxicity. These agents target the PD1 pathway. PD1-ligands (PD-L1, PD-L2) engage with PD1 resulting in reversible inhibition of T-cell activation and proliferation. HRS cells overexpress PD-L1 and PD-L2. ICIs block the PD1/PD-L1/PD-L2 engagement resulting in enhanced T-cell activation and induction of T cell-mediated antitumor response. These agents have demonstrated impressive activity, especially in combination with chemotherapy or BV, with limited toxicity. They are currently recommended for patients who have received three strategies of therapy or have relapsed post-ASCT respectively.

The role of maintenance immunotherapy for up to a year after ASCT with BV or checkpoint inhibitors has been evaluated in adult patients at high risk of subsequent relapse and demonstrated improved PFS. Its role in children is currently being evaluated. Therapeutic options, currently being evaluated in this setting include anti-CD30 chimeric antigen receptor T-cell therapy and the precise role of immunotherapy and ICIs in the setting.

In summary, current treatment algorithm for RR-HL in children is risk stratified and response adapted aimed at limiting toxicity while optimizing outcomes. Monoclonal antibodies and ICIs are expected to play a bigger role in future.

CHAPTER 12

Myelodysplastic Syndrome

Mohanaraj Ramachandran, Jagdish P Meena

CASE VIGNETTE

A 7-year-old male child presented with a history of fever on and off for 2 months. He had a history of bleeding manifestations in the form of epistaxis and petechiae for 1 month. There was no history of cough, coryza, vomiting, loose stools, abdominal pain, abdominal distension, breathing difficulty, decreased urine output, no loss of weight or loss of appetite, swelling anywhere, and no family history of similar illness. He received a platelet transfusion once before being referred to us. On examination, the child was found to have pallor. There was no lymphadenopathy, no organomegaly, no skin/nail changes, no hyper-/hypopigmentation, and no short stature. The investigations showed hemoglobin of 8.2 g/dL, total leukocyte count of 2,100/mm^3, absolute neutrophil count (ANC) of 900/mm^3, and platelet count of 40,000/μL. The renal and liver function tests were within normal limits. The lactate dehydrogenase (LDH) value was 262 IU/L. The peripheral smear showed no blasts. Bone marrow (BM) examination was suggestive of 4% blasts with marked dysplastic changes in erythroid and megakaryocyte lineage. BM biopsy was suggestive of marked hypocellularity and patchy distribution of erythropoiesis. Karyotype suggestive of normal male karyotype 46, XY.

1. What is the diagnosis in the above case?

Myelodysplastic syndrome (MDS) should be considered as a clinical possibility in the index child in view of dysplastic changes in marrow and cytopenias.

Myelodysplastic syndrome is a very rare entity in children and it is the diagnosis of exclusion. Common disorders should be ruled out before labeling as MDS. Inherited bone marrow failure syndromes (IBMFSs) can also have morphological dysplasia in the marrow and it can predispose to MDS. It is advised to do two BM examinations at least 2 weeks apart in absence of a cytogenetic marker. Following is the list of differential diagnoses for index child:

1. *Hematological disorders:*
   a. *Inherited BM failure disorders:*
      i. Fanconi anemia (FA), Diamond–Blackfan anemia
      ii. Dyskeratosis congenita (DKC)
      iii. Severe congenital neutropenia, Shwachman–Diamond syndrome (SDS)
      iv. Amegakaryocytic thrombocytopenia, thrombocytopenia with absent radii (TAR), and Seckel syndrome

b. *Severe aplastic anemia:*
      i. Paroxysmal nocturnal hemoglobinuria (PNH)
      ii. Hypoplastic prephase of B-cell precursor acute lymphoblastic leukemia
2. *Nonhematological disorders:*
   a. *Infections:*
      i. Cytomegalovirus
      ii. Epstein–Barr virus (EBV)
      iii. Herpesvirus, parvovirus, varicella virus, human immunodeficiency virus (HIV), and visceral leishmaniasis
      iv. Bacterial infections
      v. Vitamin deficiency: B_{12}, folate, and vitamin E deficiency
   b. Metabolic disorders like mevalonate kinase deficiency
   c. Rheumatic disease
   d. Pearson syndrome.

2. What is MDS?

It is a clonal hematopoietic stem cell disorder characterized by persistent and unexplained cytopenias, ineffective hematopoiesis, significant morphological dysplasia, and has increased risk of progression to acute myeloid leukemia (AML).[1]

3. What are the types of MDS and its current classification?

This entity was first described by Giovanni Antonio Di Guglielmo as chronic erythremic myelosis in 1920. Later in the 1960 and 1970s, it was called by various names like preleukemia and smoldering leukemia. In 1976, French–American–British (FAB) classification named it dysmyelopoietic syndrome, which was further modified to the current terminology of MDS.[2]

World Health Organization (WHO) classification has been updated periodically from 2001 to 2008 and 2016. This classification is suited well for the adult population, and adult MDS is not comparable with its pediatric counterpart. For example, refractory anemia is not commonly observed in children; unlike adults, they usually present with thrombocytopenia and/or neutropenia rather than anemia. Ringed sideroblasts are commonly secondary to nutritional deficiency, drug toxicity, and sideroblastic anemias in children rather than MDS.[3] Refractory cytopenia of childhood (RCC) was introduced for the first time in the 2008 classification, which remains a provisional entity in the 2016 classification. Refractory anemia with excess blasts 1 (RAEB-1) and RAEB-2 are replaced by MDS-EB-1 and EB-2 in the latest WHO classification.[4] Because of the above reasons, we may expect a change in subsequent classification, and clinically relevant pediatric MDS classification and diagnostic categories.

Refractory cytopenia of childhood is considered a low-grade MDS. MDS-EB-1 and EB-2 are considered high-grade or advanced MDS. Therapy-related MDS and MDS associated with germline predisposition are given as separate categories in classification. WHO classification is described in **Table 1**.

The index case presented with cytopenias, with no blasts in peripheral smear and 4% blasts in BM with dysplasia in two lineages (erythroid and megakaryocyte) and thus can be labeled as RCC.

TABLE 1: World Health Organization (WHO) classification of MDS.[5]

	Cytopenias	Circulating blasts	Dysplastic lineage	Ringed sideroblasts	Cytogenetics
Refractory cytopenia of childhood	1–3	• Peripheral blood: <2% • BM: <5%	1–3	None	Any
MDS-EB-1	1–3	• Peripheral blood: 2–4% • BM: 5–9%	0–3	None or any	Any
MDS-EB-2	1–3	• Peripheral blood: 5–19% • BM: 10–19%	0–3	None or any	Any

(BM: bone marrow; MDS-EB-1: myelodysplastic syndrome with excess blasts-1; MDS-EB-2: myelodysplastic syndrome with excess blasts-2)
Source: Adapted from ICMR.

4. What is the common clinical presentation of MDS?

Refractory cytopenia of childhood is the most common type of MDS seen in children. It usually presents with cytopenias. Unlike adults, where isolated anemia is common, children usually present with neutropenia and thrombocytopenia. The mean corpuscular volume (MCV) is elevated, and these patients can have elevated fetal hemoglobin (HbF) levels. Organomegaly and lymphadenopathy are not commonly seen in MDS.[1]

5. How common is MDS in children?

Myelodysplastic syndrome is rare in children. The incidence of MDS is 1–4 cases/million population. It constitutes <5% of childhood hematological malignancies. Germline syndromes and IBMFSs can predispose to MDS or AML.[1]

6. What is the difference between adult MDS and pediatric MDS?[6]

TABLE 2: Difference between adult and pediatric MDS.

	Pediatric MDS	Adult MDS
Incidence per million	1–4	>40
The median age in years	7	70
Presentation	• *Bilineage cytopenia:* Most common • Thrombocytopenia >Neutropenia and/or anemia	Isolated anemia
Associated IBMFSs and predisposition syndromes (%)	>30	<5
Familial aggregation	Present in a proportion of patients	Uncommon
Morphological subtype	RCC	RARS
BM cellularity	*Variable and hypocellular:* Common	Hyper- or normocellular

Contd...

Contd...

	Pediatric MDS	Adult MDS
Chromosomal aberrations (%)		
−7/−7q	25–30	10
−5/−5q	1	20
Molecular aberrations	Germline mutations are common, less frequent somatic mutations; absent spliceosomal mutations	Germline mutations are less common; frequent somatic mutations; spliceosomal mutations are common
The general aim of treatment	Curative	Often palliative

(IBMFSs: inherited bone marrow failure syndromes; MDS: myelodysplastic syndrome; RARS: refractory anemia with ringed sideroblasts; RCC: refractory cytopenia of childhood)

7. What are predisposing factors for MDS in children?

1. *Germline predisposition:*[7]
   a. *Familial MDS with mutated GATA2:*
      i. GATA2 mutation is the most common germline predisposing condition that was first described in 2011.[2] It is a multisystem disorder characterized by variable cytopenias, BM failure, severe immunodeficiency, and predisposition to MDS/AML. It can manifest as Emberger syndrome, which constitutes lymphedema, warts, and predisposition to MDS/AML. MonoMAC syndrome can manifest as monocytopenia, nontubercular mycobacterial infection, and also as severe immunodeficiency with dendritic cell, monocyte, B- and NK-cell lymphoid deficiency (DCML).[2]
      ii. The incidence of GATA2 mutation in advanced MDS is 15% compared to low incidence (4%) in low-grade MDS.[1] The majority (70%) of monosomy 7 positive MDS have GATA2 mutations. GATA2 mutations are at higher risk for progression to advanced MDS.
   b. *Familial platelet disorder with predisposition to myeloid malignancy (FPDMM):* This disorder is characterized by a germline mutation in RUNX1. It can present with mild to moderate thrombocytopenia with platelet function defect, which can increase the risk of bleeding tendency. They are at increased risk of transformation into AML, MDS, or T-cell acute lymphoblastic leukemia (T-ALL). MDS/AML transformation is around 20–60% which is associated with a second mutation in RUNX1 or acquisition of trisomy 21.
   c. *ANKRD26-related thrombocytopenia:* This disorder is characterized by lifelong mild to moderate thrombocytopenia. But usually, they will have normal hemostasis or mild bleeding phenotype. They are at risk for MDS and myeloid malignancies such as AML and chronic myelocytic leukemia (CML). BM examination at baseline itself will show dysmegakaryopoiesis with hypolobulated micromegakaryocytes, which makes it very difficult to differentiate the primary disorder from the development of MDS.

d. *ETV6-associated familial thrombocytopenia and hematological malignancy:* This disorder is characterized by mild to moderate thrombocytopenia with a variable predisposition to MDS, AML, and ALL. Thrombocytopenia is completely penetrant, and there is a higher risk for ALL.
e. *SAMD9 and SAMD9L mutation:* Germline SAMD9/SAMD9L mutation has been recently found to be associated with MDS. The mutation can also lead to a multisystem disorder like ATXPC syndrome, which manifests as ataxia, variable cytopenias, and MIRAGE syndrome characterized by myelodysplasia, infection, restriction of growth, adrenal hypoplasia, genital problems, and enteropathy.[8]
2. Inherited bone marrow failure syndromes.
3. Therapy-related MDS—exposure to alkylating agents, epipodophyllotoxins, and radiotherapy.

8. How to investigate MDS/hypoplastic marrow with cytopenias?

Investigations should be done to rule out the close differential diagnosis and specialized investigations pertinent to MDS as depicted below in **Table 3**.

TABLE 3: Investigation of MDS/hypoplastic marrow.

Investigations	Remarks
Hemoglobin level and red cell indices	• *Macrocytosis:* Drugs, folate/B_{12} deficiency, IBMFS, MDS, JMML • *Microcytic and ringed sideroblasts:* Mitochondrial disease, copper and vitamin B_6 deficiency • *Normocytic:* Anemia of chronic disease, IBMFS, acquired aplastic anemia—some cases
WBC, differential count, platelet count	It can give a clue about the degree of cytopenias. Monocytopenia can occur in GATA2 mutation
Peripheral smear	For morphological dysplasias
Fetal hemoglobin	Increased in MDS, JMML, IBMFS
B cell, NK cell numbers	Can be decreased in GATA2 mutation
Special tests	Chromosomal breakage study, telomere length/mutation study for telomeropathies, flow cytometric study for PNH, especially in hypoplastic marrow
BM aspirate	To assess cytologic dysplasia, blast count
BM flow cytometry	For immunophenotyping and blast count
BM biopsy	To assess cellularity, presence of reticulin fibers, marrow architecture, and dysplastic megakaryocytes. IHC—CD41/61 for micromegakaryocytes differentiates MDS from severe aplastic anemia
BM cytogenetics Karyotype +/– FISH	To detect monosomy 7, del 7q, trisomy 8, monosomy 5, del 5q, del 20q
BM molecular studies	• Targeted MDS panel for germline genetic predisposition, IBMFS • Acquired somatic mutation involving SETBP1, ASXL1, RUNX1, and RAS pathway genes can be done

(BM: bone marrow; FISH: fluorescence in situ hybridization; IBMFS: inherited bone marrow failure syndrome; IHC: immunohistochemistry; JMML: juvenile myelomonocytic leukemia; MDS: myelodysplastic syndrome; NK: natural killer; PNH: paroxysmal nocturnal hemoglobinuria; WBC: white blood cell)

9. How to differentiate hypoplastic MDS from aplastic anemia?

Differentiation of hypoplastic MDS from aplastic anemia has been given in **Table 4**.

TABLE 4: Differentiation of hypoplastic MDS from aplastic anemia.

	Severe aplastic anemia (SAA)	Refractory cytopenia of childhood (RCC)
Erythropoiesis	Lacking or single small focus with <10 cells with maturation	• Patchy distribution—left shift • Increased mitoses
Granulopoiesis	Lacking or marked decrease—very few small foci with maturation	Marked decrease—left shift
Megakaryopoiesis	• Lacking or very few megakaryocytes • No dysplastic megakaryocytes	• Marked decrease • Dysplastic changes • Micromegakaryocytes

Bone marrow and peripheral blood images of MDS showing dysplasias in various lineages are depicted in **Figures 1A to F**.

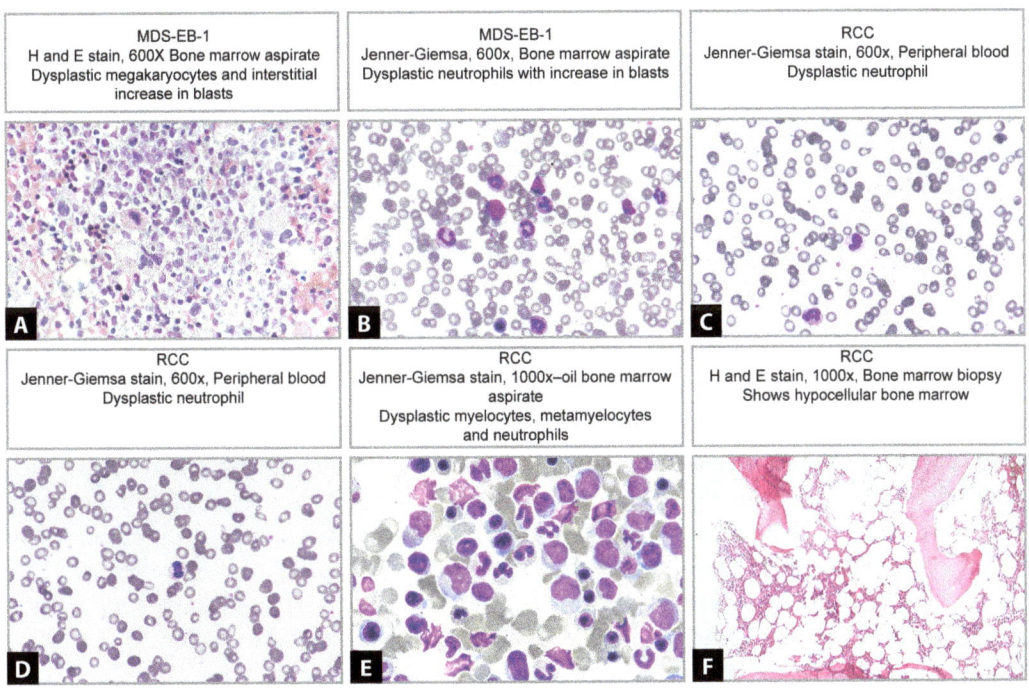

Figs. 1A to F: Histology: Bone marrow and peripheral blood images of MDS.
Courtesy: Dr Ganesh Kumar Viswanathan, Assistant Professor Hematology, AIIMS, New Delhi.

10. Can normal karyotype in the index child be compatible with the diagnosis of MDS?

Yes. The majority of children will have a normal karyotype. Monosomy 7 is the most common abnormality seen in 30% of cases. Trisomy 8 is the next common abnormality. A complex karyotype is characterized by three or more abnormalities with at least one structural alteration associated with a poor prognosis. Monosomy 5 abnormality is rarely seen in children as compared to adults.[2]

11. How to treat this child?

Treatment Options

Advanced Myelodysplastic Syndrome

Advanced MDS includes MDS-EB and MDS-EB-t, which account for 25% of cases. European working group on MDS recommends allogeneic hematopoietic stem cell transplantation (HSCT) for all advanced cases. Matched sibling donor or unrelated matched 9/10 or 10/10 human leukocyte antigen (HLA) loci by high-resolution typing is recommended. Myeloablative conditioning with Bu/Cy/Mel had a 5-year overall survival (OS) of 63%. Nonrelapse mortality (NRM) and disease relapse contribute equally to treatment failure. Children of ages >12 years are at high risk for NRM. The European Working Group of Myelodysplastic Syndrome (EWOG-MDS) recommends graft-versus-host disease (GVHD) prophylaxis with cyclosporine and methotrexate. A complex karyotype is associated with a poor prognosis.

Low-risk Myelodysplastic Syndrome RCC

Treatment of low-risk MDS RCC depends on the presence of adverse cytogenetic markers, transfusion dependency, degree of neutropenia, and the clinical course. Individuals with monosomy 7, del 7q, and complex karyotype are at higher risk for progression to advanced MDS. Transfusion dependency and severe neutropenia (ANC <1,000 or 500 in some studies) need therapeutic intervention.[1] A child with normal karyotype, transfusion independent, and ANC >1,000/mm^3 can be kept on a wait-and-watch policy.[9]

The European Working Group of Myelodysplastic Syndrome recommends a treosulfan-based regimen for RCC, which helps in initial engraftment with a low incidence of secondary graft failure with OS of 90%. Thiotepa/fludarabine-based preparation regimen had OS of 94% and event-free survival (EFS) of 88%, with 10% graft failure requiring stem cell boost and/or second HSCT. RCC with hypocellular marrow with normal karyotype can be given reduced-intensity conditioning with BM as the preferred stem cell source because of a lesser incidence of disease recurrence and a higher chance of GVHD in peripheral blood compared to the marrow. In normal and hypercellular marrow, myeloablative conditioning is preferred.[10]

The index child has transfusion dependency with low ANC (900/mm^3) and needs therapeutic intervention in the form of HSCT rather than wait-and-watch policy.

12. The index child had no suitable sibling or unrelated donor, and the family could not afford a stem cell transplant. Is there any other option for this child?

Yes. Immunosuppressive therapy may be an option for children with RCC with the absence of poor cytogenetic features with hypocellular marrow. There is an overlap of the pathophysiology of severe aplastic anemia and RCC with hypocellular marrow, which leads to the usage of immunosuppressive therapy with antithymocyte globulin and cyclosporine in those subsets of patients with failure-free survival of 57%. But the risk of disease relapse and clonal evolution persists.[6]

Hematopoietic Stem Cell Transplantation in GATA2 Haploinsufficiency

GATA2 mutation is at higher risk of progression to advanced MDS. The ideal time to perform HSCT is during the hypocellular phase of the disease before the occurrence of complications such as invasive infection and before progression to advanced MDS.[1]

Donor workup, including complete blood count with differential and genetic workup, should be done to rule out germline predisposition conditions. IBMFS FA, DKC, and SDS should be given reduced-intensity conditioning.[11]

13. How to treat MDS-EB?

Allogeneic stem cell transplant is the only curative option in advanced MDS. The role of AML-like induction therapy in MDS-EBt is controversial. The OS rate is around 30% for those who are treated only with chemotherapy without HSCT. Though chemotherapy decreases relapse rates, it increases toxicity. Bu-Cy-Mel is a commonly used conditioning regimen. Complex karyotype, monosomy, and AML evolved from MDS have a poor prognosis and high relapse rates.

14. How is t-MDS/AML treated?

It usually occurs months to years after treatment of the primary disorder. Incidence is 5–11% for those who are treated for solid tumors and 1–5% for ALL. Alkylating agents have a latency period of 5–7 years and are associated with chromosome 5 or 7 abnormalities. Etoposide has a short latency period and is associated with mixed lineage leukemia (MLL) translocation. Studies have shown that about 30% of adult t-MDS/AML have somatic mutations in TP-53. Treatment includes cytarabine-based induction chemotherapy followed by HSCT with a busulfan-based preparative regimen. OS ranges from 13 to 36% across studies, and disease recurrence plays a major role in treatment failure.[3]

Outcome of Pediatric Myelodysplastic Syndrome

Prognosis depends upon the MDS type. Children with low-grade MDS with hypocellular marrow have a relatively stable course for months to years. International prognostic scoring systems (IPSS) based on BM blasts, karyotype abnormalities, and cytopenias are not validated in children. Two or more lineage cytopenias and blast count of >5% in BM are associated with poor prognosis. Survival rates varied across studies and ranged from 3 years OS, about 50% in HLA-matched family donors, 35% in matched unrelated donors, and 20–30% in secondary MDS. Recently, outcomes improved to 5 years OS of 63% after HSCT in both related and unrelated donors, and the relapse rate post-transplant varies between 4% in low grade and 29% in advanced cases.[4]

■ REFERENCES

1. Locatelli F, Strahm B. How I treat myelodysplastic syndromes of childhood. Blood. 2018;131(13):1406-14.
2. Hofmann I. Pediatric myelodysplastic syndromes. J Hematopathol. 2015;8(3):127-41.
3. Galaverna F, Ruggeri A, Locatelli F. Myelodysplastic syndromes in children. Curr Opin Oncol. 2018;30(6):402-8.

4. Fish JD, Lipton JM, Lanzkowsky P. Lanzkowsky's Manual of Pediatric Hematology and Oncology, 7th edition. Amsterdam, Netherlands: Elsevier; 2021.
5. Indian Council of Medical Research. (2019). MSS_Myelodysplastic_Syndrome_MDS.pdf [online]. Available from https://main.icmr.nic.in/sites/default/files/guidelines/MSS_Myelodysplastic_Syndrome_MDS.pdf [Last accessed October, 2022].
6. Glaubach T, Robinson LJ, Corey SJ. Pediatric myelodysplastic syndromes: they do exist! J Pediatr Hematol Oncol. 2014;36(1):1-7.
7. Park M. Myelodysplastic syndrome with a genetic predisposition. Blood Research. 2021;56(S1):S34-8.
8. Thomas ME, Abdelhamed S, Hiltenbrand R, Schwartz JR, Sakurada SM, Walsh M, et al. Pediatric MDS and bone marrow failure-associated germline mutations in SAMD9 and SAMD9L impair multiple pathways in primary hematopoietic cells. Leukemia. 2021;35(11):3232-44.
9. Niemeyer CM. Pediatric MDS Including Refractory Cytopenia and Juvenile Myelomonocytic Leukemia. In: Carreras E, Dufour C, Mohty M, Kröger N (Eds). The EBMT Handbook: Hematopoietic Stem Cell Transplantation and Cellular Therapies, 7th edition. Cham (CH): Springer; 2019.
10. Niemeyer CM, Baumann I. Classification of childhood aplastic anemia and myelodysplastic syndrome. Hematology Am Soc Hematol Educ Program. 2011;2011:84-9.
11. Nakano TA, Lau BW, Dickerson KE, Wlodarski M, Pollard J, Shimamura A, et al. Diagnosis and treatment of pediatric myelodysplastic syndromes: a survey of the North American Pediatric Aplastic Anemia Consortium. Pediatr Blood Cancer. 2020;67(10):e28652.

EXPERT OPINION

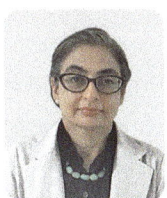

Tulika Seth
Professor
Department of Hematology AIIMS, New Delhi, India

1. When to suspect MDS in children? How to approach the management of MDS in children?

Myelodysplastic syndrome is very rare in children, some important differentials to consider before making a diagnosis of MDS are B_{12} deficiency, Down's syndrome, and IBMFSs. There are familial disorders in which MDS, aplastic anemia or leukemias, and other hematologic disorders may cluster. Children with bicytopenia or pancytopenia without any other diagnosis and sustained over several weeks need a BM test. The BM and, many times, the peripheral smear also will have features of dyspoiesis, may reveal blasts, and often are associated with a cytogenetic or molecular abnormality. Postchemotherapy for solid malignancy is another etiology associated with MDS. Another important differential to consider in a child with cytopenias and cellular BM is autoimmune lymphoproliferative syndrome (ALPS).

2. Is there a subset of MDS patients who can be observed and followed up without doing transplants? When to treat MDS?

The groups of childhood MDS are usually associated with high-risk cytogenetic (monosomy 7, etc.) or molecular abnormalities (SAMD9/SAMD9L, GATA2, etc.). Children with Down's syndrome may be observed with MDS, particularly if they present in infancy where a transient myeloproliferative disorder may be seen, though these children also have a risk of development of AML.

3. How to bridge MDS to transplant?

In MDS patients, there is no randomized controlled trial (RCT) to guide the need for bridging to transplant. In most cases, the patient is directly taken for transplant. If there is a delay in donor availability or other problems which impede the transplant, then bridging may be undertaken with hypomethylating agents while waiting for the procedure.

4. What conditioning regimen do you recommend for a child with MDS? Suppose a child does not have a suitable sibling or unrelated donor. Is there any other option for this child? Share your post HSCT experience.

The conditioning will depend if this is related to an underlying IBMFS, therapy-related MDS, or *de novo* MDS. If the BM prior to transplant is hypercellular, then a myeloablative regimen is preferred; if hypocellular, then a reduced intensity regimen is required. It is important to check the donor by molecular tests for familial or inherited disorders, even if phenotypically normal.

5. What are management options for t-MDS/AML?

Therapy-related MDS/AML often does not respond to chemotherapy induction, and these patients may develop organ toxicity or infections which can delay definitive treatment. Transplantation is the best option, and here again, proceeding for an allogeneic transplant without chemotherapy if a donor and other factors permit should be attempted.

CHAPTER 13: Langerhans Cell Histiocytosis

Shilpa Khanna Arora, Rachna Seth

CASE VIGNETTE

A 2-year-old boy, presented with complaints of recurrent episodes of cough with fever for 1 year. There was history of repeated episodes of hospitalizations for the same complaints, during one of which he developed pneumothorax needing intercostal drainage and mechanical ventilation. There was history of scaly and itchy skin lesions over the body for past 1 year. The patient also developed a swelling above right eye that was gradually increasing in size. There was history of progressive pallor needing blood transfusion. There was no history of jaundice, polyuria, or polydipsia. He received antitubercular therapy (ATT) for 6 months but the symptoms continued to persist. The child was born out of nonconsanguineous marriage and was developmentally normal.

At presentation, he had respiratory distress and mild pallor. A swelling above right eye was present. The skin showed rash and hypopigmented lesions. Respiratory system examination revealed intercostal retractions with bilateral normal vesicular breath sounds. Liver was enlarged 5 cm below right costal margin and the spleen was not palpable. Cardiovascular and neurological systems were unremarkable.

Investigations revealed hemoglobin of 10.2 g/dL with normal leukocyte count and thrombocytosis. Liver function tests were normal. Chest X-ray revealed diffuse bilateral interstitial infiltrates with a reticulonodular pattern. Contrast enhanced computed tomography (CECT) chest revealed bilateral ground glass opacities with a reticulonodular pattern and some cystic changes. Skin biopsy showed presence of atypical histiocytes that were positive for immunohistochemical staining with CD1a, langerin (CD207), and S-100 making a diagnosis of Langerhans cell histiocytosis (LCH) **(Figs. 1A to D)**.

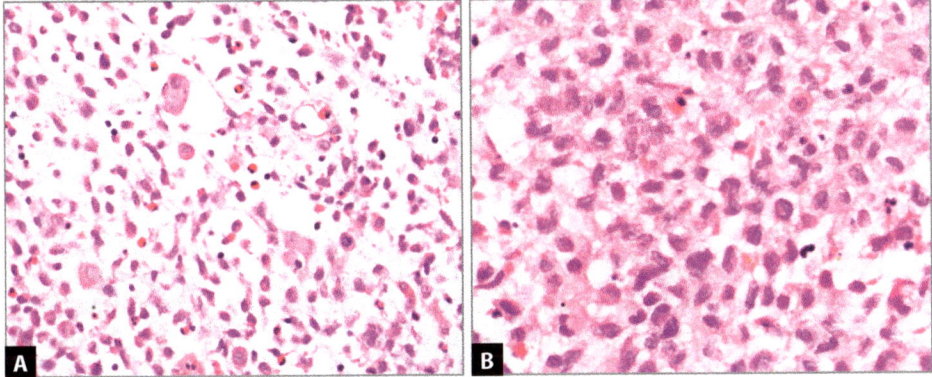

Figs. 1A and B: (A) Biopsy shows large round to ovoid histiocytes along with multinucleated histiocytes and eosinophils. (B) The histiocytes have irregular nuclear contours, some showing a nuclear groove.

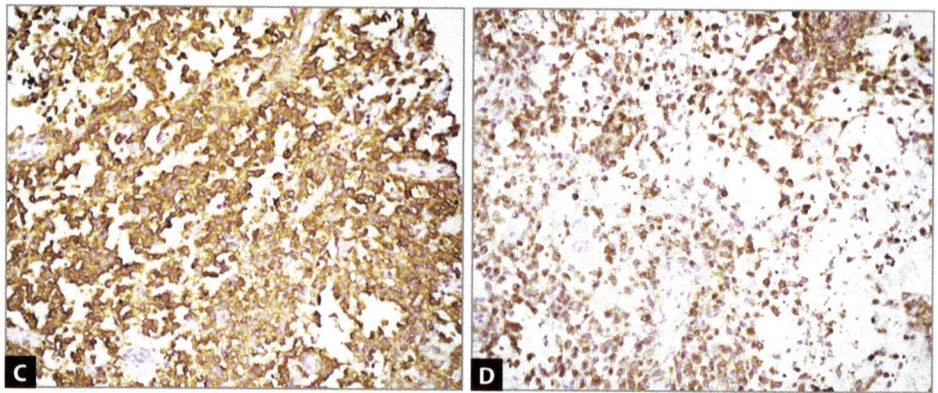

Figs. 1C and D: These atypical histiocytes are immunopositive for CD1a and langerin.

1. How common is LCH?

Langerhans cell histiocytosis is a rare disease. The incidence of LCH has been variably reported to be between 2 and 10 cases per million children under-15 years of age with a male-to-female ratio of 1:2.[1] Though the median age of occurrence has been reported as 30 months, it may occur at any age. Its incidence is reported to be 1–2 cases per million in adults but is speculated that it is under reported.[2,3]

2. What is the current understanding about pathogenesis of LCH?

The pathologic dendritic cells constitute <10% of the LCH lesion. The rest of it is constituted by inflammatory cells like macrophages, eosinophils, and lymphocytes including activated T-cells. CD1a positive LCH cells and CD3 positive T-cells have been implicated in orchestrating the cytokine storm in this immune dysregulation. Clonal origin of LCH cells was discovered in 1994 following observation of nonrandom inactivation of X chromosomes in these lesions.[4] Genetic studies discovered the presence of BRAF V600E mutation in >50% of LCH lesions in 2010.[5] This mutation results in constitutive activation of the tyrosine receptor kinase involved in RAS–RAF–MEs signal transduction pathway. Subsequently, other activating mutations in BRAF and mitogen-activated protein kinase (MAPK) pathway were recognized. This pathway is involved in numerous cell functions and its constitutive activation has been seen in almost 7% of neoplastic disorders including melanoma, hairy cell leukemia, thyroid cancer, etc.

According to "misguided myeloid differentiation" hypothesis, the state of differentiation of the precursor cell in which somatic MAPK activating mutations occur, determine the clinical extent and severity of the disease. Mutation occurring in pluripotent hematopoietic stem cell precursor lead to high-risk LCH, those occurring in more committed (tissue-restricted) precursors lead to multifocal low-risk LCH, and the ones occurring in local precursor cell result in a single lesion.[3] Considering the pathogenesis, LCH is regarded as an inflammatory neoplastic disorder.[1]

3. How does LCH Present?

Most common presenting symptoms of LCH are skin rash or painful bone lesions. Other symptoms can be fever, weight loss, jaundice, diarrhea, edema, dyspnea, polydipsia, and polyuria. Though any organ or system can be affected, most frequently affected are skeleton (80%), skin (33%), and pituitary (25%). Others are liver, spleen, hematopoietic system and lungs (15% each), lymph nodes (5–10%), and central nervous system (CNS) (2–4%).[6] Liver, spleen, and bone marrow are regarded as high-risk organs, whereas skin, bone, lymph nodes, and pituitary gland are regarded as low-risk organs, depending on the risk of death (Histiocyte Society). Lung is no longer regarded as a risk organ as death in pulmonary LCH, if occurs, is secondary to its "mechanical complications" like pneumothorax, or as a late event due to chronic emphysematous changes. Other reasons cited for not regarding it as a risk organ are frequent association of pulmonary involvement with involvement of other risk organs, low relative hazard ratio in a multivariate analysis, and also, the evaluation of disease activity and therapy response in this organ is very difficult and subjective.[7]

Central nervous system involvement in LCH has been reported to occur variably in 3.4–57% cases.[8] It may be in the form of active disease (AD) associated with focal mass lesions and lesions leading to progressive neurodegeneration or it may lead to chronic long term sequel persisting despite resolution of AD. Neurodegenerative LCH has been described to occur in two clinical forms, viz., LCH-associated abnormal CNS imaging (LACI) in asymptomatic patients having radiologic findings, and LCH associated abnormal CNS symptoms (LACS) in those manifesting abnormal cognitive and psychological features.[9] Anterior pituitary dysfunction in LCH is more common in childhood-onset disease and in multisystem (MS) disease. It most commonly results in deficiency of antidiuretic hormone, followed by growth hormone, gonadotropin, and thyrotropin.

Multisystem LCH is more common in younger children in comparison to older children and adults. Clinical course of LCH is highly variable from a self-limiting to a fulminant one leading to death. Almost 30–40% patients eventually develop permanent sequelae.

4. How do you diagnose LCH?

Diagnosis of LCH can be confirmed by histopathological examination in the background of clinical setting of LCH. Biopsy from LCH lesion demonstrates the presence of characteristic pathologic dendritic cells with variable number of T-lymphocytes, eosinophils, and macrophages. LCH dendritic cell is characterized by abundant eosinophilic-to-amphophilic cytoplasm and an indented/grooved nucleus (kidney shaped). Giant cells composed of fused dendritic cells may also be seen occasionally. Immunohistochemical evaluation reveals expression of CD1a and/or CD207. Electron microscopy reveals the presence of rod/tennis racket shaped cytoplasmic organelles known as Birbeck granules which are thought to be involved in receptor mediated endocytosis. Demonstration of CD207 expression confirms the presence of Birbeck granules, hence electron microscopic examination is no longer considered as gold standard for diagnosis. Expression of CD207 is considered to be an event occurring late in LCH dendritic cell differentiation as a variable expression of CD207+ is sometimes reported in CD1a+ and BRAF-V600E+ histiocytes in the lesions. BRAF-V600E can be detected by immunostain (VE-1 antibody) and/or polymerase chain reaction (PCR).

Rarely, the risk involved in doing a biopsy may outweigh the need for a tissue diagnosis, e.g., in case of isolated vertebra plana without a soft tissue component.[7] In such a situation, patient can be closely observed and biopsy may be done in case of progression, especially if systemic therapy is warranted.

The index child had skin, lungs, and liver involvement (based on clinical assessment).

5. How was this child evaluated?

A detailed history with respect to symptoms was taken (onset, duration, and progression of symptoms, for any swelling, pain, skin rash, seborrhea, ear discharge, fever, poor appetite, loss of weight, poor weight gain, failure to thrive, polydipsia, polyuria, loose stools, dyspnea, exposure to smoke, irritability, lethargy, behavioral changes, or neurological deficits. Vitals and anthropometry were recorded. Sexual maturity rating (SMR) staging was prepubertal. Scalp lesions were noted. The child was also evaluated for presence of pallor, jaundice, edema, lymphadenopathy, orbital, or other skeletal or other soft tissue swelling/abnormalities. Aural and oral cavity examination, detailed systemic examination to look for any respiratory distress, ascites, liver and spleen size, and neurological sign/deficits was done. This child underwent detailed laboratory evaluation as mentioned above, followed by positron emission tomography-CT (PET-CT). At our center, PET-CT is done at baseline and at subsequent time points for response evaluation.

Fludeoxyglucose (FDG) PET-CT of the index case revealed metabolically active reticular thickening with ground glass haziness and some cystic lesions in both lung fields and a lytic lesion in right frontal bone **(Figs. 2A to E)**. *Based on the clinical, laboratory investigations,*

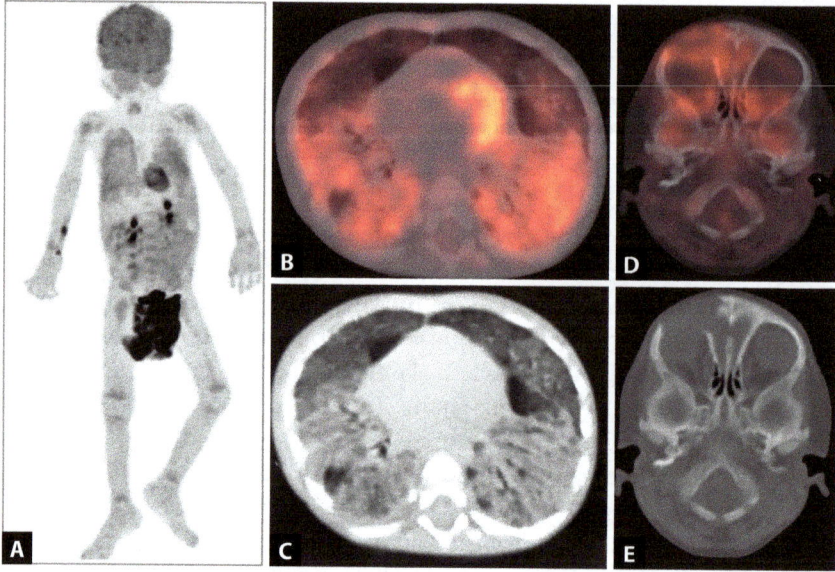

Figs. 2A to E: (A) Baseline FDG PET: maximum intensity projection, (B and C) fused transaxial PET/CT and CT sections showing extensive FDG avid reticular thickening and ground glass haziness with few cystic lesions and areas of consolidation involving bilateral lungs and (D and E) lytic lesions in right frontal bone. (CT: computed tomography; FDG: fludeoxyglucose; PET: positron emission tomography)

histopathology, and imaging findings, a diagnosis of MS LCH with risk organ involvement (skin, lung, bone, and liver) was made in the index case.

The diagnostic evaluation in a suspected case of LCH includes certain mandatory investigations and some system specific investigations that must be guided by detailed clinical evaluation **(Table 1)**. Bone marrow evaluation is indicated for patients having cytopenias and for all children <2 years of age.[2]

TABLE 1: Laboratory evaluation in LCH.

Mandatory Investigations	
All cases	Biopsy from suspected lesion (bone, skin, lymph node, liver, etc.)
	Complete blood count, ESR
	Liver function tests, proteins
	Kidney function test and electrolytes
	PT, APTT, fibrinogen
	Alkaline phosphatase
	Ferritin
	• Urine specific gravity and osmolality • Serum osmolality
	USG abdomen
	CXR
	PET/skeletal radiographic survey
System-specific investigations	
Indication	**Investigation**
Cytopenias	Bone marrow aspiration and biopsy to rule out other causes
Liver dysfunction	Liver biopsy only if clinically significant liver involvement and the results are likely to affect further management (to differentiate between active LCH and sclerosing cholangitis)

Respiratory symptoms or abnormal CXR	• CT chest
	• Lung function tests
	• If CT abnormal but findings not characteristic of LCH or suspected atypical infection/ other pathology
	  – BAL >5% CD1a-positive cells diagnostic in nonsmokers
	  – Lung biopsy, if BAL not diagnostic

Suspected craniofacial bone lesions	MRI brain/face
Suspected vertebral lesions	MRI of spine (to exclude spinal cord compression and evaluate soft tissue masses)
Visual or neurological abnormalities	• MRI brain • Detailed neurological assessment • Neuropsychiatric evaluation
Endocrine abnormality—short stature, growth failure, polyuria, polydipsia, hypothalamic syndromes, precocious, or delayed puberty	• Endocrine assessment (including water deprivation test and dynamic tests of the anterior pituitary) • MRI brain

Contd...

Contd...

System-specific investigations	
Indication	Investigation
Aural discharge or suspected hearing impairment/mastoid involvement	• Formal hearing assessment • MRI brain • CT temporal bone
Unexplained chronic diarrhea, failure to thrive or malabsorption	Endoscopy and biopsy

(APTT: activated partial thromboplastin time; BAL: bronchoalveolar lavage; CXR: chest X-ray; ESR: erythrocyte sedimentation rate; LCH: Langerhans cell histiocytosis; MRI: magnetic resonance imaging; PET: positron emission tomography; PT: prothrombin time; USG: ultrasonography)

6. What are the indications of doing a bone marrow examination in a patient of LCH?

Bone marrow aspiration or biopsy is a painful procedure and is also associated with risks involved during sedation in children. It is not indicated in all cases of LCH. It is required to be done only in patients having cytopenias to rule out other causes for the same **(Table 2)**.

7. What is the role of PET/CT, conventional imaging and whole body MRI in LCH?

Fludeoxyglucose PET/CT can detect LCH lesions not visualized on other imaging modalities and helps to distinguish metabolically active lesions from inactive ones. It has been shown to be superior to conventional imaging in LCH for diagnosing as well as monitoring response to therapy and detecting relapse. Two organ systems where PET/CT might miss the lesions are CNS and lungs.[10] Contrast-enhanced MRI is a good modality for identifying CNS lesions not apparent on PET/CT. Pituitary involvement often goes undetected on PET/CT scan and is easily demonstrated on MRI by observing for loss of bright spot or presence of thickening of the pituitary stalk. However, as diabetes insipidus is a common manifestation of AD as well as a long-term complication of pituitary involvement in LCH, characterizing these findings on MRI as active versus in AD is difficult. MRI, unlike PET/CT, may also detect tumorous involvement of meninges, pineal gland, choroid plexus as well as neurodegenerative involvement of cerebellum, basal ganglia or brain stem. High-resolution computed tomography (HRCT) chest is a better modality for evaluation of pulmonary disease than PET/CT and demonstrates reticulonodular infiltrates in initial stages and cystic changes in advanced disease. These findings are classically symmetrical, and involve the costophrenic angles in children unlike in adults where there is sparing of costophrenic angles and lower lung fields. Chest X-ray may demonstrate presence of bilateral interstitial infiltrates with a reticulonodular pattern, often with peribronchial thickening; cystic changes and pneumothoraces may be seen in advanced disease. But HRCT is often indicated in absence of CXR findings in a child with persistent respiratory symptoms and a strong clinical suspicion of pulmonary LCH.

8. Is there any role of BRAF V600E mutation studies in this child?

Recurrent *BRAF* V600E mutations have been identified in approximately 50% of LCH patients, more so in MS LCH than in SS LCH. Presence of this mutation has been correlated with high-risk features, increased resistance to the first-line therapy and decreased progression free survival (PFS).[9] BRAF V600E mutation can be detected in peripheral blood by next-generation sequencing (NGS) or by droplet digital PCR (ddPCR). Whereas, in formalin fixed paraffin embedded (FFPE) samples, it can be detected by immunohistochemistry (IHC) using BRAF mutation-specific antibody or by NGS after DNA extraction. It is speculated that cell-free (cf) *BRAF* V600E analysis in plasma using ddPCR can serve as a promising biomarker in LCH for diagnosing, monitoring response as well as predicting relapse.[11]

9. What will be you approach to management of this child?

Management of LCH depends on its clinical manifestations and organ dysfunction. The clinical classification of LCH **(Table 2)** helps in guiding the same.

TABLE 2: Clinical classification of LCH.

Classification	System Involved
Single system (SS) LCH	One organ/system involved (uni- or multifocal): • Bone unifocal (single bone) or multifocal (>1 bone) • Skin • Lymph node (excluding draining LN of another LCH lesion), single (one group) or multiple (>1 group) • Lungs • Central nervous system • Other (e.g., thyroid and thymus)
Multi system (MS) LCH	Two or more organs/systems involved It can be with "risk organ" involvement (MS RO+) or without (MS RO-)
Definition of risk organ involvement (have significantly higher risk of mortality than other sites)	Hematopoietic involvement (with/without BM): ≥2 of following: • Hb <10 g/dL (infants <9 g/dL), not attributable to other/nutritional cause • Total leukocyte count (TLC) <4,0 ×10^9/L • Platelet count <100 × 10^9/L Splenic involvement: • Palpable >2 cm below costal margin in the midclavicular line Liver involvement: • Palpable >3 cm below costal margin in the midclavicular line • Dysfunction – total protein <5.5 g/dL, albumin <2.5 g/dL (not due to other causes) • Histopathology suggestive of active disease
Special sites	Vertebral lesions with significant intraspinal soft tissue component
	"CNS risk lesions" lesions in the facial bones and skull base with intracranial soft tissue extension (associated with an increased risk of development of diabetes insipidus)

The management protocol for LCH followed at our institute is based on LCH III study of the Histiocyte Society **(Flowchart 1)**.[12] We are in the process of integrating our current protocol with the LCH IV protocol **(Flowchart 2)**.[7]

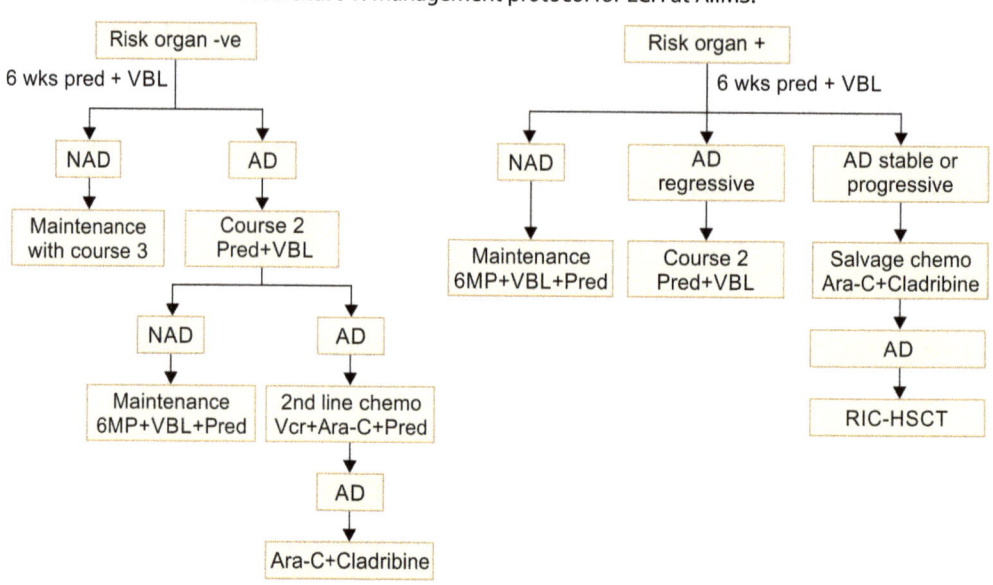

Flowchart 1: Management protocol for LCH at AIIMS.

(AD: active disease; Ara-C: cytarabine; NAD: no active disease; Pred: prednisolone; RIC-HSCT: reduced intensity conditioning hematopoietic stem cell transplant; VBL: vinblastine; wks: weeks; 6MP: 6 mercaptopurine)

The LCH III study, which was carried out from 2001 to 2008, divided the patients into three groups as follows: (1) "risk group" patients (MS-LCH with risk organ involvement); (2) "low risk group" patients (MS-LCH without risk organ involvement); and (3) multifocal bone disease and "special sites" (patients with single-system LCH who have an indication for systemic therapy). All group 1 (MS LCH RO+) patients were randomized to receive not receive methotrexate in addition to 1–2, 6 week courses of vinblastine and prednisone in induction but the additional methotrexate was not found to be beneficial. Another significant finding of LCH III was that longer duration (12 months) of continuation therapy was associated with superior survival and lower relapse risk in RO-patients in comparison to shorter duration (6 months) of maintenance.

The ongoing LCH IV study divides the treatment into 7 strata **(Flowchart 1)**. Stratum I: First-line treatment for MS-LCH patients (group 1) and patients with SS-LCH with multifocal bone or "CNS-risk" lesions (group 2); Stratum II: Second-line treatment for nonrisk patients; Stratum III: Salvage treatment for risk LCH; Stratum IV: Stem cell transplantation for risk LCH (patients with dysfunction of risk organs who fail first-line therapy); Stratum V: Monitoring and treatment of isolated tumorous and neurodegenerative CNS-LCH; Stratum VI: Natural history and management of "other" SS-LCH (not needing systemic therapy at the time of diagnosis); and Stratum VII: Long-term follow-up (all patients).

Flowchart 2: LCH IV strata.[7]

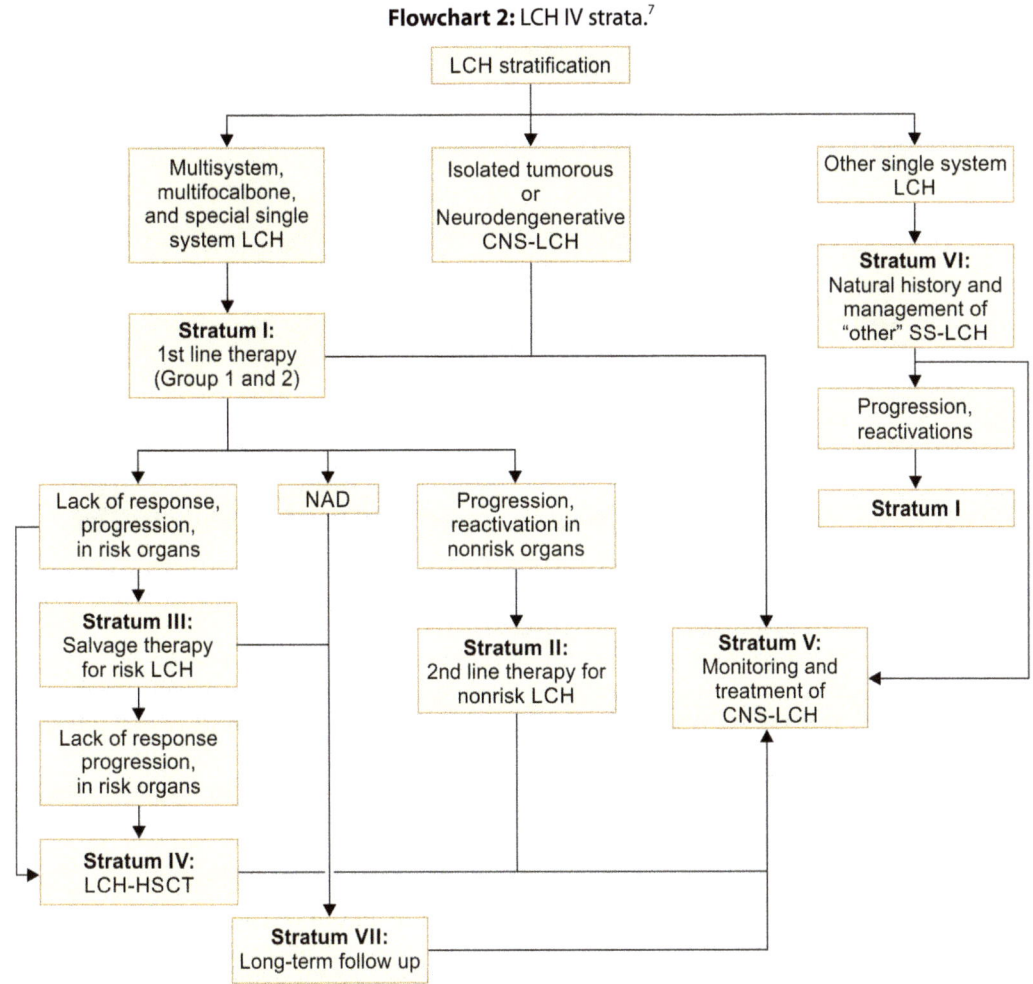

(CNS: central nervous system; HSCT: hematopoietic stem cell transplant; LCH: Langerhans cell histiocytosis; NAD: no active disease; SS: single system)

10. **The index case is MS LCH with risk organ involvement. How will you manage this child?**

*The index case was initiated on initial course 1 consisting of weekly vinblastine (6 mg/m^2) and prednisolone for 4 weeks (40 mg/m^2/day in three divided doses) followed by tapering in next 2 weeks. Response assessment PET/CT done after 6 weeks revealed partial response with uptake persisting in lungs and bone **(Fig. 3)** signifying AD regressive. Hence, he was given course 2 consisting of weekly vinblastine with prednisolone 3 days per week for a duration of 6 weeks. Repeat PET/CT done after total 12 weeks of vinblastine and prednisolone showed partial response with some persistent residual disease in lungs and bone in this child.*

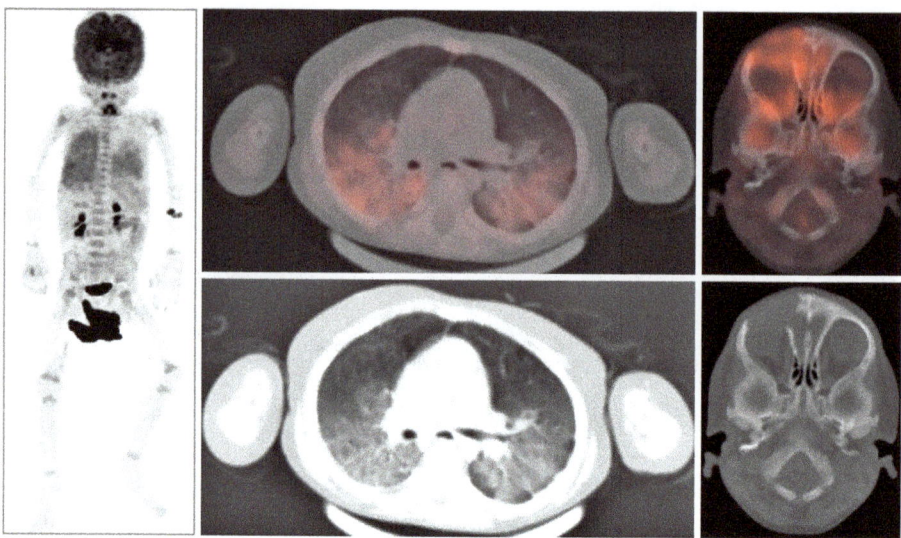

Fig. 3: FDG PET after 6 weeks of therapy: Transaxial fused PET/CT and CT sections shows FDG avid reticular thickening with few cystic lesions and areas of consolidation involving bilateral lungs and lytic lesions in right frontal bone with soft tissue component suggestive of partial response.
(CT: computed tomography; FDG: fludeoxyglucose; PET: positron emission tomography)

11. When will you assess response to treatment and what is the best modality to assess response?

As per LCH III response, evaluation is carried out at 6/12 weeks depending of disease extent and clinical response. The *disease state is categorized* as nonactive disease (NAD) or AD.

Nonactive disease—resolution of all signs/symptoms (no evidence of disease)

Active disease—AD if present, further classified as better, stable, or worse
- Better (regressive disease)—regression of signs/symptoms, no new lesions
- Stable (stable disease)—persistence of signs or symptoms, no new lesions
- Worse (progressive disease)—progression of signs or symptoms and/or appearance of new lesions

Based on disease state categories, *response categories* are defined in LCH IV protocol as better, intermediate, or worse as follows:
- Better—if NAD or AD better
- Intermediate—stable (unchanged) disease
- Worse—progressive disease

The response categories help in guiding further therapy. *In the index case, the response after total of 12 weeks of therapy was AD intermediate (with persistent residual disease in nonrisk organs—lungs and bone). Hence he was shifted to Stratum II, i.e., second-line treatment for nonrisk LCH and started on second-line chemotherapy, i.e., prednisolone, vincristine, and cytarabine. Repeat response evaluation was carried out after 12 weeks which showed evidence of stable disease. Repeat evaluation after 24 week initial course again showed stable disease (AD intermediate). Thus, a decision was taken to shift him to salvage therapy (even though it is suggested to do so only for risk LCH as per LCH IV, stratum III) with cladribine (5 mg/m^2/day × 5 days) and cytarabine (500 mg/m^2/dose BD × 5 days)* **(Flowchart 3)**. *After* two courses, disease continued to be stable hence he was given three more courses of same chemotherapy. After total five courses of cladribine-cytarabine, PET-CT showed complete metabolic response **(Fig. 4)** and hence he was shifted to maintenance chemotherapy. The child is currently in 10th month of maintenance and doing well. In case, there would have been disease progression any time after two courses of stratum III therapy, the patient would have required hematopoietic stem cell transplant (HSCT) **(Flowchart 3)**.

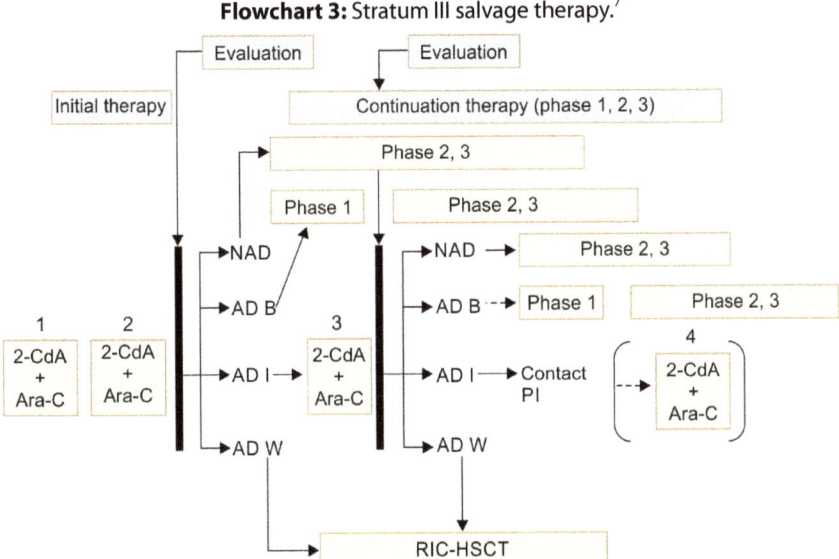

Flowchart 3: Stratum III salvage therapy.[7]

(AD B: AD better; AD I: AD intermediate; AD W: AD worse; Ara-C: cytarabine; NAD: nonactive disease)

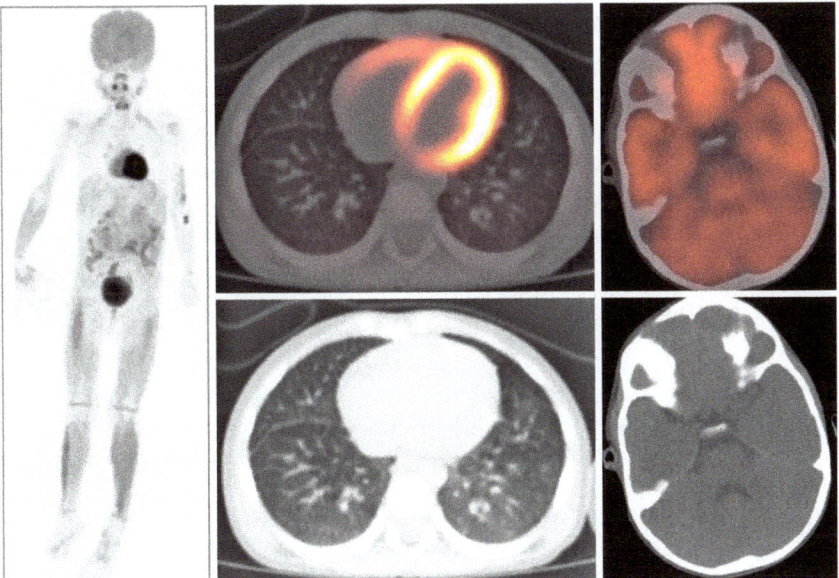

Fig. 4: PET CT after five courses of cladribine and cytarabine: No metabolically active residual disease with decrease in ground glass haziness with evidence of near complete healed lytic lesion in the right frontal bone. (CT: computed tomography; PET: positron emission tomography)

12. Is there any role of newer drugs/targeted therapy in LCH?

Mitogen-activated protein kinase pathway inhibition in adults with LCH and Erdheim-Chester Disease (ECD) has been tried in some clinical trials. Vemurafenib, a BRAF inhibitor, has shown promising results but unfortunately, the results are not long lasting and it is associated with significant toxic effects such as rash, arthralgia, pyrexia, nausea, vomiting, diarrhea, fatigue, and secondary malignancy like squamous-cell carcinoma of skin.[3] MEK inhibitor trametinib has also shown some efficacy but is associated with side effects like rash, ophthalmologic inflammation, drug reaction with eosinophilia and systemic symptoms (DRESS), rhabdomyolysis, and pneumonitis.

The proportion of pathognomonic dendritic cells in an LCH lesion is <10% and the rest of it is constituted by inflammatory cells. Hence, anti-inflammatory agents have a potential role in blocking the recruitment and activation of inflammatory T-cells.[3] Anti-inflammatory drugs such as thalidomide and indomethacin have shown some clinical efficacy in early trials.

13. Is there any role of bone marrow transplant in difficult to treat LCH?

Hematopoietic stem cell transplant has shown promising results in patients with refractory disease with severe organ dysfunction by immunomodulatory mechanisms.[13] Initial efforts with myeloablative conditioning (MAC) were associated with high transplant-related mortality, hence reduced intensity conditioning (RIC) has been tried. RIC HSCT is being evaluated in LCH IV as stratum IV strategy for MS-LCH patients with severe organ dysfunction (hematological and/or hepatic), who fail to respond to front-line therapy (Stratum I) OR to cladribine/cytarabine salvage (Stratum III). Novel-targeted therapies MAPK pathway inhibitors are being utilized as bridging measures to stabilize the disease activity before proceeding with HSCT.[13]

14. What are the sequelae of LCH?

Almost half of the LCH survivors have at least one permanent long-term effect. Those with MS disease and who have multiple reactivations are more likely to develop sequelae. Most commonly reported of these are diabetes insipidus and skeletal abnormalities in about 20%, followed by growth retardation, hearing loss, and neurodegeneration in around 10%, and biliary cirrhosis, and respiratory insufficiency in around 5% of survivors.[8] Neurodegenerative syndrome may occur years after the primary diagnosis. Damage to bile ducts in LCH can result in progressive sclerosing cholangitis and biliary cirrhosis that can lead to liver dysfunction and failure requiring liver transplantation.

REFERENCES

1. Mc Clain KL, Allen CE, Visser JH, Hicks MJ. Histiocytosis. In: Blaney SM, Adamson PC, Helman LJ (Eds). Pizzo and Poplack's Pediatric Oncology, 8th edition. Philadelphia: Wolters Kluwer Health; 2021. pp. 568-81.
2. Allen CE, Ladisch S, McClain KL. How I treat Langerhans cell histiocytosis. Blood. 2015;126(1):26-35.
3. Allen CE, Merad M, McClain KL. Langerhans-Cell Histiocytosis. N Engl J Med. 2018;379:856-68.
4. Willman CL, Busque L, Griffith BB, Favara BE, McClain KL, Duncan MH, et al. Langerhans'-cell histiocytosis (histiocytosis X)—a clonal proliferative disease. N Engl J Med. 1994;331:154-60.

5. Badalian-Very G, Vergilio JA, Degar BA, MacConaill LE, Brandner B, Calicchio ML, et al. Recurrent BRAF mutations in Langerhans cell histiocytosis. Blood. 2010;116:1919-23.
6. Haupt R, Minkov M, Astigarraga I, Schäfer E, Nanduri V, Jubran R, et al. Langerhans cell histiocytosis: guidelines for diagnosis, clinical work-up, and treatment for patients till the age of 18 years. Pediatr Blood Cancer. 2013;60:175-84.
7. Children's Cancer Research Institute. LCH-IV International Collaborative Treatment Protocol for Children and Adolescents with Langerhans Cell Histiocytosis. Available from: https://www.uhs.nhs.uk/Media/UHS-website-2019/Docs/PaediatricOncology/Solids/LCH-IV-protocol-vs-1-4-Nov-2016.pdf. [Accessed 3 Nov 2022].
8. Rodriguez-Galindo C, Allen CE. Langerhans cell histiocytosis. Blood. 2020;135(16):1319-31.
9. Yeh EA, Greenberg J, Abla O, Longoni G, Diamond E, Hermiston M, et al; North American Consortium for Histiocytosis. Evaluation and treatment of Langerhans cell histiocytosis patients with central nervous system abnormalities: current views and new vistas. Pediatr Blood Cancer. 2018;65(1):65.
10. Ferrell J, Sharp S, Kumar A, Jordan M, Picarsic J, Nelson A. Discrepancies between F-18-FDG PET/CT findings and conventional imaging in Langerhans cell histiocytosis. Pediatr Blood Cancer. 2021;68(4):e28891.
11. Cui L, Zhang L, Ma HH, Wang CJ, Wang D, Lian HY, et al. Circulating cell-free BRAF V600E during chemotherapy is associated with prognosis of children with Langerhans cell histiocytosis. Haematologica. 2020;105(9):e444-7.
12. Gadner H, Minkov M, Grois N, Pötschger U, Thiem E, Aricò M, et al; Histiocyte Society. Therapy prolongation improves outcome in multisystem Langerhans cell histiocytosis. Blood. 2013;121(25):5006-14.
13. Kudo K, Maeda M, Suzuki N, Kanegane H, Ohga S, Ishii E, et al. Hematopoietic stem cell transplantation in children with refractory langerhans cell histiocytosis. *Blood.* 2018;132 (Supplement 1):4657.

EXPERT OPINION

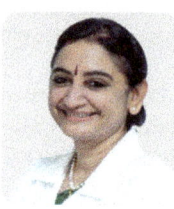

Revathi Raj
Senior Consultant, Pediatric Hemtaology-Oncologist
Apollo Specialty Cancer Hospital, Chennai, India

Langerhans cell histiocytosis presenting in infancy is a challenging disorder and the best approach is the one which reduces immediate and late regimen-related side effects. In all children, the initial approach recommended is prednisolone at 40 mg/m^2 for 4 weeks followed by a 2 week taper along with weekly vinblastine injections at 6 mg/m^2 intravenously. The children need prophylaxis with cotrimoxazole and aciclovir during chickenpox season. Calcium and vitamin D supplementation are recommended to help bone mineralization.

The interim PET is invaluable in LCH as the response to the initial 6 weeks of prednisolone and vinblastine guides the physician to plan further therapy. The lung is now not considered a risk organ, however, this child had significant hepatomegaly and the liver is a risk organ in LCH. MRI whole body can be used as a follow-up imaging modality to limit radiation exposure.

Children showing complete metabolic response in the interim PET can go on to 3 weekly vinblastine and prednisolone pulses and as per current recommendations, prolonged therapy for 1 year helps to reduce relapse rates.

At the end of 6 weeks, in children with risk organ involvement and partial or no response on PET-CT scan, the ideal option would be to obtain BRAF V600E mutation status and start the child on oral trametinib. Targeted therapy has changed the algorithm for children with LCH as it has minimal side effects with maximum efficacy and should be recommended as the standard of care. However, the huge costs involved on a monthly basis preclude its use in a resource limited setting.

In children showing partial or no response with risk organ involvement, the recommendation would be to start six cycles of modified Cladribine and Cytarabine salvage chemotherapy. The dose reduction in the modified protocol reduces morbidity and prevents mortality. The risk of end-organ damage and late effects and the need for HSCT could be avoided with early intervention.

In children with relapsed refractory disease, the use of bisphosphonates helps to reduce bone-related morbidity. Pulse dexamethasone and lenalidomide combination could be offered if there are financial constraints and this regimen results in durable remissions in two-thirds of these patients at a fraction of the cost of trametinib or other intensive salvage regimens.

In the era of targeted therapy with trametinib, the role of HSCT is limited with only a few case reports in published literature. In summary, interim PET-guided risk stratification and therapy has paved the way for systematic management in children with LCH. Early introduction of salvage regimens and targeted therapy will prevent organ damage and the need for HSCT. Supportive care in the form of infection prophylaxis, calcium, and vitamin D replacement, bisphosphonates help to reduce morbidity. Whole body MRI imaging is a useful tool for follow-up rather than X rays or CT scans in these children to avoid cumulative radiation exposure.

CHAPTER 14

Non-Langerhans Cell Histiocytosis

Debasish Sahoo, Rachna Seth

CASE VIGNETTE 1

An 11-year-old girl presented with history of intermittent, high-grade fever for 5 months, not associated with any localizing symptoms. On examination, she had tenderness on deep palpation of long bones; her physical examination was otherwise unremarkable. Her complete blood count, serum electrolytes, and renal function tests and liver function tests were within normal limits. The urine investigations were normal. Her skeletal survey revealed well-defined geographic lytic lesions without sclerosis in multiple bones including in ribs, clavicle, sternum, and scapulae.

1. What are the common differential diagnoses in such a situation?

Some common differential diagnoses are Langerhans cell histiocytosis (LCH), fibrous dysplasia, metastatic disease, hyperparathyroidism, and multifocal osteomyelitis.

The lesions were *fluorodeoxyglucose (FDG) avid on positron-emission tomography/computed tomography (PET-CT)* **(Fig. 1)**. *A CT-guided biopsy which was done from bony lesion*

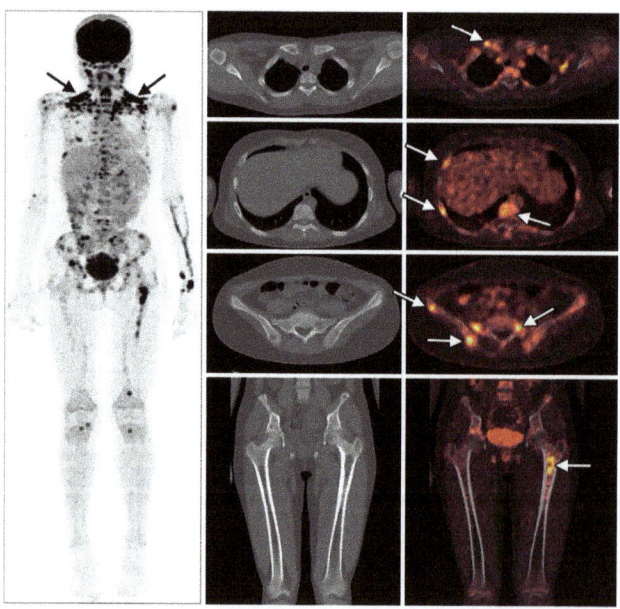

Fig. 1: PET-CT showing multiple lytic lesions with FDG uptake.
(FDG: fluorodeoxyglucose; CT: computed tomography; PET: positron-emission tomography)

revealed a foamy histiocytic infiltrate with pale eosinophilic abundant cytoplasm in a background of fibroblastic proliferation, and lymphocytic infiltrate. The histiocytic cells were CD1a and S100 negative but showed positivity for CD68 **(Fig. 2)**. A diagnosis of Erdheim–Chester disease (ECD) was made.

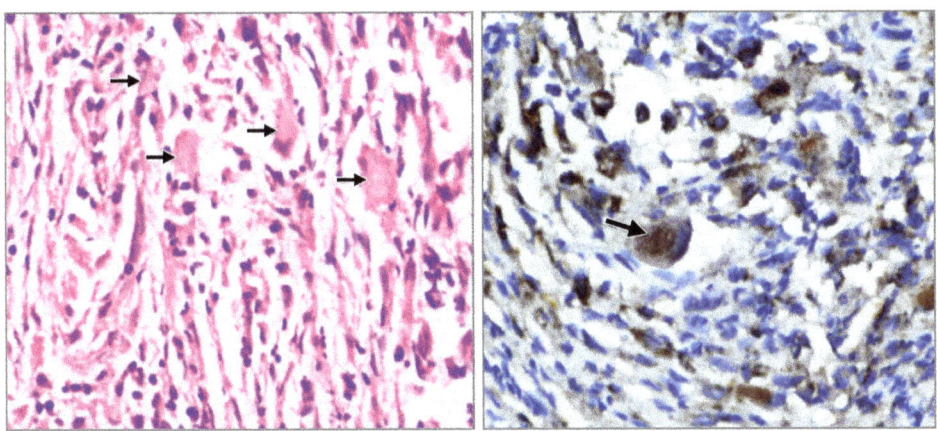

Fig. 2: Hematoxylin and Eosin-stained sections showing foamy histiocytic infiltrate on the left panel (black arrows) with pale eosinophilic abundant cytoplasm in a background of fibroblastic proliferation and lymphocytic infiltrate. The histiocytic cells were CD1a and S100 negative but were positive for CD68.

2. How will you differentiate ECD from LCH?

Though both LCH and ECD are histiocytosis, there are wide differences in their ontogeny, histopathological features, epidemiology, and clinical features **(Table 1)**.

TABLE 1: Differentiating Erdheim–Chester disease (ECD) from Langerhans cell histiocytosis (LCH).[1]

Characteristic	LCH	ECD
Cell of origin	Dendritic	Mononuclear-phagocyte
Population	Children	Adults
CD68	+	+
CD1a	+	–
S100	+	–
Factor XIIIa	–	+
Fascin	–	+
Cytology: Nuclear grooves, pseudoinclusions or dendrite-like cytoplasmic processes	+	–
Touton giant cells	–	+
Birbeck granules	+	–
T6 protein	+	–
Bone involvement	Osteolytic, axial	Osteosclerosis/appendicular
Lung involvement	Peribronchial	Lymphangitic
Skin involvement	Common	Uncommon

However, it is to be noted that 10–20% of patients with ECD have coexistent LCH lesions, commonly pulmonary or cutaneous.

3. What are the various non-LCH and describe their current classification?

Histiocytosis represents an abnormal clonal proliferation of histiocytes. They can originate at various stages of differentiation and maturation of macrophages **(Fig. 3)**.

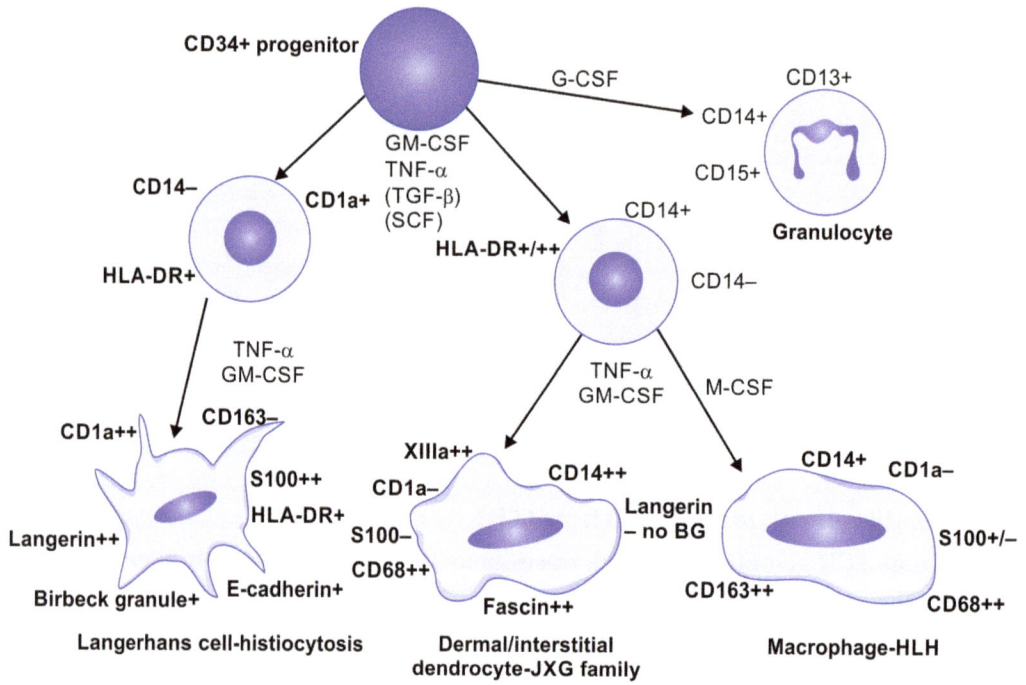

Fig. 3: Origin of various histiocytoses.
(G-CSF: Granulocyte-colony stimulating factor; GM-CSF: granulocyte-monocyte-colony stimulating factor; HLH: hemophagocytic lymphohistiocytosis; JXG: juvenile xanthogranuloma; HLA-DR: human leukocyte antigen-DR isotype; BG: Birbeck granule)

Based on the ontogeny, cell of origin, genetic aberration and the histology, and histiocytosis have been classified into the following groups: L group, C group, R group, M group, and H group **(Fig. 4)**. They have a varied clinical presentation and course.

L group	C group	R group	M group	H group
• LCH • ECD • Indeterminate cell histiocytosis	• Juvenile xanthogranuloma	• Rosai-Dorfman disease	• Histiocytic sarcoma • Langerhan cell sarcoma • Dendritic cell sarcoma	• Primary HLH • Secondary HLH

Fig. 4: Revised classification of histiocytoses.
(HLH: hemophagocytic lymphohistiocytosis; ECD: Erdheim–Chester disease; LCH: Langerhans cell histiocytosis)

BRAF, a serine/threonine protein kinase, is a proto-oncogene which regulates cell proliferation and survival. $BRAF^{V600E}$ mutation is an activating mutation which results in stimulation of RAS-RAF-MEK-ERK pathway, independently of RAS activation **(Fig. 5)**. The incidence of $BRAF^{V600E}$ mutation positivity is found to be higher in ECD compared to other

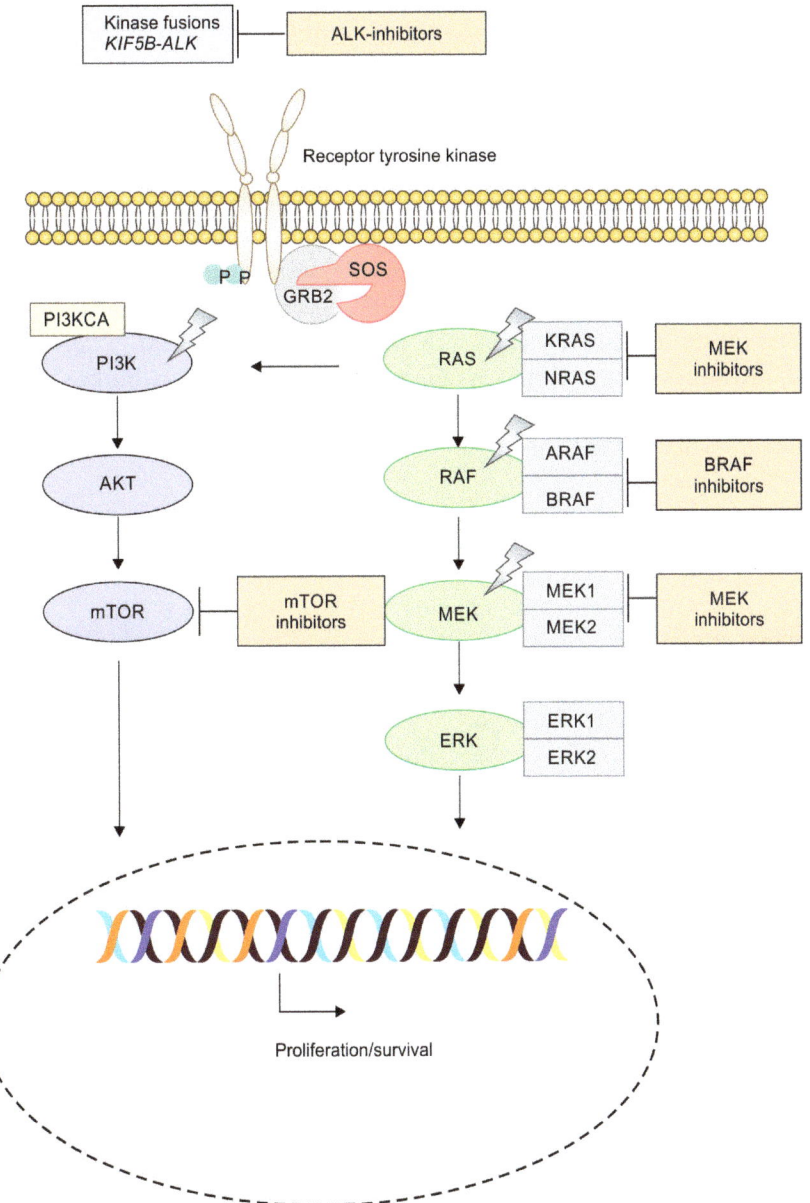

Fig. 5: MAPK pathway signaling in Erdheim–Chester disease (ECD) with therapeutic targets.
Source: Adapted from Goyal G, Heaney ML, Collin M, Cohen-Aubart F, Vaglio A, Durham BH, et al. Erdheim–Chester disease: Consensus recommendations for evaluation, diagnosis, and treatment in the molecular era. Blood. 2020;135(22):1929-45.

histiocytosis.[2] In multisystemic, severe forms of this disease, targeted treatments with the BRAF inhibitors, vemurafenib, and dabrafenib, have been successfully used. In wild-type BRAF patients, cobimetinib, a MEK inhibitor, has also been used with success.

4. Why is ECD referred to as an "inflammatory myeloid neoplasm"?

It is postulated that ECD shares a common pathogenic pathway with myeloproliferative neoplasms (MPN) or myelodysplastic syndromes (MDS). In a review of 189 ECD and mixed histiocytosis, it was found that 10% had over-lapping myeloid neoplasms.[3] The JAK2V617F mutation was the most frequent in myeloid neoplasms, followed by NRAS, TET2, ASXL1, and U2AF1 mutations. Similarly, next-generation sequencing (NGS) revealed that 42% of ECD patients harbor additional mutations like TET2, ASXL1, DNMT3A, and NRAS, which are commonly seen in myeloid neoplasms.

It is obvious from the study of inflammatory markers levels in patients with ECD that inflammation is a key driver in its pathogenesis. However, the link between clonal oncogenesis and this inflammation is not fully clear, only speculated (**Fig 6**). $BRAF^{V600E}$ mutation has been associated with increased expression of tumor suppressors such as p16Ink4a.[2] Senescent cells induce a complex inflammatory response. The pathogenesis and thus the targeted therapy of ECD are similar to that of LCH.

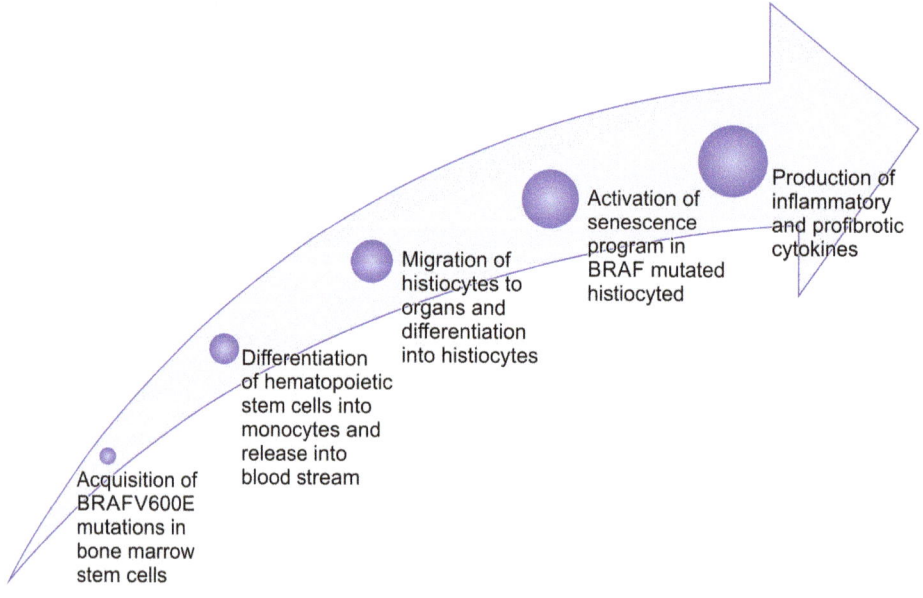

Fig. 6: Ontogenesis of mutated histiocytes in Erdheim–Chester disease (ECD).

5. Are there established criteria for diagnosis of ECD? Is biopsy always necessary?

There is limited evidence for making a diagnosis of ECD. Clinical, radiological, and distinct histopathological findings can often be used to clinch the diagnosis. Radiographically, we typically find symmetric diaphyseal and metaphyseal osteosclerosis in the bones of the lower limb, best visualized by bone scan. However, 4% of ECD patients may lack these findings.

CT abdomen is usually (in 68% of cases) demonstrative of a "hairy kidney" secondary to dense infiltration of perinephric fat. Histopathology involves demonstration of foamy or lipid-laden histiocytes with surrounding fibrosis. Touton giant cells are often present. On immunohistochemical staining, ECD histiocytes are positive for CD68, CD163, and factor XIIIa, and negative for CD1a and Langerin (*see* **Table 1**). Positivity for S100 has been observed rarely.[3] It is noteworthy that even with typical clinical profile and radiological findings, biopsy is necessary to confirm the diagnosis and establish BRAF mutational status. Recently, cell-free DNA (cfDNA) testing in plasma or urine has been used to detect $BRAF^{V600E}$ mutation.[1] Alternative mutations of the MAP-ERK and PI3K-AKT pathways (*KRAS, NRAS, ARAF, MAP2K1, and PIK3CA*)[1] can be analyzed if the $BRAF^{V600E}$ mutation is absent. Analysis of NGS is usually recommended for analysis of the above alternative mutations, detection of which can drive the choice of targeted therapies.

6. What are the current recommendations for BRAFV600E testing in ECD?

It is strongly encouraged to confirm negative $BRAF^{V600E}$ testing in ECD using more than one genotyping modality and/or genotyping from more than one anatomic site (particularly when bone lesions are found to be BRAF wild-type). This is because the highly variable histiocyte content in many ECD biopsy samples influences BRAF mutational testing results. In addition, the frequency of bone biopsies required to identify BRAF mutations in ECD presents an additional challenge. In addition to molecular tests,[4] immunohistochemistry (IHC) analysis of paraffin sections using the BRAFV600E mutant specific antibody (VE1) is possible. In several comparisons of BRAF mutational testing using IHC versus high-resolution melt curve and Sanger sequencing analysis in paraffin-embedded specimens, IHC had sensitivity and specificity of 95%. Whenever possible, VE11 IHC staining should be confirmed with molecular testing.

7. What are the common presentations of ECD?

Patients of ECD typically present with the symmetrical long bone osteosclerosis as described above.[5] Proximal and distal tibia, distal femur, and also the bones of the upper limbs are usually involved, whereas the axial skeleton and mandible (common LCH localizations) are typically spared. Bone pain is the leading symptom of bone involvement. However, despite the high prevalence of skeletal infiltration, 60% of patients are asymptomatic.

8. Is ECD a multi-system disease like LCH?

In addition to skeletal involvement, ECD is shown to involve almost every organ system.
- *Central nervous system (CNS):* Patients with ECD can have parenchymal lesions, meningeal lesions, supratentorial lesions of the white matter, intra- or extramedullary spinal cord masses, and cerebellar/brainstem atrophy.
- *Head and neck:* Proptosis may be seen (secondary to soft tissue retro-orbital infiltration). Craniofacial bones, especially the skull base and paranasal sinuses may be involved.
- *Endocrine:* Both the anterior and posterior pituitary hormone deficiencies have been described. Adrenal insufficiency secondary to adrenal infiltration has also been documented.

- *Cardiovascular:* Pericardial thickening and effusion, myocardial infiltration causing pseudotumoral atrial wall thickening, and infiltration of the right atrioventricular sulcus and coronary artery sheathing have been seen. Valvular disease or conduction disturbances are rare. Circumferential infiltration ("coated aorta") affecting almost any aortic segment is common.
- *Lung:* Lung infiltration is usually asymptomatic, presenting as interlobular septal thickening, ground-glass, or centrilobular opacities on high-resolution CT. On pulmonary function tests, the pattern is mainly restrictive.
- *Renal:* Diffuse calycectasia and hydroureteronephrosis, due to infiltration of perinephric fat with varying degrees of chronic kidney disease.

9. What is the treatment for ECD?

In view of very few RCTs, treatments have been based on an anecdotal evidence base and retrospective data. Corticosteroids, vinca alkaloids, cyclophosphamide, doxorubicin, cyclosporin, autologous haematopoietic stem cell transplantation, and radiation therapy have been used with uncertain sustained benefit. A systematic review of 2015 concluded that efficacy of all treatment modalities remains undefined, due to the frequent concomitant administration of more than one drug and short follow-up.[6,7] Current options for ECD include interferon-alpha (IFN-α), anticytokine directed therapy (anakinra, infliximab, and tocilizumab), cladribine, tyrosine kinase inhibitors, and BRAF and MEK inhibitors.

CASE *(Continued)*

The index case was given a trial on the LCH III protocol (multifocal bone disease; group 3), to which she responded and went into complete remission, which she continued to be in, 3 years post-treatment completion.

9a. What has been the experience with LCH-based protocols in pediatric ECD?

There are three case-reports in children among which two showed sustained remission on LCH-II[8] and LCH-III,[9] respectively and the other progressed and was subsequently treated with IFN-α.[10]

9b. If this child were BRAF^{V600E} mutation positive, if given a choice, what would be the appropriate choice—BRAF inhibitor or pegylated IFN-α?

The answer perhaps is PEG IFNα. BRAF inhibitors are currently recommended as first line in *BRAF^{V600E}* carriers with severe and diffuse disease and as second-line in other cases. Its most impressive responses have been in multisystemic and refractory disease despite IFN-α therapy (especially CNS, cardiovascular ECD). The largest experience of treatment of ECD has been with use of IFN-α. As retrospective studies have shown that treatment with IFN-α was a major independent predictor of survival, its preferable pegylated formulation is now recommended as first-line therapy for nonlife-threatening manifestations, considering the better toxicity profile, and ease of administration of the pegylated formulation.

9c. Does zoledronic acid has a role?

Bisphosphonates have been shown to be effective in osseous-only ECD and is particularly effective in pain relief. However, there are no large studies. Possible mechanisms include direct action on the macrophage cell line, inhibition of the osteocyte apoptosis and enhancement of osteocyte activity, anti-angiogenesis by prolonged suppression of vascular endothelial growth factor (VEGF), transient suppression of platelet-derived growth factor (PDGF), and cytostatic effects on tumor cell through the action on the mevalonate pathway and adenosine triphosphate metabolism[11]

CASE VIGNETTE 2

A 6-year-old boy presented with insidious onset bilateral neck swellings of 4 months duration. On examination, he had bilateral massive adenopathy, firm, nontender nodes with no overlying skin changes. Pemberton's sign was negative and there were no features of superior mediastinal syndrome. Rest of his systemic examination was unremarkable. Lymph node biopsy showed the presence of emperipolesis, with notable sinus infiltration of large histiocytic cells with pale cytoplasm. On IHC, these cells displayed a positive reaction to CD68 and S100 protein, whereas reaction to CD1a was negative. The child was diagnosed to have Rosai–Dorfman disease (RDD).

10. Is the phenomenon of emperipolesis specific to RDD? How does it differ from phagocytosis and entosis?

Histiocytic emperipolesis is the hallmark of RDD. However, megakaryocytic emperipolesis has been reported in hematolymphoid disorders such as Hodgkin's disease, acute and chronic myeloid leukemia, non-Hodgkin's lymphoma, myeloproliferative disorders, and myelodysplastic syndrome. Emperipolesis is the active penetration of one cell by another which remains intact. The engulfed cell exists temporarily within another cell with its structure normal and intact, while in phagocytosis, the engulfed cell is usually dead or dying and is destroyed by lysosomal enzymes. In entosis, epithelial cells are involved rather than professional phagocytes.[12] Phagocytosis is driven by cytoskeletal rearrangements within the host cell while the engulfment in entosis is through a mechanism involving adherens junctions and Rho-mediated contractile force.

11. How does RDD commonly present?

Massive, bilateral, and painless cervical lymphadenopathies are the hallmarks of RDD; Majority (80–90%) have cervical nodal involvement followed closely by inguinal (26%), axillary (24%), and mediastinal (15%) group of lymph nodes.[13]

12. How common is the extra-nodal presentation of RDD?

Extranodal involvement in RDD may be present in up to 40% of cases. The common extranodal sites include skin, CNS, orbit and eyelid, upper respiratory tract, and the gastrointestinal tract.[13]

13. The pathogenesis of most histiocytic disorders involves common pathways. How does the pathogenesis of RDD differ from the rest?

Monocytes produce macrophage colony-stimulating factor (M-CSF) when recruited to inflammatory lesions and are then stimulated to differentiate into RDD cells. Subsequently, via the PI3K/Akt/mTORC1 (mammalian target of rapamycin complex 1) and Ras/Raf/MEK/ERK/mTORC1 pathway, these RDD cells promote the production of TNF-α, interleukin-1β (IL-1β), and IL-6. Simultaneously, the inhibition of glycogen synthase kinase-3β (GSK3β) by mTORC1 could augment the expression of phosphatase and tensin homolog (PTEN) and epithelial-mesenchymal transition (EMT), but hinder the release of myeloid-related protein (MRP) 8 and MRP14 by obstructing the formation of microtubules. The accumulation of MRP8 in monocytes could reduce cholesterol efflux and result in the formation of foamy histiocytes **(Flowchart 1)**.

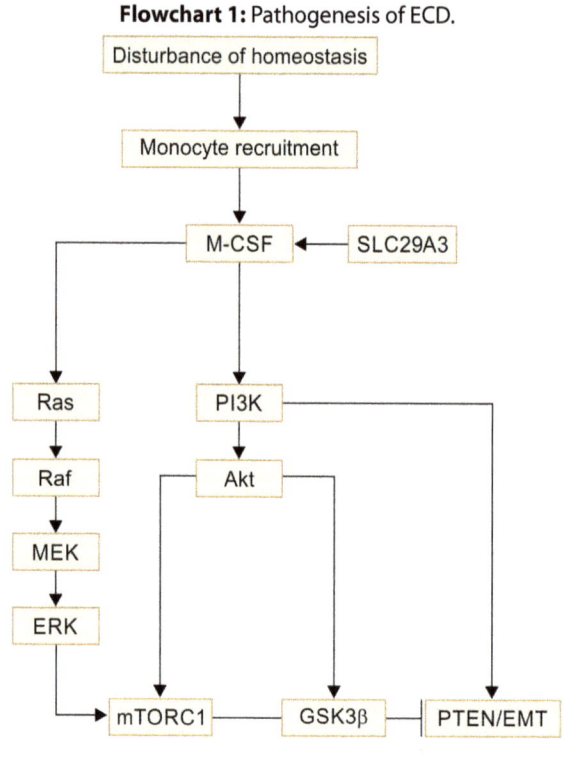

Flowchart 1: Pathogenesis of ECD.

(IL-1β: interleukin-1β; M-CSF: colony-stimulating factor; mTORC1: mammalian target of rapamycin complex 1; GSK3β: glycogen synthase kinase-3β (GSK3β); PTEN: phosphatase and tensin homolog; EMT: epithelial-mesenchymal transition; ECD: Erdheim–Chester disease)

15. How common is CNS involvement in RDD? What is its closest differential?

Central nervous system is affected in 5% of RDD and may be mistaken for meningioma because lesions are typically dural-based, uniformly enhanced, and can have a dural tail on imaging. Digital subtraction angiography may help to distinguish between meningioma and RDD, based on the absence of arterial-venous shunting and hypervascularity expected with meningioma.[14]

16. Have any inherited conditions been demonstrated to be predisposing to RDD?

Germline mutations in SLC29A3 have been reported in patients with familial RDD.[15] Heterozygous germline mutations in the FAS gene TNFRSF [responsible for autoimmune lymphoproliferative syndrome (ALPS) type 1], may be associated with RDD.[16]

17. What have been the treatment strategies used in RDD?

A total 20% of cases show spontaneous regression without therapy. Treatment is advised only in patients who are symptomatic or have vital organ (such as, CNS) involvement.

For patients with localized disease, simple observation can be recommended. In case of airway compromise or superior vena cava syndrome, surgery is the approach of choice. If surgery is not feasible, one may try radiotherapy for local lesions. The role of chemotherapy is doubtful, however, combination of chemotherapy, including steroids, vinca alkaloids, antimetabolites, alkylating agents, and alpha interferon have been used. Complete responses, however, are uncommon with any approach.

At our center, patients who require treatment for RDD are started on steroids (prednisolone at 1–2 mg/kg/day) for 6–8 weeks, while monitoring for steroid toxicity. Response assessment is done by PET-CT. Subsequently steroids are tapered to a low dose and stopped. In case of inadequate response or steroid toxicity, alternative agents like 6-mercaptopurine and weekly methotrexate are used for a prolonged duration with clinical and radiological assessment.

18. What is the prognosis of RDD?

Patients with nodal RDD usually do well. Complications arise due to emergencies rather than the disease itself. Patients with disseminated/extranodal RDD usually have an unpredictable course. They have diseases which are more aggressive to begin with and have a propensity to relapse.[17]

The prognosis of ECD patients has been traditionally described to be poor with a mean survival of 32 months. Majority of the patients die from either renal, cardiovascular, pulmonary, or neurological complications. Recent reports describe an overall 5-year survival of 68% with interferon therapy.[18]

19. Can more than one form of histiocytoses co-occur?

"Mixed histiocytosis" is an emerging group of syndromes defined by the overlap of LCH and another histiocytic disorder of different type. Despite its assumed rarity, it has accounted for up to a fifth of systemic histiocytosis in some series.[19] It has been described concurrently in patients at different sites of biopsy, or in the same lesion or as one disease preceding another. The prominent patterns include LCH/ECD, LCH/JXG, LCH/RDD, or ECD/RDD. The most prevalent of these is LCH/ECD. A multicenter study of 23 patients reported an association between LCH and ECD, linked to the BRAFV600E mutation. The BRAFV600E mutation was found in 11/16 LCH lesions (69%) and 9/11 ECD lesions (82%).[20]

REFERENCES

1. Weitzman S, Jaffe R. Uncommon histiocytic disorders: the non-Langerhans cell histiocytoses. Pediatr Blood Cancer. 2005;45(3):256-64.
2. Haroche J, Charlotte F, Arnaud L, von Deimling A, Hélias-Rodzewicz Z, Hervier B, et al. High prevalence of BRAF V600E mutations in Erdheim-Chester disease but not in other non-Langerhans cell histiocytoses. Blood. 2012;120:2700-3.
3. Papo M, Diamond EL, Cohen-Aubart F, Emile JF, Roos-Weil D, Gupta N, et al. High prevalence of myeloid neoplasms in adults with non-Langerhans cell histiocytosis. Blood. 2017;130:1007-13.
4. Ziai J, Hui P. BRAF mutation testing in clinical practice. Expert Rev Mol Diagn. 2012;12(2):127-38.
5. Michaloglou C, Vredeveld LCW, Soengas MS, Denoyelle C, Kuilman T, van der Horst CMAM, et al. BRAFE600-associated senescence-like cell cycle arrest of human naevi. Nature. 2005;436:720-4.
6. Goyal G, Heaney ML, Collin M, Cohen-Aubart F, Vaglio A, Durham BH, et al. Erdheim-Chester disease: consensus recommendations for evaluation, diagnosis, and treatment in the molecular era. *Blood.* 2020;135 (22):1929-45.
7. Cives M, Simone V, Rizzo FM, Dicuonzo F, Lacalamita MC, Ingravallo G, et al. Erdheim-Chester disease: a systematic review. Crit Rev Oncol Hematol. 2015;95(1):1-11.
8. Clerico A, Ragni G, Cappelli C, Schiavetti A, Gonfiantini M, Uccini S. Erdheim-Chester disease in a child. Med Pediatr Oncol. 2003;41(6):575-7.
9. Gupta AK, M AW, Meena JP, Arunraj ST , Mridha A, Naranje P, et al. A rare presentation of Erdheim Chester disease in a pediatric patient subsequently cured on the LCH III protocol. Cancer Reports. 2021;4:e1304.
10. Song SY, Lee SW, Ryu KH, Sung SH. Erdheim-Chester disease with multisystem involvement in a 4-year-old. Pediatr Radiol. 2012;42(5):632-5.
11. Srikulmontree T, Massey HD, Roberts WN. Treatment of skeletal Erdheim-Chester disease with zoledronic acid: case report and proposed mechanisms of action. Rheumatol Int. 2007;27(3):303-7.
12. Püschel F, Muñoz-Pinedo C. In the Hunger Games, the Winner Takes Everything. Trends Biochem Sci. 2017;42(10):763-4.
13. Foucar E, Rosai J, Dorfman R. Sinus histiocytosis with massive lymphadenopathy (Rosai-Dorfman disease): review of the entity. Semin Diagn Pathol. 1990;7(1):19-73.
14. Nasany RA, Reiner AS, Francis JH, Abla O, Panageas KS, Diamond EL. Rosai-Dorfman-Destombes disease of the nervous system: a systematic literature review. Orphanet J Rare Dis. 2022;17(1):92.
15. Morgan NV, Morris MR, Cangul H, Gleeson D, Straatman-Iwanowska A, Davies N, et al. Mutations in SLC29A3, encoding an equilibrative nucleoside transporter ENT3, cause a familial histiocytosis syndrome (Faisalabad histiocytosis) and familial Rosai-Dorfman disease. PLoS Genet. 2010;6(2):e1000833.
16. Wilson NR, Fang H, Loghavi S, Wang W, Tang G, Haltom RO, et al. Treating Rosai–Dorfman disease and RAS-associated autoimmune leucoproliferative disorder with malignant transformation. Br J Haematol. 2021;192:667-71.
17. Pulsoni A, Anghel G, Falcucci P, Matera R, Pescarmona E, Ribersani M, et al. Treatment of sinus histiocytosis with massive lymphadenopathy (Rosai-Dorfman disease): report of a case and literature review. Am J Hematol. 2002;69(1):67-71.
18. Arnaud L, Hervier B, Neel A, Hamidou MA, Kahn JE, Wechsler B, et al. CNS involvement and treatment with interferon- are independent prognostic factors in Erdheim-Chester disease: a multicenter survival analysis of 53 patients. Blood. 2011;117(10):2778-82.
19. Bonometti A; for Associazione Italiana Ricerca Istiocitosi AIRI ONLUS. The triptych of mixed histiocytosis: a systematic review of 105 cases and proposed clinical classification. Leuk Lymphoma. 2021;62(1):32-44.
20. Hervier B, Haroche J, Arnaud L, Charlotte F, Donadieu J, Néel A, et al. Association of both Langerhans cell histiocytosis and Erdheim-Chester disease linked to the BRAFV600E mutation. Blood. 2014;124:1119-26.

EXPERT OPINION

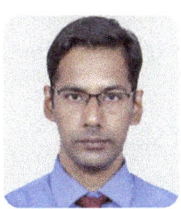

Sidharth Totadri MD DM (Pediatric Hematology Oncology)
European Hematology Exam Certified (2017)
Associate Professor
Pediatric Hematology Oncology Unit
Department of Pediatrics
Christian Medical College, Vellore, India

Langerhans cell histiocytosis is a well-known clinic-pathological entity defined by CD1a+/S100+/CD207+ positive histiocytic cells infiltrating a wide range of organ/s such as skin, bone, reticuloendothelial system, and CNS. The term "non-LCH histiocytosis" encompasses a myriad group of disorders that are infrequently encountered in comparison to LCH and are immunophenotypically distinct from the LCH cells. The cells of origin for histiocytic disorders are macrophages (called histiocytes when they are tissue-resident) and dendritic cells. The 2016 revised World Health Organization classification of lymphoid neoplasms describes a category of "histiocytic and dendritic cell neoplasms" which includes diseases such as disseminated juvenile xanthogranuloma (JXG), and ECD in addition to LCH. Based on the clinical and biological nature of the disorders, the histiocyte society provides a more comprehensive classification comprised of the L (LCH and LCH-like), C (cutaneous histiocytosis), R [Rosai–Dorfman–Destombes disease (RDD)], M (malignant histiocytosis), and H groups (hemophagocytic lymphohistiocytosis). Typically, the first three groups are what one would refer to as non-LCH histiocytosis.

Erdheim–Chester Disease

Erdheim–Chester disease resembles LCH in its clinical presentation with bilateral and symmetrical osteosclerotic lesions that involve long. A multisystem disease is seen in >50% of the patients. Skin rash, exophthalmos, diabetes insipidus, and CNS disease can mimic LCH. Xanthelasma, cardiovascular, retroperitoneal, and renal disease are unique to ECD. The frequency of the *BRAF-V600E* mutation is reported to be 50–75% in ECD, and akin to LCH, it is now established to be a clonal disorder with constitutive activation of the MAPK signaling pathway. Pathological diagnosis is characterized by the identification of foamy macrophages and Touton giant cells. Unlike LCH the cells are CD1a and CD207 negative and show variable S100 positivity. The positive immunohistochemical markers include CD68, CD163, factor XIIIa, and fascin. An ^{18}F–FDG–PET-CT can be used for staging and response assessment. Neuroimaging and cardiac assessment are strongly recommended at diagnosis. Molecular testing for the *BRAF-V600E* mutation is strongly recommended as it offers scope for targeted therapy. The conventional first-line drugs used for ECD include subcutaneous IFN-α, cladribine, and anakinra followed by second-line agents such as steroids, imatinib, and low-dose methotrexate. BRAF inhibitors such as vemurafenib for patients with the *BRAF-V600E* mutation and MEK inhibitors such as cobimetinib have shown promising results, with the former recently being approved for use in ECD in the United States of America.

Juvenile Xanthogranuloma

Juvenile xanthogranuloma is the most common non-LCH histiocytosis encountered in clinical practice. The proposed pathological basis for JXG is ERK activation. The prototype presentation is an infant or young child with varying numbers of cutaneous papules and nodules, with a predilection for the head and neck region. The natural course of cutaneous JXG is benign with a spontaneous resolution with or without scarring. The challenge arises when there is systemic JXG, which is observed in <10% of the patients. Systemic JXG can potentially involve soft tissue, CNS, liver, spleen, and lungs, and up to half the patients may lack cutaneous lesions. Children with JXG must be screened for features of neurofibromatosis-1 (NF-1) and can develop juvenile myelomonocytic leukemia on follow-up, particularly if having NF-1. Typical cutaneous JXG may be clinically diagnosed and followed up till resolution. Biopsy if there is suspicion of LCH or other cutaneous disorders, or if there is evidence of systemic disease. Historically, ECD has been considered to be part of the JXG spectrum and the entities are similar in histopathology and IHC. Clinical presentation, radiology, and the presence of the *BRAF-V600E* mutation (not described in JXG) can distinguish ECD and systemic JXG. Solitary symptomatic JXG lesions can be treated with surgical resection. LCH-based therapy with vinblastine/steroids and cladribine has been reported to be of benefit in systemic JXG. Targeted therapy with MEK inhibitors such as cobimetinib is being tested in JXG.

Rosai–Dorfman–Destombes Disease

The archetypal clinical presentation of RDD or sinus histiocytosis with massive lymphadenopathy is a young male with bilateral, progressively enlarging, and painless lymphadenopathy. The pathophysiology remains ambiguous but is conceivably related to a cytokine-mediated activation and accumulation of histiocytes in the affected tissues triggered by diverse immune triggers. RDD is associated with lymphomas, bone marrow transplant, inherited conditions such as ALPS, collagen vascular diseases, and IgG4-related disease. Besides lymphadenopathy, other manifestations include B-symptoms akin to lymphoma and extranodal involvement which is reported from almost all organs, including the CNS, skin, soft tissue, eye, respiratory tract, and abdomen. Histopathology demonstrates sinus expansion by histiocytes which are large with pale cytoplasm and a large nucleus and nucleolus. Similar to ECD and JXG, RDD histiocytes are CD1a/CD207 negative but uniformly stain positive for S100 in addition to fascin and CD68. Emperipolesis or the presence of intact leukocytes within the cytoplasm of the histiocytes is often associated with RDD. Absence does not rule out RDD as it may be focally present and presence is not pathognomonic as it may occur in other histiocytic disorders too. Strong clinical suspicion is needed for diagnosis of RDD, particularly in extranodal sites where the morphology may not be as typical as in lymph nodes. In patients with a limited nodal or cutaneous disease and minimal symptoms, a wait-and-watch strategy can be adopted, as a spontaneous resolution can occur. However, patients can have a prolonged waxing and waning clinical course with mortality occurring in 5–10% of patients. Surgery can be used as a curative modality for a unifocal disease and for the emergent treatment of lesions causing end-organ compromise or cord compression. Steroids such as prednisolone can be used for systemic therapy with a slow tapering strategy after achieving a good clinical response. Chemotherapeutic agents such as vinca alkaloids, oral methotrexate/6-mercaptopurine, and lymphoma-like regimens such as CHOP (cyclophosphamide, adriamycin, vincristine, and prednisolone) have been tried with variable benefit in refractory or relapsed cases. Radiotherapy may have a role in refractory disease with compressive complications.

CHAPTER 15

Autoimmune Lymphoproliferative Disorders

Kanwaljeet Kaur Chopra, Aditya Kumar Gupta

CASE VIGNETTE

Patient A, an 8-year-old boy presented with a history of cervical lymphadenopathy (LAP) for 9 months, low-grade fever, on and off for 7 months along with bleeding gums for 3 days at presentation. There was no loss of appetite, weight loss, or night sweats. Born to nonconsanguineous marriage as a preterm, the child was the second of a twin delivery with a birth weight of 1 kg. There was no family history of malignancy, LAP, or blood transfusions. The twin brother and elder sister were healthy.

On examination he was hemodynamically stable, with right cervical LAP of 3 × 3 cm (firm, nontender, mobile, nonmatted). There was no hepatosplenomegaly. Rest of the examination was normal.

Blood counts showed pancytopenia with hemoglobin (Hb) of 9.9 g/dL, total leucocyte count (TLC) of 2,000/cumm, absolute neutrophil count (ANC) 400/cumm, and platelet counts of 17,000/cumm. The lymph node biopsy showed florid lymphoid hyperplasia. There was generalized LAP on the imaging by a positron emission tomography (PET) scan. The bone marrow aspirate showed hematopoietic elements of all three series and no evidence of malignancy. Work-up also ruled out tuberculosis (TB), human immunodeficiency virus (HIV), Ebstein-Barr virus (EBV), cytomegalovirus (CMV), Castleman disease, lymphoma, immune thrombocytopenia (ITP), and hemophagocytic lymphohistiocytosis (HLH).

The peripheral blood sample analysis by flow cytometry showed $CD3^-$, $CD4^-$, $CD8^-$, T-cell receptor (TCR)$\alpha\beta^+$ cells to be 14.1%. The child was diagnosed with an autoimmune lymphoproliferative syndrome (ALPS). The clinical exome sequencing however, was negative for any specific mutations.

The child was started on prednisolone at 1 mg/kg/day. The cytopenias improved on prednisolone therapy. However on tapering of steroids after 5 m, the cytopenias recurred, so steroids were continued for another month and thereafter tapered successfully. Concomitantly he was started on mycophenolate mofetil (MMF). Currently he is on MMF at 30 mg/kg/day for the past 4 years. On follow-up with clinical examination the child has been normal with normal complete blood count (CBC) and liver function test (LFT).

1. What is ALPS?

Autoimmune lymphoproliferative syndrome represents a clinical syndrome caused by the persistence of autoreactive lymphoid cells due to failure of apoptosis, leading to chronic nonmalignant LAP, splenomegaly, and recurring multilineage cytopenia.

2. What are the clinical features found in ALPS?

Autoimmune lymphoproliferative syndrome is more common in males and the clinical manifestations usually occur early in life. Lymph node enlargement and enlargement of the liver and spleen occurring between 30 and 36 months of life are characteristic.[1,2] Half of the cases have liver enlargement.[3] Rarely splenomegaly may be the only manifestation.[4] The LAP in ALPS typically fluctuates and involves the cervical, axillary, and inguinal chains, although other lymph nodes may be involved too. LAP unlike splenomegaly becomes less pronounced after adolescence and massive splenomegaly may also be associated with hypersplenism.[4]

Autoimmunity is the second most common finding and occurs in 70% of patients.[1,2] The autoimmune manifestations may manifest after 2-3 years from the onset of lymphoproliferative symptoms. However, patients of older age may initially present with autoimmune manifestations.[1,2] It results in episodes of pallor and icterus associated with hemolytic anemia, spontaneous bruises, and mucocutaneous hemorrhages because of thrombocytopenia or bacterial infections associated with neutropenia. Cytopenia are typically most severe in early childhood and tend to improve in adolescents and young adults.

3. What is the pathophysiology of ALPS?

In healthy individuals, peripheral T cells that react with self-antigens undergo repeated stimulation, which leads to increased Fas ligand production. Under normal conditions, T-cell activation induces expression of Fas ligand on T cells, which can bind to Fas receptors on the same or nearby cells. A process known as activation-induced cell death is subsequently triggered that prevents the expansion of autoreactive T cells, which can otherwise lead to autoimmune diseases.[5]

In ALPS self-reactive T cells accumulate. These are negative for CD4 and CD8, i.e., double negative and α/β TCR positive. The elevated double-negative T cells (DNTs) in ALPS were initially thought to be an epiphenomenon, but they have been reported to stimulate abnormal B-cell proliferation and hence autoimmunity. These DNTs are highly proliferative owing in part to the upregulation of mammalian target of rapamycin (mTOR) and other growth pathways.[6]

4. When to suspect ALPS?

- Clinical picture consistent with ALPS as above. Less common presentations include glomerulonephritis, autoimmune hepatitis, connective tissue changes resembling systemic lupus erythematosus (SLE), uveitis, urticarial rash, thyroiditis, and Guillain-Barre syndrome. A positive family history for nonmalignant and noninfectious LAP and/or splenomegaly with or without autoimmune cytopenia may be positive in some cases.[7]
- ALPS should also be suspected in patients with a history of previous lymphoma and now presenting with nonmalignant LAP and cytopenias.[8]
- ALPS is also the underlying cause in nearly 50% of patients with Evans syndrome (ES) (presence of ≥2 cytopenia), even in those without significant lymphoproliferation.[9,10] Emperipolesis (lymphophagocytosis) was thought to be pathognomonic for Rosai-Dorfman disease (RDD); however, lymph node biopsies from ALPS patients can demonstrate emperipolesis, as well as other RDD features.[11] Accordingly, testing for ALPS should be considered in any child diagnosed with RDD.

5. What are the diagnostic criteria for ALPS?

Revised diagnostic criteria for ALPS based on First International ALPS Workshop are given in **Table 1**.[12]

TABLE 1: Revised diagnostic criteria for ALPS based on First International ALPS Workshop.

Required criteria	Additional criteria
• Chronic (>6 months), nonmalignant, noninfectious lymphadenopathy, and or splenomegaly • Elevated CD3$^+$ TCR αβ$^+$ CD4$^-$ CD8$^-$ DNT cells (>1.5% of total lymphocytes or >2.5% of CD3$^+$ lymphocytes) in the setting of normal or elevated lymphocyte counts	*Primary* • Defective lymphocyte apoptosis in two separate assays • Somatic or germline pathogenic mutation in FAS, FASLG, or CASP10 *Secondary* • Elevated plasma sFASL levels (>200 pg/mL), plasma IL-10 levels (>20 pg/mL), serum or plasma vitamin B$_{12}$ levels (>1,500 ng/L) or plasma IL-18 levels >500 pg/mL • Typical immunohistologic findings as reviewed by a hematopathologist • Autoimmune cytopenias (hemolytic anemia, thrombocytopenia, or neutropenia) with elevated IgG levels (polyclonal hypergammaglobulinemia) • Family history of a nonmalignant/noninfectious lymphoproliferation with or without autoimmunity

Definitive diagnosis: Both required criteria plus one primary accessory criterion
Probable diagnosis: Both required criteria plus one secondary accessory criterion
(DNT: double-negative T cell; Ig: immunoglobulin; IL: interleukin; TCR: T-cell receptor)

Double-negative T cells should only be tested in an experienced clinical laboratory and must include testing for the TCRα/β receptor, as other nonpathogenic lymphocyte subsets are CD3$^+$/CD4$^-$/CD8$^-$. The reference range of DNT test results can vary between laboratories. Hence, caution should be exercised in interpretation. Finally, lymphopenic patients and those on high-dose steroids or sirolimus should not undergo DNT testing due to risks of false positives or negatives, respectively.[13] DNT cells >3% of the total lymphocytes or >5% of T-lymphocytes are essentially pathognomonic for ALPS.

In the Fas-mediated apoptosis assay, the lymphocytes are separated and tested for the ability to undergo apoptosis upon ligation with cell surface Fas.

T-cell expansion in the paracortical areas with florid follicular hyperplasia, and progressive transformation of germinal centers may be seen on histopathological examination.

Several types of ALPS have been identified based on the genetic defect identified **(Table 2)**.[12]

TABLE 2: Types of ALPS on the basis of genetic defect.

ALPS-FAS	FAS (germline)
ALPS-sFAS	FAS (somatic)
ALPS-FASL	FASL
ALPS-CASP10	CASP10
ALPS-U	Unknown/undefined
ALPS-related diseases	
CEDS	*CASP8:* These patients also show defective T, B, and NK-cell activation, with consequent recurrent bacterial and viral infections
RALD	*NRAS, KRAS:* May present with atypical features such as elevations in cells of myeloid origin (monocytosis and granulocytosis) and showed partial overlap with JMML as well as lymph node histopathology not typical of ALPS

(ALPS: autoimmune lymphoproliferative syndrome; CEDS: caspase 8 deficiency state; JMML: juvenile myelomonocytic leukemia; RAS: rat sarcoma; RALD: RAS-associated leukoproliferative disease)

Revised classification of ALPS and ALPS-related diseases based on the gene defect identified.

CASP8 mutated patients were earlier classified as ALPS because they also present with LAP and defective Fas-mediated apoptosis. However, in ALPS the apoptotic defects occur in T-lymphocytes, whereas in *CASP8* mutated subjects defective apoptosis is noted in B, T, and natural killer (NK) lymphocytes. Also the *CASP8* mutated subjects are at significant risk of severe herpes virus infection. The patients with *CASP8* mutations are now classified as having caspase 8 deficiency state (CEDS).

6. Is ALPS a hereditary disease?

More than 300 families with hereditary ALPS have been described and nearly 500 patients from these families have been studied and followed worldwide. Germline *FAS* mutations are autosomal dominant. However, somatic *FAS* mutations are more common. There are two types of genetic defects in ALPS.[13]

1. *The dominant negative mutations:* Most often *FAS* defects are dominant negative heterozygous missense mutations. The gene product of the mutated allele inhibits the function of the wild-type allele—all in the same cell leading typically to the complete absence of FAS activity.
2. *Haploinsufficiency:* It arises from a *de novo or inherited loss-of-function mutation* in the variant allele, such that it produces little or no gene product (often a protein). Haploinsufficient mutations usually lead to decreased activity in contrast to dominant negative mutation as the other, standard allele still produces normal amount of product. However, the total gene product is less than normal.

The patients with FAS mutations have variable severity of clinical picture suggesting variable penetrance of the genetic defect. Higher disease penetrance is noted in families with dominant negative mutations versus those with haploinsufficiency.[14]

Regarding the role of genetic counseling, if the defect is identified in the index patient, then the family should be offered genetic testing. However, in the absence of clinical features suggestive of ALPS and if DNT percentage, vitamin B_{12}, and interleukin (IL)-10 are normal the genetic tests for the family member are not done.

7. How common is the risk of malignancy in ALPS patients?

A higher risk of Hodgkin and non-Hodgkin lymphoma (HL and NHL), has been reported in those with ALPS-*FAS* mutations. Patients with ALPS have a risk of 10–20% for the development of secondary malignancies, which does not diminish with age, extends across mutation types, and is most prevalent in *FAS*-mutant ALPS.[15] Clinically normal relatives with *FAS* mutations are also at higher risk of malignancy.

In an ALPS patient the risk of developing HL is 50-fold and that of NHL is 14-fold that of the general population. The median age at lymphoma diagnosis has been reported as 17 years (range, 5–50 years). These patients respond to conventional chemotherapy and radiotherapy.

8. Is ALPS associated with increased risk of infections?

The immune system including T, B, and NK cells is preserved in ALPS. Some studies report reduced responses of B cells to polysaccharide antigens.[16] However, neutropenia due to immune cytopenia, steroids, rituximab, and splenectomy may increase the risk of infections.

9. Enumerate the differential diagnoses and work-up of ALPS.

Differential Diagnoses

The differential diagnoses of ALPS include:
- *Immune thrombocytopenic purpura (ITP):* Autoimmune cytopenias noted in ALPS often present with bleeding, whereas ITP, usually presents without significant bleeding.
- *Lymphoproliferative disorders:* Pretreatment biopsy of bone marrow and/or lymph node is useful to differentiate ALPS from Castleman disease and Rosai–Dorfman disease.
- *Ras-associated lymphoproliferative disorder (RALD):* Presents with lymphoproliferation, autoimmune cytopenias, and hypergammaglobulinemia. DNTs may be mildly elevated or normal.
- Common variable immunodeficiency (CVID) can present with lymphoproliferation and autoimmune disease.[17] All patients with CVID and cytopenias should be tested for ALPS.
- ES, defined by autoimmune destruction of at least two hematologic cell types.[18] Although few authors have[19] reported that a significant percentage of children diagnosed with ES have ALPS, the French noted fewer ALPS patients among ES cases.[20]
- Dianzani autoimmune lymphoproliferative disease is characterized by autoimmunity, LAP and/or splenomegaly, and defective apoptosis, without elevation in TCR-DNT cells. The genetic defect is not known, but the defective FAS function displayed by relatives of these patients.
- Chronic active EBV infection,[21] CMV infection.

Work-up

The work-up should include the ruling out of infections that can present with cytopenias, LAP, and hepatosplenomegaly. Doppler ultrasound of portal vein, splenic, and hepatic veins should be done to rule out any other cause of hepatosplenomegaly.

Work-up for chronic single lineage or multiple lineage autoimmune cytopenias:
- DNTs by flow cytometry (ALPS)
- Direct Coombs test (DCT) and Indirect Coombs Test (ICT)
- Bone marrow aspiration (BMA) and biopsy
- Antinuclear antibody (ANA) (SLE), antiphospholipid antibodies
- Quantitative immunoglobulins (CVID)—consider specific antibody titers (CVID)
- T-cell subsets (CD3/CD4, CD3/CD8)
- HIV.

10. How to follow-up ALPS patients?

Chronic generalized adenopathy in ALPS patients can fluctuate over time in its size by up to 20–30% and create some concern of evolving lymphoma if one or more regional group of nodes enlarges unusually. Hence, these patients need close clinical observation and follow-up. Important clues for lymphoma are itching, fever, sweating at night, loss of weight, and significant change in disease pattern. The questionable nodes may require biopsy. In ALPS LAP there is polyclonal expansion of abnormal cells whereas in lymphomas there is monoclonal expansion of similar cells.

Role of PET computed tomography (CT) is being explored to determine whether qualitative or quantitative fluorodeoxyglucose (FDG) localization can help differentiate ALPS patients with benign adenopathy from those with ALPS-associated lymphomas. The studies shows mixed results regarding use of FDG PET to discriminate between ALPS-associated adenopathy and ALPS-associated lymphoma.[22] Due to very high false-positive rate, some groups do not perform routine serial PET scans of ALPS patients.

11. What is the management of ALPS?[23]

Indications of treatment: Indication for therapy are refractory cytopenias because of significant hypersplenism or immune cytopenias. Asymptomatic LAP and splenomegaly often improve with age without any immunosuppressive treatment.

The occurrence of autoimmunity implies the need for immunosuppressive therapy which portends a poor prognosis and the treatment can last for years (long-term) or be intermittent.

The treatment of the disease has changed over time with MMF and sirolimus demonstrating activity against the disease and safety too.

Short-term Steroids and Intravenous Immunoglobulins

- *Immune suppression with corticosteroids.* High-dose pulse therapy with 5–10 mg/kg of intravenous (IV) methylprednisolone followed by 1–2 mg/kg/day of oral prednisolone therapy tapered over 8–12 weeks works in most patients. However, IV methylprednisolone at doses as high as 30 mg/kg/day for 1–3 days may have to be used in some critical patients

Autoimmune Lymphoproliferative Disorders

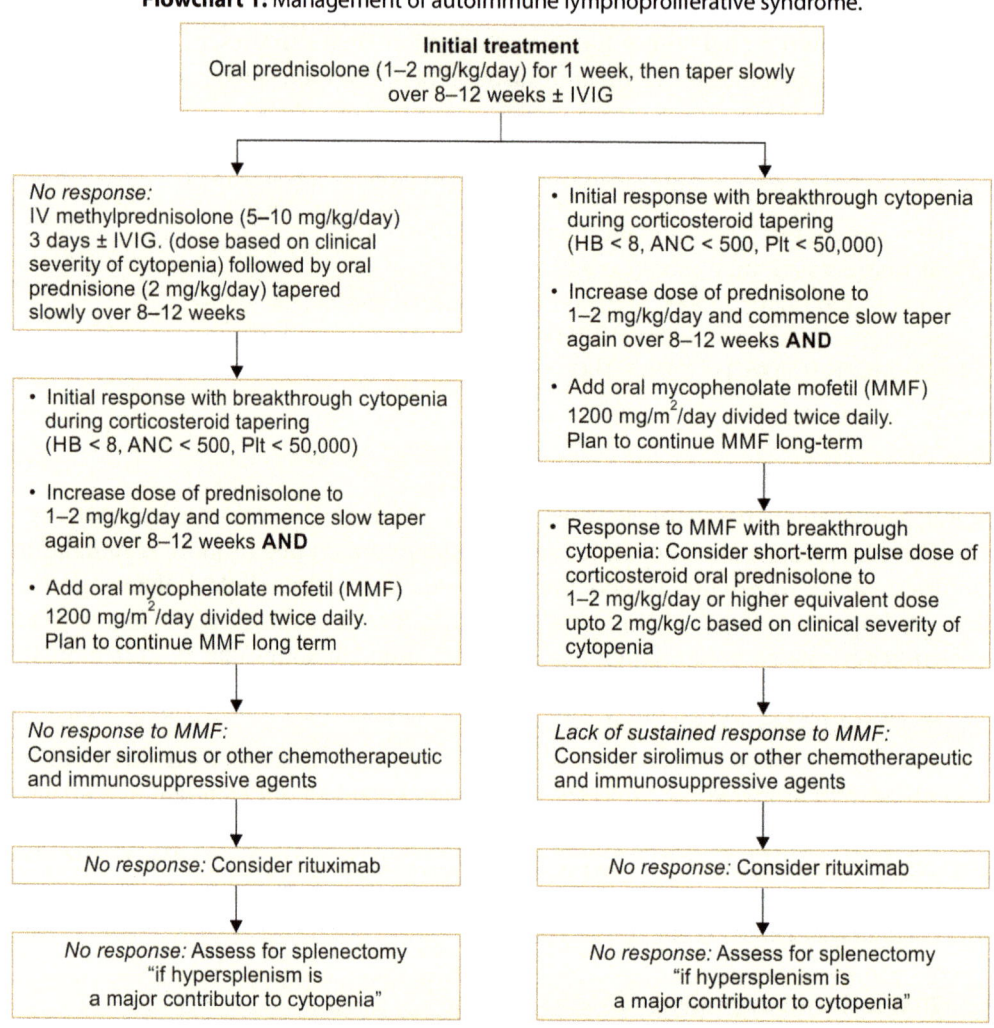

Flowchart 1: Management of autoimmune lymphoproliferative syndrome.

(IV: intravenous; IVIG: intravenous immunoglobulins)

with profoundly refractory cytopenia (e.g., Hb < 5 g requiring intensive care for hypoxia). Some patients may develop organ dysfunction from autoimmunity. Most patients respond to short corticosteroid pulses. However, high dose/long-term steroids have significant toxicities.

- *Intravenous immunoglobulin (IVIG) G* (1–2 g/kg) given concomitantly with pulse dose methylprednisolone *may benefit some patients with severe autoimmune hemolytic anemia (AIHA).*

Steroid-sparing Measures: Mycophenolate Mofetil and Sirolimus[23]

- MMF does not improve lymphoproliferation or reduce DNTs. MMF is a well-tolerated medication with common side effects being neutropenia and diarrhea. The recommendations for MMF are to use it only in the context of a steroid-sparing measure and not as a first-line upfront therapy. MMF should be added if patient does not tolerate

tapering of steroids. MMF should be started while patient still on tapering of steroids for at least 2 weeks to reach the required drug levels. The dose of MMF is 600 mg/m² BD.
- Sirolimus is uniquely active in ALPS with most patients showing rapid, complete responses.²⁴ In patients who had failed other treatments, sirolimus inhibited autoimmune disease, lymphoproliferation, and also eliminated the abnormal DNTs. The mTOR signaling pathway is abnormally activated in ALPS therefore treating ALPS patients with sirolimus a well-tolerated targeted therapy. Side effects include hypercholesterolemia, hypertension, and mucositis.

The loading dose of sirolimus is 3 mg/m² followed by once daily at 2.5 mg/m²/day up to a maximum daily dose of 4 mg. The target 24-hour trough drug level is 5–15 ng/mL. Levels are done at least twice per week until the levels stabilize and weekly or monthly thereafter.

Other drugs, including hydroxychloroquine, azathioprine, 6-mercaptopurine and dapsone have reported in some children and adults with ALPS. Rituximab in dose of 375 mg/m²/week, for four doses has been used in children with refractory, chronic cytopenias. Thrombocytopenia is more likely to respond than AIHA. An additional infection risk, especially in those with splenectomy may make it a reserved option. Patients with ALPS have a very high risk of developing postsplenectomy sepsis, even with antibiotic prophylaxis and vaccination. Accordingly, splenectomy should be avoided except in the case of uncontrolled hypersplenism that fails other medical management.

12. What are long-term outcome of ALPS patients and role of hematopoetic stem cell transplant (HSCT)?

The chronic cytopenias tend to improve with age, and often continue responding to intermittent short-term steroids. Only a few selected ALPS patients with lymphoma, polyarteritis nodosa, or very severe phenotype because of homozygous *FAS* mutation and refractory cytopenias may require HSCT.

In the case of matched sibling donor (MSD) HSCT, an asymptomatic sibling with the same mutation as the index patient is not a suitable donor.

■ REFERENCES

1. Neven B, Magerus-Chatinet A, Florkin B, Gobert D, Lambotte O, De Somer L, et al. A survey of 90 patients with autoimmune lymphoproliferative syndrome related to TNFRSF6 mutation. Blood. 2011;118(18):4798-807.
2. Price S, Shaw PA, Seitz A, Joshi G, Davis J, Niemela JE, et al. Natural history of autoimmune lymphoproliferative syndrome associated with FAS gene mutations. Blood. 2014;123(13):1989-99.
3. Matson DR, Yang DT. Autoimmune lymphoproliferative syndrome: an overview. Arch Pathol Lab Med. 2020;144(2):245-51.
4. Bleesing JJH, Nagaraj CB, Zhang K. (2006). Autoimmune lymphoproliferative syndrome. [online]. In: GeneReviews® [Internet]. Seattle (WA): University of Washington, Seattle. Available from https://www.ncbi.nlm.nih.gov/books/NBK1108/ [Last accessed October, 2022].
5. Green DR, Droin N, Pinkoski M. Activation-induced cell death in T cells. Immunol Rev. 2003;193:70-81.
6. Völkl S, Rensing-Ehl A, Allgäuer A, Schreiner E, Lorenz MR, Rohr J, et al. Hyperactive mTOR pathway promotes lymphoproliferation and abnormal differentiation in autoimmune lymphoproliferative syndrome. Blood. 2016;128(2):227-38.

7. Jackson CE, Fischer RE, Hsu AP, Anderson SM, Choi Y, Wang J, et al. Autoimmune lymphoproliferative syndrome with defective Fas: Genotype influences penetrance. Am J Hum Genet. 1999;64(4):1002-14.
8. Rao VK, Oliveira JB. How I treat autoimmune lymphoproliferative syndrome. Blood. 2011;118(22):5741-51.
9. Seif AE, Manno CS, Sheen C, Grupp SA, Teachey DT. Identifying autoimmune lymphoproliferative syndrome in children with Evans syndrome: a multi-institutional study. Blood. 2010;115(11):2142-5.
10. Iyengar SR, Ebb DH, Yuan Q, Shailam R, Bhan AK. Case records of the Massachusetts General Hospital. Case 27-2013. A 6.5-month-old boy with fever, rash, and cytopenias. N Engl J Med. 2013;369(9):853-63.
11. Maric I, Pittaluga S, Dale JK, Niemela JE, Delsol G, Diment J, et al. Histologic features of sinus histiocytosis with massive lymphadenopathy in patients with autoimmune lymphoproliferative syndrome. Am J Surg Pathol. 2005;29:903-11.
12. Oliveira JB, Bleesing JJ, Dianzani U, Fleisher TA, Jaffe ES, Lenardo MJ, et al. Revised diagnostic criteria and classification for the autoimmune lymphoproliferative syndrome (ALPS): Report from the 2009 NIH InternationalWorkshop. Blood. 2010;116(14):e35-e40.
13. Teachey DT. New advances in the diagnosis and treatment of autoimmune lymphoproliferative syndrome. Curr Opin Pediatr. 2012;24(1):1-8.
14. Kuehn HS, Caminha I, Niemela JE, Rao VK, Davis J, Fleisher TA, et al. FAS haploinsufficiency is a common disease mechanism in the human autoimmune lymphoproliferative syndrome. J Immunol. 2011;186(10):6035-43.
15. Straus SE, Jaffe ES, Puck JM, et al. The development of lymphomas in families with autoimmune lymphoproliferative syndrome with germline Fas mutations and defective lymphocyte apoptosis. Blood. 2001;98(1):194- 200.
16. Neven B, Bruneau J, Stolzenberg MC, Meyts I, Magerus-Chatinet A, Moens L, et al. Defective anti-polysaccharide response and splenic marginal zone disorganization in ALPS patients. Blood. 2014;124(10):1597-609.
17. Savasan S, Warrier I, Buck S, Kaplan J, Ravindranath Y. Increased lymphocyte Fas expression and high incidence of common variable immunodeficiency disorder in childhood Evans' syndrome. Clin Immunol. 2007;125:224-9.
18. Evans RS, Takahashi K, Duane RT, Payne R, Liu C. Primary thrombocytopenic purpura and acquired hemolytic anemia; evidence for a common etiology. AMA Arch Intern Med. 1951;87:48-65.
19. Teachey DT, Manno CS, Axsom KM, Andrews T, Choi JK, Greenbaum BH, et al. Unmasking Evans syndrome: T-cell phenotype and apoptotic response reveal autoimmune lymphoproliferative syndrome (ALPS). Blood. 2005;105(6):2443-8.
20. Aladjidi N, Leverger G, Leblanc T, Picat MQ, Michel G, Bertrand Y, et al.; Centre de Référence National des Cytopénies Auto-immunes de l'Enfant (CEREVANCE). New insights into childhood autoimmune hemolytic anemia: A French national observational study of 265 children. Haematologica. 2011;96(5):655-63.
21. Szcwzawińska-Poplonyk A, Grześk E, Schwartzmann E, Materna-Kiryluk A, Małdyk J. Autoimmune Lymphoprliferative Syndrome vs. Chronic Active Epstein-Barr Virus Infection in Children: A diagnostic challenge. Front Pediatr. 2021;9:798959.
22. Rao VK, Carrasquillo JA, Dale JK, Bacharach SL, Whatley M, Dugan F, et al. Fluorodeoxyglucose positron emission tomography (FDG-PET) for monitoring lymphadenopathy in the autoimmune lymphoproliferative syndrome (ALPS). Am J Hematol. 2006;81(2):81-5.
23. Rao VK. Approaches to managing autoimmune cytopenias in novel immunological disorders with genetic underpinnings like autoimmune lymphoproliferative syndrome. Front. Pediatr. 2015;3(65):1-6.
24. Bride K, Teachey D. Autoimmune lymphoproliferative syndrome: more than a FAScinating disease. F1000Res. 2017;6:1928.

EXPERT OPINION

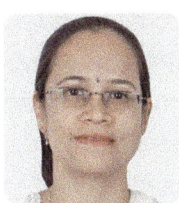

Manisha Madkaikar MD
Director, ICMR National Institute of Immunohematology,
KEM Hospital, Mumbai, India

1. Over the past two decades how has our understanding regarding the pathophysiology of ALPS evolved?

In 1967, Canale and Smith first described five patients with LAP, splenomegaly, and autoimmune cytopenias that mimicked malignant lymphoma. Investigation of two similar patients with progressive lymphoproliferative disease and autoimmunity by Sneller et al. in 1992 revealed an increase in a normally rare population of T cells characterized by the surface phenotype TCR ab$^+$ CD4$^-$ CD8$^-$ or DNTs. The first disease-causing mutations were identified in *FAS* gene in 1995. Since then multiple genetic etiologies have been identified resulting in FAS-mediated apoptotic defect and ALPS. Recent International Union of Immunological Societies (IUIS) classification of ALPS has listed mutations in five genes namely, *FAS, FASLG, FADD, CASP8,* and *CASP10*.

The mode of inheritance of ALPS is controversial. Both autosomal dominant and autosomal recessive types of inheritance have been described. Though heterozygous mutation in FAS is sufficient to explain a disease, a severe phenotype usually requires a double hit either in the same gene or other FAS-related gene.

With the advent of next-generation sequencing (NGS) technique, many new mutations have been identified in patients with autoimmunity and benign lymphoproliferation. Though they have overlapping clinical phenotype they often do not fit into diagnostic criteria for ALPS and often have hypogammaglobulinemia and susceptibility to infections. They can have elevated DNTs, but usually they are <6% of the total T cells. Some of the common ALPS-like disorders include LPS-responsive beige-like anchor protein (LRBA) deficiency, CTLA4 deficiency, activated phosphoinositide 3-kinase δ syndrome (APDS), etc.

2. Is there a role for screening the family members if the mutation is detected?

There is no simple answer to this question. In autosomal recessive diseases especially with variants of unknown significance identified by NGS, it is advisable to do familial segregation studies and show that unaffected parents are asymptomatic carriers. In patients with heterozygous mutations initially it was recommended to screen the family members to identify yet asymptomatic members who can be counseled for the disease. However, it is increasing seen that *FAS* mutations have variable penetrance (<60%) and the family members can remain asymptomatic throughout their life and hence screening of asymptomatic family members is no more recommended.

3. What is the natural history of ALPS without treatment? Is there a subset of patients in whom the disease can spontaneously regress?

Benign lymphoproliferation in the form of LAP and splenomegaly usually regress with age. However, risk of malignant transformation remains and needs to be monitored regularly. Autoimmune cytopenia occur in >80% of ALPS-FAS patients and often represent a therapeutic challenge.

Treatment of isolated benign lymphoproliferation for cosmetic reasons is not usually indicated.

4. What are the precautions to be taken when interpreting the report of DNTs?

Elevated DNTs are one of the important laboratory abnormality seen in ALPS. However, it is not pathognomonic of ALPS. Many ALPS-like diseases have elevated DNTs and hence molecular confirmation is required for final diagnosis.

The levels of DNTs may fluctuate and can be affected by immunosuppressive therapy and hence must be interpreted carefully.

Other biomarkers like sFASL levels, B12, IL-10, and IL-18 levels are useful in evaluation of these patients especially in patients with borderline elevated DNTs.

5. What is your approach to the treatment of ALPS?

The following points should be considered in the treatment of ALPS:
- Do not treat isolated LAP unless it is cosmetically disfiguring/causing obstructive symptoms.
- Avoid splenectomy as far as possible as incidence of postsplenectomy pneumococcal sepsis is high.
- Autoimmune cytopenias in ALPS have been classically treated as sporadic immune cytopenias, using corticosteroids and IVIG as first-line options.
- Due to refractoriness to these treatments, cytopenias in ALPS often require the use of second-line agents.
- Rituximab though effective, is not usually recommended due to a consistent increase in the risk of severe infections.
- MMF proved to be an effective steroid-sparing agent, without evidence of significant toxicities or infections.
- If facilities for drug monitoring are available, sirolimus may be considered as a first-line treatment option and, once complete remission is achieved, its serum levels may be maintained at a lower therapeutic range (i.e., 2–5 ng/mL).
- ALPS patients exhibit an increased risk of lymphoma; therefore, periodic surveillance with CT and PET scans should be carried out, and lymph node biopsies must be performed in case of clinical or radiological suspect of malignancy.

6. In a child with malignancy and ALPS how would you approach the treatment? Is there a role of hematopoietic stem cell transplant for ALPS?

Conventional multiagent chemotherapy and radiation are usually effective and no specific treatment protocols are available for ALPS-related lymphoma.

Hematopoetic stem cell transplant may be considered in early onset ALPS especially with homozygous mutations in FAS or FASL.

7. When do you try to stop treatment? What are the chances of recurrence after the treatment is stopped?

The treatment followed for cytopenias is similar to other immune cytopenias. However, chances of recurrence are high.

Sirolimus may be considered as a first-line treatment option and, once complete remission is achieved, its serum levels may be maintained at a lower therapeutic range (i.e., 2–5 ng/mL) to avoid relapse.

CHAPTER 16

Oncologic Emergencies

Prasanth Srinivasan, Rachna Seth

■ INTRODUCTION

The overall survival of childhood cancers has improved dramatically over the past few decades. This is attributed to advances in diagnostics and therapeutics and improvement in supportive care. One of the important factors leading to improvement in childhood cancer survival is timely recognition and treatment of oncological emergencies.[1] Among the wide spectrum of oncologic emergencies, we will be discussing the four important emergencies, viz., tumor lysis syndrome (TLS), superior mediastinal syndrome (SMS), hyperleukocytosis, and febrile neutropenia (FN).

CASE VIGNETTE 1

Tumor Lysis Syndrome

A, a 3-year-old boy, symptomatic for the past 2 weeks with subacute febrile illness with pallor and bleeding manifestations, which required multiple blood component support and bone pain.
- *On examination (O/E):* Vitals—heart rate (HR): 92/min, respiratory rate (RR): 28 breaths/min, blood pressure (BP): 92/68 mm Hg, temperature: 101.2°F, capillary filling time (CFT): 3 seconds, and SpO_2: 97% with room air
- *General physical examination (GPE):* Pallor and petechial spots, generalized lymphadenopathy, and bony tenderness.
- *Per abdomen (P/A) examination:* Liver—5 cm below right costal margin (RCM), Spleen—6 cm below left costal margin (LCM), and bilateral (B/L) testis—within normal limit (WNL).
- *Other system:* WNL
- *Presumptive diagnosis:* Acute leukemia.

1. What are the immediate potential life-threatening emergencies in this child?
- Tumor lysis syndrome
- Superior mediastinal syndrome/superior vena cava syndrome (SVCS)
- Hyperleukocytosis
- Life-threatening major bleeds
- Severe anemia.

2. What is tumor lysis syndrome?

Tumor lysis syndrome is characterized by the constellation of metabolic derangements caused by massive and abrupt release of intracellular metabolites into blood after lysis of malignant cells. It usually occurs after initiation of cytotoxic chemotherapy but can also occur spontaneously in tumors with high proliferative rate, large tumor burden, or high sensitivity to chemotherapy **(Flowchart 1)**.

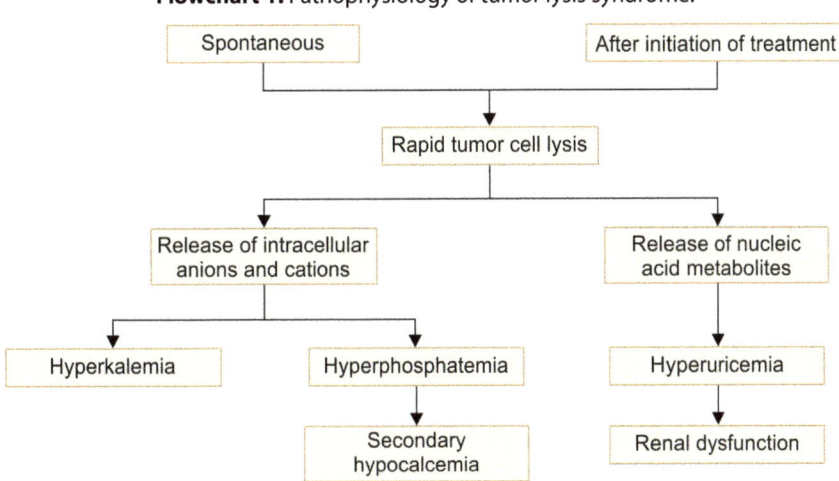

Flowchart 1: Pathophysiology of tumor lysis syndrome.

3. What are the clinical features which suggest the diagnosis of TLS?

Most of the times, patients with TLS are asymptomatic in the beginning. When the metabolic abnormalities overwhelm, the patient will manifest the clinical features of the underlying metabolic derangements. It is prudent to actively screen all the patients with newly diagnosed malignancies associated with increased risk of TLS rather than waiting for the symptoms of TLS to develop **(Table 1)**.

TABLE 1: Clinical features of tumor lysis syndrome.

Metabolic derangements	Clinical features
Hyperkalemia	• *Electrocardiogram (ECG) changes and arrhythmias:* Tall T waves, prolonged PR interval, absent P waves, wide QRS complex, ST-T wave changes, ectopic beats, ventricular fibrillation, and sudden death • Muscular cramps, paresthesias
Hyperphosphatemia	Nausea, vomiting, diarrhea, lethargy, and seizures
Hypocalcemia	• *Cardiac arrhythmia:* QTc prolongation, hypotension • Perioral numbness, tetany, muscular cramps, seizures • Sudden death
Hyperuricemia	Renal dysfunction—through crystal dependent and independent mechanism
Uremia	Oliguria, anuria, fluid overload, hypertension

CASE (Continued)

The resident in emergency room (ER) sent the emergency laboratories for the child A—whose reports as follows:
- *Complete blood count (CBC):* Hemoglobin (Hb)—7.2 g/dL, Total leukocyte count (TLC)—68,000/mm³ with 68% blasts (lymphoblasts), and platelets—12,000/mm³
- *Serum electrolytes:* K—4.2 mEq/dL, PO$_4$—4.2 mg/dL, Ca—9.1 mg/dL, and uric acid—3.5 mg/dL
- *Renal function test (RFT):* Urea—32 mg/dL and serum creatinine—0.5 mg/dL
- *Lactate dehydrogenase (LDH):* 750 U/L
- *Urine output:* 2 mL/kg/hour.

4. Does the child A have TLS?

Howard modification of Cairo-Bishop definition of TLS:[2]

Definition of laboratory TLS: Two or more of the following should be present simultaneously during the same 24 hours within 3 days before or up to 7 days after the initiation of chemotherapy.
- *Hyperuricemia:* Uric acid >8.0 mg/dL in adults or above upper limit of normal (ULN) range in children.
- *Hyperphosphatemia:* Phosphorus >4.5 mg/dL in adults or >6.5 mg/dL in children.
- *Hyperkalemia:* Potassium >6.0 mEq/L.
- *Hypocalcemia:* Corrected calcium <7.0 mg/dL or ionized calcium <1.12.

Definition of clinical TLS: Laboratory TLS + any one of the following:
- *Renal dysfunction:* Serum creatinine >1.5 times ULN or increase in serum creatinine of 0.3 mg/dL or oliguria (urine output of <0.5 mL/kg/hour for 6 hours)
- *Cardiac:* Cardiac arrhythmias or sudden death
- *Neurological:* Seizures.

CASE (Continued)

As per the abovementioned definition, the child A does not fulfill the criteria for both laboratory as well as clinical TLS.

5. What is the risk of the child A to develop TLS?

The risk factors for developing TLS depend on:
- *Malignancy specific risk:* Tumor type and tumor burden, tumor infiltrating kidneys
- *Patient specific risk:* Age, preexisting renal dysfunction, and volume depleted state
- *Treatment specific risk:* Efficacy and potency to cytoreductive therapy and coadministration with nephrotoxic drugs.[3]

Based on these risk factors, the patients are classified into three risk groups as given in **Table 2**.[4,5]

TABLE 2: Risk stratification of tumor lysis syndrome.

Risk category	Malignancies
Low risk	- Solid tumors - Hodgkin's lymphoma - AML with TLC <25,000/mm^3 and LDH <2 × ULN - CML
Intermediate risk	- ALL with TLC <100,000/mm^3 and LDH <2 × ULN - AML with TLC <25,000/mm^3 and LDH >2 × ULN - AML with TLC 25,000/mm^3: 100,000/mm^3 - DLBCL and ALCL
High risk	- Burkitt's leukemia/lymphoma - ALL with TLC <100,000/mm^3 and LDH >2 × ULN - ALL with TLC ≥100,000/mm^3 - AML with TLC ≥100,000/mm^3

(ALCL: anaplastic large cell lymphoma; ALL: acute lymphoblastic leukemia; AML: acute myeloid leukemia; CML: chronic myeloid leukemia; DLBCL: diffuse large B-cell lymphoma; LDH: lactate dehydrogenase; ULN: upper limit of normal)

Since initial clinical features of TLS are nonspecific, it is necessary to identify the high-risk patients and initiate preventive measures in order to avoid development of clinical TLS.

CASE *(Continued)*

As per the abovementioned risk stratification criteria, the child A will belong to high-risk category for developing TLS.

6. What all preventive measures should be initiated for the child A?

Early and aggressive intervention decreases the morbidity and mortality associated with TLS. Identification of patient at-risk and prevention of TLS by adequate prophylaxis is the best management.

- *Continuous monitoring:* Close monitoring of urine output, serum electrolytes (sodium, potassium, calcium, and phosphorus), urea, creatinine, and uric acid every 6–8 hours during the initial 2–3 days of cytotoxic chemotherapy.
- *Hydration:* Hyperhydration is the cornerstone of both prevention and treatment of TLS. Hyperhydration improves the intravascular volume, renal blood flow, and glomerular filtration, which in turn promotes the excretion of uric acid, phosphate, and potassium.

  Hyperhydration usually refers to fluid rate of 3 L/m^2/day to achieve a target urine output of >3 mL/kg/hour or 100 mL/m^2/hour and urine specific gravity of <1.010. This could be either oral or intravenous (IV) hydration depending on the oral acceptance of the child.

  Choice of IV fluid, isotonic versus hypotonic, remains controversial. Conventionally, hypotonic fluids were used for hyperhydration. They were associated with increased incidence of hyponatremia, further complicated by the development of syndrome of inappropriate antidiuretic hormone secretion (SIADH) associated with vincristine. Recent studies demonstrated that using isotonic fluid for hyperhydration resulted in modest decrease in the incidence of hospital-acquired hyponatremia without causing increased incidence of hypernatremia or acute kidney injury (AKI). This needs further evaluation.[6,7]

Potassium and calcium should not be added to hydration fluid.

If the child has severe anemia (Hb <6 g/dL), hydration is started at lower rate while correcting the anemia with packed red cell transfusion.

- *Diuresis:* Use of diuretics may be necessary when the child develops fluid overload or when the urine output is suboptimal despite adequate hydration. Loop diuretics (furosemide @0.5 mg/kg/dose) or osmotic diuretic (mannitol @0.5 g/kg/dose) are more commonly utilized for this purpose. Diuretics are contraindicated when the child has obstructive uropathy or hypovolemia.
- *Alkalinization:* Urinary alkalinization is done with IV sodium bicarbonate. This helps in solubilizing uric acid. However, this approach needs caution especially while using along with hypouricosuric agents. Because, at a pH of >7.5, xanthine and hypoxanthine crystals are formed and at pH >8.0, $CaPO_4$ may crystallize in the kidneys, which can lead to worsening of nephropathy. The resultant alkaline pH causes binding of calcium with albumin leading to symptomatic hypocalcemia. Despite being a subject of controversy, alkalinization of urine can be utilized to prevent hyperuricemia provided strict monitoring of urine pH is done to maintain pH <7.5.[8]
- *Uric acid lowering agents:* Hyperuricemia is the most important predictor of adverse renal events. Therefore, uric acid lowering agents became an integral part of preventive as therapeutic strategies in the management of TLS **(Table 3)**.
  - *Allopurinol:* Allopurinol is a competitive inhibitor of xanthine oxidase which blocks further conversion of xanthine and hypoxanthine to uric acid. Multiple studies have shown that use of allopurinol has reduced the incidence of obstructive uropathy caused by uric acid crystallization. Studies have shown that allopurinol effectively prevented an increase in serum uric acid in 92% of children when used prophylactically.[9]
  - *Febuxostat:* Febuxostat is a novel non purine xanthine oxidase inhibitor which does not require any dose adjustment in renal failure and is associated with low risk of hypersensitivity reactions. FLORENCE trial compared efficacy of febuxostat with that

TABLE 3: Uric acid lowering agents.

Drug	Dose	MOA	Side effects and limitations
Allopurinol	300 mg/m²/day	Competitive inhibition of xanthine oxidase → reduced conversion of xanthine and hypoxanthine to uric acid	• Hypersensitivity reaction—skin rash • GI intolerance • Needs 50% dose reduction in renal dysfunction • No effect on already formed uric acid → may take several days to decrease the uric acid level • Precipitation of xanthine and hypoxanthine crystals • Interactions with other drugs—6-MP, azathioprine

Contd...

Contd...

Drug	Dose	MOA	Side effects and limitations
Febuxostat	10 mg/day	Inhibition of xanthine oxidase → reduced conversion of xanthine and hypoxanthine to uric acid	• Lesser risk of hypersensitivity reaction • Does not need dose reduction in renal failure • No effect on already formed uric acid → may take several days to decrease the uric acid level • Precipitation of xanthine and hypoxanthine crystals • Interactions with other drugs—6-MP, azathioprine • Costlier compared with allopurinol
Rasburicase	• 0.05–0.2 mg/kg (or) • 1.5 mg single dose	Conversion of uric acid into more soluble allantoin, which is readily excreted	• Hypersensitivity reaction—skin rash • Hemolysis in patients with G6PD deficiency—contraindicated • Costlier

(G6PD: glucose-6-phosphate dehydrogenase; MOA: mechanism of action; MP: mercaptopurine)

of allopurinol among 346 adults with intermediate and high risk of TLS. Febuxostat achieved significantly lower mean serum uric acid in comparison to allopurinol, with no difference in clinical TLS and renal failure rates.[10] However, there is little evidence on the role of febuxostat in the management of TLS among children.

- *Rasburicase:* Rasburicase is recombinant urate oxidase cloned from *Aspergillus flavus* which converts uric acid into more soluble allantoin, which is readily excreted. Rasburicase rapidly decreases the serum uric acid levels compared to allopurinol (4 hours vs. 1–2 days). After its efficacy been proved in adults who received rasburicase in compassionate use study, its role in pediatric patients was explored in many studies. Recently published meta-analysis of seven studies suggests that urate oxidase is effective in reducing the serum uric acid levels with little effect on clinical TLS, renal failure, and mortality.[11] Single fixed dose of 1.5 mg or 0.15 mg/kg showed high response rate with rapid lowering of serum uric acid compared to the Food and Drug Administration (FDA) approved regimen (0.2 mg/kg × 5–7 days) with significant reduction in cost of treatment of pediatric TLS.[12] Pharmacoeconomic studies conducted by Candrilli et al. and Anneman et al. suggest that prophylactic rasburicase in initial management of high-risk patients may be a cost-effective approach than management of AKI with renal replacement therapy (RRT).[9]

Risk-based preventive measures of TLS have been given in **Table 4**.[9]

TABLE 4: Risk-based tumor lysis syndrome prophylaxis.

Low risk	Intermediate risk	High risk
Monitoring	• Monitoring • Hydration ± Diuretics • Uric acid lowering agent: Allopurinol • (Rasburicase—only if uric acid is elevated)	• Monitoring • Hydration ± Diuretics • Uric acid lowering agent: Allopurinol • Rasburicase

CASE (Continued)

As per the abovementioned risk-based prophylactic strategy, child A (who has high risk for developing TLS) was carefully monitored for the biochemical abnormalities and was started on IV hydration in view of inadequate oral acceptance along with allopurinol and rasburicase.

His bone marrow was hypercellular with near complete replacement with blasts. Flow cytometry was suggestive of B-cell acute lymphoblastic leukemia (ALL). Following which, he was started on prephase steroids.

On D3 of induction, his biochemical parameters are as follows:
- *Serum electrolytes:* K—6.2 mEq/dL, PO_4—7.2 mg/dL, Ca—6.1 mg/dL, and uric acid—9.5 mg/dL
- *RFT:* Urea—32 mg/dL and serum creatinine—0.5 mg/dL.

7. How will you manage child A, who has now developed laboratory TLS?

The child A fulfilled the criteria for laboratory TLS on D3 of induction. This child requires stringent monitoring preferably in a pediatric intensive care unit/high-dependency unit (PICU/HDU) setting along with multidisciplinary care involving pediatric oncologist, nephrologist, and intensivist.

Vigorous monitoring of urine output, serum electrolytes (sodium, potassium, calcium, and phosphorus), urea, creatinine, and uric acid along with continuous electrocardiogram (ECG) monitoring should be done.

Hyperhydration with or without diuretics to achieve a target urine output of >3 mL/kg/hour or 100 mL/m^2/hour along with allopurinol and rasburicase are the initial step in the management of TLS.

Management of electrolyte abnormalities has been given in **Table 5**.

TABLE 5: Management of dyselectrolytemia associated with tumor lysis syndrome.

Electrolyte abnormality	Management
Hyperkalemia	- *In case of ECG changes:* IV calcium gluconate 1 mEq/kg (maximum dose: 10 mEq) slow IV over 20 minutes under ECG monitoring - Salbutamol nebulization (2.5 mg/dose over 20 minutes) - IV insulin (0.1 U/kg) + 25% dextrose (2 mL/kg) over 20 minutes - IV sodium bicarbonate 1–2 mEq/kg (maximum dose: 10 mEq) slow IV over 20 minutes - Sodium polystyrene sulfonate (1 g/kg/dose) with 50% sorbitol/lactulose Q4–6H

Hyperphosphatemia	- Hydration
	- Oral phosphate binders:
	  – Aluminum hydroxide (50–150 mg/kg/day)
	  – Sevelamer (20–40 mg/kg/dose Q8H)

Hypocalcemia	- *Asymptomatic:* Not treated - *Symptomatic:* IV calcium gluconate 1 mEq/kg (maximum dose: 10 mEq) slow IV over 20 minutes under ECG monitoring

(ECG: electrocardiogram; IV: intravenous)

CASE (Continued)

The child A was shifted to HDU where he was carefully monitored for the biochemical abnormalities, ECG abnormalities, and urine output. He did not have any ECG changes of hyperkalemia or hypocalcemia. He also had urine output of 2.2 mL/kg/hour during the first 6 hours after shifting to HDU. He was continued on IV hydration along with allopurinol and a second dose of rasburicase. He received salbutamol nebulization, insulin + dextrose along with sodium polystyrene sulfonate for his hyperkalemia and oral sevelamer for his hyperphosphatemia. He did not receive calcium correction, as he had only asymptomatic hypocalcemia.

After 6 hours of HDU stay, his clinical condition worsened with fluid overload and urine output of 0.6 mL/kg/hour with repeat biochemical parameters as follows:
- *Serum electrolytes:* K—5.2 mEq/dL, PO_4—7.9 mg/dL, Ca—5.8 mg/dL, and uric acid—3.2 mg/dL
- *RFT:* Urea—96 mg/dL and serum creatinine—1.1 mg/dL
- *Arterial blood gas (ABG):* pH—7.121 and HCO_3—14.

8. How will you manage child A, who has now developed clinical TLS?

The child A fulfilled the criteria for clinical TLS with refractory electrolyte abnormalities not responding to adequate medical management. So, the child would be requiring RRT for further stabilization.

Renal replacement therapy: With the introduction of rasburicase, the requirement of RRT has decreased to around 1.5% of pediatric patients with TLS. Pediatric nephrology team should be involved early for timely initiation of RRT.

Indications of RRT: Indications of RRT are similar to those of AKI due to other causes but with lower threshold due to ongoing rapid tumor cell lysis.
- Refractory hyperkalemia, hyperphosphatemia—not responding to medical management
- Severe metabolic acidosis
- Volume overload—not responding to medical management
- Overt uremic symptoms.[13]

Choice of RRT technique depends on the laboratory parameters, tumor cell proliferative rate, and clinical condition of the patient such as volume status and hemodynamic stability.

Peritoneal dialysis is not recommended in patients with TLS, unless other modalities are not available. Although intermittent hemodialysis (IHD) may be effective for children with refractory hyperkalemia and hyperphosphatemia, it is associated with rebound hyperkalemia and hyperphosphatemia in children with rapid turnover of malignant cells. Moreover, IHD may not be feasible in critically ill children with hemodynamic instability. Continuous renal replacement technique [continuous venovenous hemofiltration (CVVH), continuous arteriovenous hemofiltration (CAVH), sustained low efficiency daily diafiltration (SLEDD), etc.] results in effective management of metabolic abnormalities without any increased risk of hemodynamic instability or rebound hyperkalemia and hyperphosphatemia.[14]

CASE (Continued)

The child A underwent two courses of IHD along with other supportive measures. His prephase steroids was withheld temporarily. His biochemical parameters gradually improved with adequate urine output and his induction chemotherapy was restarted.

9. What is the prognostic significance of TLS?

The development of clinical TLS especially those with AKI are associated with increased risk of mortality compared to those who had only laboratory TLS. The renal function is usually recovered fully after TLS-related AKI. But, the long-term effect of TLS and AKI on renal function is not known.[14]

CASE VIGNETTE 2

Hyperleukocytosis

B, a 3-year-old boy, symptomatic for the past 2 weeks with subacute febrile illness with pallor and bleeding manifestations, which required multiple blood component support and bone pain. He developed headache, blurring of vision, and vomiting for the past 1 day and his parents also noticed that he is lethargic for the past 6 hours. He was brought to emergency in postictal state following one episode of self-abortive generalized tonic-clonic seizure which lasted for around 2 minutes.
- *O/E:* Vitals—PR: 67/min, RR: 16/min with shallow respiratory efforts, BP: 122/88 mm Hg, temperature: 100.2°F, CFT: 3 seconds, and SpO_2: 92% with room air
- *GPE:* Pallor and petechial spots and generalized lymphadenopathy and bony tenderness.
- *P/A:* Hepatosplenomegaly. B/L testis—WNL
- *Central nervous system (CNS):* Glasgow coma scale (GCS)—E2M4V3, B/L pupils—equally reactive to light (ERTL), and no focal deficits.

Presumptive Diagnosis: Acute Leukemia

10. What could be the possible causes for the recent onset neurological worsening in child B?

- Intracranial hemorrhage
- CNS leukemic deposits
- CNS leukostasis
- Acute CNS infection.

CASE *(Continued)*

The child B was stabilized with intubation and mechanical ventilation along with other anti-raised intracranial tension (ICT) measures. He was started on antiepileptics and osmotherapy with hypertonic saline. His hemodynamic status was stable.

The resident in ER sent the emergency laboratories for the child B—whose reports as follows:
- *CBC:* Hb—7.2 g/dL, TLC—268,000/mm³ with 88% blasts (lymphoblasts), platelets—12,000/mm³
- Prothrombin time/international normalized ratio (PT/INR)—29 seconds/2.1 and activated partial thromboplastin time (aPTT)—42 seconds
- *Serum electrolytes:* Na—134 mEq/dL, K—6.2 mEq/dL, PO_4—7.2 mg/dL, Ca—6.1 mg/dL, and uric acid—9.5 mg/dL
- *RFT:* Urea—32 mg/dL and serum creatinine—0.5 mg/dL
- *ABG:* pH—7.321, HCO_3—14, pCO_2—37, and pO_2—105.

The child B who presented to emergency with neurological dysfunction was identified to have acute leukemia with hyperleukocytosis.

11. What is hyperleukocytosis?

Hyperleukocytosis is defined as peripheral blood (PB) leukocyte count exceeding an arbitrary threshold of 100,000/mm^3. The life-threatening consequences of hyperleukocytosis are due to the complications that arise out of high white blood cell (WBC) count and not the high count itself. Even WBC counts below this cut off can also lead to hyperleukocytosis-related complications especially among children with acute myeloid leukemia (AML) (due to large size and increased adhesiveness of myeloblasts).

Pathophysiology

Pathophysiology of hyperleukocytosis has been given in **Flowchart 2**.

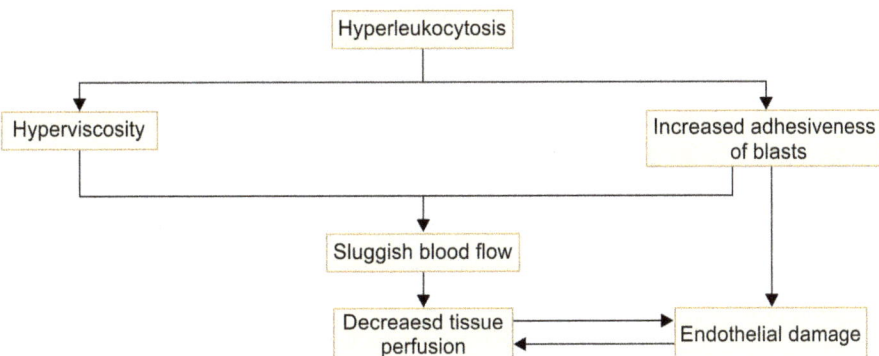

Flowchart 2: Pathophysiology of hyperleukocytosis.

12. What are the clinical features of hyperleukocytosis?

The major complications of hyperleukocytosis that lead to clinical manifestations of hyperleukocytosis include **(Table 6)**:[15]

TABLE 6: Clinical features of hyperleukocytosis.

Leukostasis	CNS	Confusion, lethargy, irritability, altered sensorium, seizures, focal neurological deficits, and raised ICT
	Pulmonary	Dyspnea, hypoxia, pulmonary hemorrhage, and respiratory failure
	Eyes	Retinal hemorrhage
	Vascular system	Priapism, dactylitis, and limb ischemia
DIC		Skin and mucosal hemorrhage (CNS, lung, GI, etc.)
TLS		Hyperkalemia, hypocalcemia, hyperphosphatemia, hyperuricemia, renal dysfunction, cardiac arrhythmias, and seizures

(CNS: central nervous system; DIC: disseminated intravascular coagulation; GI: gastrointestinal; ICT: intracranial tension; TLS: tumor lysis syndrome)

- *Leukostasis:*
  - Due to hyperviscosity caused by increased WBC count
  - Decreased deformability of blasts leading to increased adhesion to vascular endothelium
  - Cytokine-mediated endothelial damage
- *Disseminated intravascular coagulation (DIC):*
  - Increased release of tissue factor
  - Endothelial damage
  - Inhibition of fibrinolyis
- *Tumor lysis syndrome:* High tumor burden → rapid turnover of leukemic blasts.

The clinical manifestations of leukostasis are difficult to differentiate from infectious and hemorrhagic complications of acute leukemia. Therefore, the clinical diagnosis of leukostasis is made empirically when children with acute leukemia with hyperleukocytosis present with pulmonary or neurological symptoms.

CASE (Continued)

The child B who presented to emergency with neurological dysfunction was identified to have hyperleukocytosis with probable CNS leukostasis, DIC (with possible intracranial hemorrhage), and laboratory TLS.

13. What are the malignancies associated with increased risk of hyperleukocytosis?

Around 5–20% of pediatric leukemias present with hyperleukocytosis. The common etiologies associated with hyperleukocytosis and the risk factors are given in **Table 7**.

TABLE 7: Risk factors for hyperleukocytosis.

Malignancy	Incidence	Risk factor
AML	10–25%	• Age <1 year • AML—M3 (microgranular variant) • AML—M4 and M5 • KMT2A rearrangements • inv 16 • FLT3-ITD
ALL	8–13%	• Infant ALL • T-ALL • KMT2A rearrangements • Ph + ALL/Ph-like ALL • TCF3-PBX1—t(1;19) • Hypodiploid ALL
CML		• Blast crisis • Accelerated phase

(ALL: acute lymphoblastic leukemia; AML: acute myeloid leukemia; CML: chronic myeloid leukemia; FLT3-ITD: FMS-like tyrosine kinase-internal tandem duplication; KMT2A: histone-lysine N-methyltransferase 2A; TCF3-PBX1: transcription factor 3-PBX homeobox 1 fusion)

14. Can we predict the severity of hyperleukocytosis associated leukostasis based on WBC count or peripheral blast count?

Novotny et al. predicted the clinical probability of leukostasis based on severity of clinical signs and symptoms (overall severity of symptoms, pulmonary, and neurological symptoms) using graded scoring system. They documented that among patients with AML M1/M2 and chronic myeloid leukemia (CML) who scored as highly probable leukostasis had higher WBC counts and higher PB blast count compared to those with lower probability scores. However, no such association was noted among those with AML M4/M5.[16] On the other hand, Piccirillo et al. demonstrated that there was no correlation between Novotny score and WBC count and PB blast count but for immunophenotype (AML—M4/M5 >AML non-M4/M5 >ALL).[17]

This shows that nature of blasts predicts the severity of leukostasis rather than the absolute number of blasts, as reflected by monocytic leukemia which are known to cause severe symptoms even at lower counts due to increased adhesiveness and tissue invasion of monoblasts.

15. How will you further evaluate child B after stabilization with initial resuscitation measures?

Hyperleukocytosis is an oncological emergency because of increased risk of early mortality which warrants an immediate intervention. All children who present with hyperleukocytosis should be evaluated for associated complications including TLS profile, coagulation profile, fundus examination (to look for papilledema, retinal hemorrhage, and leukostasis), chest X-ray (CXR) (to look for pulmonary infiltrates, any evidence of infection, mediastinal mass, pleural/pericardial effusion), and CT chest/brain (as per requirement).

Timely initiation of definitive therapy is as important as cytoreduction for the abatement of the complications of hyperleukocytosis. So, accurate characterization of blasts is also an important parallel priority. Careful examination of peripheral smear with immunocytochemistry, if required, can give a clue to probable lineage. Immunophenotyping from PB almost always provides the final diagnosis promptly without any need for bone marrow examination.[18]

CASE (Continued)

The child B was further evaluated as follows:
- PB flow cytometry: s/o B-ALL
- Fundus: Showed papilledema with retinal leukemic deposits
- CXR: No e/o mediastinal mass or pulmonary infiltrates
- Computed tomography (CT) brain—showed multiple focal supratentorial hemorrhages.

16. How will you further manage child B?

Initial management includes hyperhydration, prevention/management of TLS, and blood component therapy. Definitive management includes reduction of tumor load with the help of pharmacological agents or mechanical methods.

- *Hydration:* Hyperhydration is the initial step in the management of hyperleukocytosis. Hyperhydration usually refers to fluid rate of 3 L/m²/day to achieve a target urine output of >3 mL/kg/hour or 100 mL/m²/hour and urine specific gravity of <1.010. Potassium and calcium should not be added to hydration fluid. The role of urinary alkalinization is controversial. If the child has severe anemia (Hb <6 g/dL), hydration is started at lower rate. Unless there is coexisting TLS and fluid overload, diuretics should be avoided, as it can lead to hemoconcentration and worsening of hyperviscosity related symptoms.
- *Prevention/treatment of TLS:* Close monitoring of urine output, serum electrolytes (sodium, potassium, calcium, and phosphorus), urea, creatinine, and uric acid every 6–8 hours
    - Uric acid lowering agent:
        - Allopurinol
        - Rasburicase (prophylactic—as risk for TLS is high; therapeutic—after documentation of laboratory TLS)
    - Correction of metabolic abnormalities
    - Early initiation of RRT, if required.
- *Blood component therapy:* Platelet concentrates should be transfused in children with hyperleukocytosis with platelet count threshold of <50,000/mm³ among those with DIC and active/life-threatening hemorrhage and <20,000/mm³ among those without any evidence of DIC or active/life-threatening hemorrhage.[15]

    Coagulopathy should be corrected with fresh frozen plasma (FFP) or cryoprecipitate transfusion with target fibrinogen level of >100–150 mg/dL.

    Packed red cell transfusion should be avoided, because hyperleukocytosis is usually compensated by decrease in erythrocrit, which may be increased by packed red blood cell (PRBC) transfusion and worsening of hyperviscosity related complications.
- *Cytoreduction:* Definitive management includes cytoreduction which could be either nonspecific or specific for the underlying etiology. Cytoreduction could be achieved using:
    - Pharmacological agents
    - Mechanical cytoreduction
        - *Pharmacological cytoreduction:* Reduction of leukemic blast count by using pharmacological agents. It could be either nonspecific or specific as follows:
            - *Nonspecific cytoreduction:* Nonspecific cytoreduction could be instituted even before accurate diagnosis of the underlying malignancy **(Table 8)**.

TABLE 8: Nonspecific cytoreduction.

Drug	Dose	Mechanism of action	Remarks

Hydroxyurea[15,19]	50–75 mg/kg/day in 2–3 divided doses	Inhibition of ribonucleoside diphosphate reductase → inhibition of DNA synthesis → cytoreduction	• It reduces TLC by 50–80% by 24–48 hours without any worsening of TLS.
			• It can be used as bridging therapy in patients:
			  – With a not yet diagnosed hematological malignancy
			  – With contraindications to induction chemotherapy
			• Role is well established in:
			  – Adults >children
			  – CML, AML >ALL

Contd...

Contd...

Drug	Dose	Mechanism of action	Remarks
Steroids[19,20] • Specific—ALL • Nonspecific—irrespective of underlying malignancy	Dexamethasone—10 mg/m²/day	Dexamethasone inhibits upregulation of adhesion molecules in leukemic and endothelial cells (selectins, VCAM-1, IL-8 receptors, CD-18).	• Observational study by Azoulay et al. demonstrated beneficial effect of dexamethasone among patients with AML-M5 with hyperleukocytosis and pulmonary dysfunction[21] • Needs more evidence

(AML: acute myeloid leukemia; CML: chronic myeloid leukemia; DNA: deoxyribonucleic acid; IL-8: interleukin 8; TLS: tumor lysis syndrome; VCAM-1: vascular cell adhesion molecule 1)

TABLE 9: Comparison between standard dose and low dose cytoreduction.

Standard dose	Low dose
• Induces a rapid and sustained remission[22,23] • Increased risk of TLS	• Gradual cytoreduction to a safer level → standard dose can be started without any risk of TLS • No effect on early mortality[24]

(TLS: tumor lysis syndrome)

- *Specific cytoreduction:* Specific cytoreduction could only be initiated after establishing accurate diagnosis. It could be either standard dose or low dose **(Table 9)**.

CASE *(Continued)*

The child B who presented to emergency with hyperleukocytosis with probable CNS leukostasis, DIC (with possible intracranial hemorrhage), and laboratory TLS was diagnosed to have B-ALL. After his initial stabilization, he was started on hyperhydration with allopurinol and rasburicase. He received multiple random donor platelets (RDPs) and FFP transfusion to correct his coagulopathy. As he was hemodynamically stable, PRBC transfusion was not given. He was promptly started on hydroxyurea and dexamethasone as soon as PS—was suggestive of possible ALL.

17. How will you monitor the child B, following the stabilization and initial management of hyperleukocytosis?

Continuous monitoring of clinical and laboratory parameters is of prime importance while managing a child with hyperleukocytosis. Vigilant monitoring of vital signs, neurological, pulmonary, and hemodynamic status is mandatory. Close monitoring of urine output, CBC, coagulation profile, serum electrolytes (sodium, potassium, calcium, and phosphorus), urea, creatinine, and uric acid every 6–8 hours should be done.

CASE *(Continued)*

After the initiation of dexamethasone, he developed with clinical TLS with renal dysfunction, which was managed with RRT. Even after 12 hours of specific cytoreduction with dexamethasone, the child A had no improvement of sensorium with repeat CBC as follows:
CBC: Hb—6.0 g/dL, TLC—233,000/mm³ with 76% blasts (lymphoblasts), platelets—57,000/mm³.

18. How will you manage the child B, who has now developed severe anemia also?

The child B with hyperleukocytosis with probable CNS leukostasis, DIC (with possible intracranial hemorrhage), and clinical TLS who persisted to have neurological dysfunction despite receiving 12 hours of specific cytoreduction with pharmacological agents (dexamethasone and hydroxyurea). The child has now developed severe anemia which would further preclude hyperhydration, as it can precipitate congestive cardiac failure.

The child B is now a candidate for mechanical cytoreduction (leukapheresis or exchange transfusion), that can help to alleviate hyperleukocytosis related hyperviscosity symptoms without increasing the risk of fluid overload.

Mechanical cytoreduction: It is a form of nonspecific cytoreduction, which is useful when marked reduction of leukocyte count, (preferentially to <100,000/mm^3) or 50% reduction in blast count needs to be achieved over short duration.[25]

- Indications:
  - Symptomatic hyperleukocytosis irrespective TLC
  - Asymptomatic hyperleukocytosis
    - TLC >100,000/mm^3—AML
    - TLC >400,000/mm^3—ALL, CML[26]
- Contraindications:[25]
  - AML-M3—increased risk of ICH/worsening DIC
  - Cardiovascular comorbidities
  - Hemodynamic instability
  - Coagulation disorders.

Types of mechanical cytoreduction **(Tables 10)**:[18,19]
- Leukapheresis:
  - *Equipment:* Continuous-flow blood cell separator
  - *Vascular access:* Central venous catheter unless bilateral cubital or cephalic veins are appropriate for peripheral large bore cannulation
  - *Anticoagulant:* Acid citrate dextrose at a ratio of 1:12
  - *RBC sedimentation agent:* 6% hydroxyethyl starch (HES)
  - Single session of leukapheresis—reduces the peripheral WBC count by 20–50% → equivalent to an 85% decrease of the circulating WBC mass
  - Recruits WBC/blasts from extravascular sites to blood stream—to be removed by another session of leukapheresis/induction chemotherapy/cytoreductive agent
  - *Complications:* Venous access related bleeding, infection, thrombosis, pneumothorax, hypocalcemia, loss of other blood products (platelets, red blood cells), nausea, vomiting, fainting or dizziness, seizures, skin rash, hives, and flushing
- Exchange transfusion:
  - *Technique:* Manual aspiration of child's blood followed by manual transfusion of reconstituted PRBC + FFP back to the child
  - *Vascular access:* Arterial line (for aspiration) + Venous line (for transfusion)
  - *Exchange volume:* 2 × blood volume

TABLE 10: Advantages and disadvantages of leukapheresis and exchange transfusion.

	Leukapheresis	Exchange transfusion
Advantages	• Rapid physical removal of circulating blasts • Multiple procedures may recruit marginated blasts into the intravascular space • Lower or no need for transfusion of erythrocytes, platelets and plasma • Little influence on coagulation • Can be performed in all children	• Rapid physical removal of circulating blasts • Multiple procedures may recruit marginated blasts into the intravascular space • No special equipment necessary
Disadvantages	• Special equipment and trained staff necessary • Labor and cost intensive • Quick rebound of blasts cells • Need for vascular access	• Cannot be performed in children (>15–20 kg) • Need for vascular access • Quick rebound of blasts cells possible • Need for massive transfusion of erythrocytes and plasma, platelets transfusion • Severe coagulation disturbance

TABLE 11: Evidence for and against leukapheresis.

	Author	Results
For	Giles et al., 2001	Leukapheresis was associated with reduced 2-week mortality rate ($p = 0.006$) and possibly with the increased CR rate ($p = 0.06$). However, there was no improvement in overall survival
	Maurer et al., 1988	Suggested an advantage for leukapheresis in pediatric ALL. They observed that a group of selected children with severe hyperuricemia and renal dysfunction may benefit from leukapheresis
	Bug et al., 2007	Leukapheresis significantly lowered the risk of early death, without any effect on long-term outcome
Against	McCarthy et al., 1997	Among, 48 unselected adult and pediatric patients with WBC >100 x 10^9/L who were leukoreduced, there was no statistical difference in early mortality rate compared with similar unselected patients who were not leukoreduced
	Porcu et al., 1997	Leukapheresis did not impact early mortality in adult patients, especially those presenting with symptoms of leukostasis
	Oberai et al., 2014	Early mortality related to hyperleukocytosis in AML is not influenced by the universal or selected use of leukapheresis

(ALL: acute lymphoblastic leukemia; AML: acute myeloid leukemia; CR: complete response; WBC: white blood cell)

- *PRBC: FFP ratio:* 2:1 to 3:1
- *Aliquot volume:* 10–50 mL depending upon the weight of the child

All the available retrospective studies have documented no effect of leukapheresis on long-term survival and conflicting results for the effect of leukapheresis on early mortality **(Table 11)**. Due to lack of randomized controlled trials (RCTs) comparing these modalities, optimal strategy to manage these patients remains controversial. The recent meta-analysis of 13 retrospective studies comprising 1,743 adult patients with AML and hyperleukocytosis reported no added benefit of leukapheresis in reducing early mortality.[27] Lack of convincing evidence along with logistic and technical difficulties demerit the routine use of mechanical cytoreduction for children with hyperleukocytosis.

CASE (Continued)

The child B underwent one session of leukapheresis following which his TLC fell to 142,000/mm³. He continued to receive other cytoreductive measures. His TLC further dropped to 78,000/mm³ along with gradual improvement in neurological status. He was gradually weaned off from mechanical ventilation and subsequently extubated. He continued to receive the induction chemotherapy as per unit protocol.

19. What is the prognostic significance of hyperleukocytosis?

Hyperleukocytosis is associated with significant early mortality and morbidity due to the accompanying neurological, pulmonary, and metabolic complications. The long-term outcome of children who present with hyperleukocytosis also remain inferior.[18] Whether hyperleukocytosis itself or the underlying disease biology is responsible for the inferior prognosis is still not known.

CASE VIGNETTE 3

Superior Mediastinal Syndrome

C, a 13-year-old boy, symptomatic for the past 2 weeks with subacute febrile illness without any pallor and bleeding manifestations. His parents also noticed that he had developed recent onset facial puffiness with respiratory distress with noisy breathing while lying down over the past 24 hours. He presented to emergency with the following complaints:
- *Vitals:* HR—122/min, RR—44/min with suprasternal and subcostal retractions and stridor, BP—102/68 mm Hg, temperature—100.2°F, CFT—3 seconds, and SpO_2—91% with room air
- *O/E:* GPE—no pallor and petechial spots, generalized lymphadenopathy, and no bony tenderness. Facial puffiness, conjunctival congestion, and neck engorgement
- *Respiratory system (RS):* Trachea—shifted to left side, right-sided chest fullness, dull note over right hemithorax, and air entry decreased on right side
- *P/A:* Hepatosplenomegaly. B/L testis—WNL.
- *Cardiovascular system (CVS):* S1, S2—normal, not muffled, no murmur
- CNS—no focal deficits.

Presumptive Diagnosis: Lymphoma

The child C was stabilized with head-end elevation and oxygen supplementation. IV cannula was placed in lower limb in view of suspected SMS/SVCS and he was started on hyperhydration and allopurinol. His hemodynamic status was stable.

The resident in ER sent the emergency laboratories for the child C—whose reports are as follows:
- *CBC:* Hb–9.2 g/dL, TLC—8,000/mm³ with no atypical cells, platelets—222,000/mm³
- *Serum electrolytes:* K—4.2 mEq/dL, PO_4—4.2 mg/dL, Ca—9.1 mg/dL, and uric acid—3.5 mg/dL

- *RFT:* Urea—32 mg/dL and serum creatinine—0.5 mg/dL
- *LDH:* 750 U/L
- *CXR:* As shown in **Figure 1**.

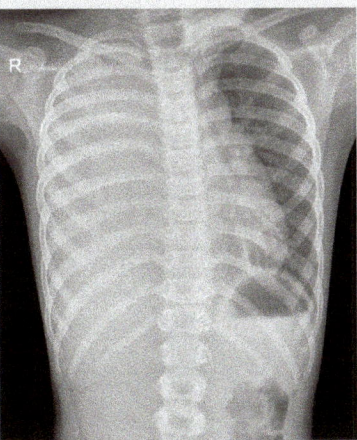

Fig. 1: Chest X-ray of child C.

The child C who presented to emergency with respiratory dysfunction was identified to have mediastinal mass.

20. What are the differential diagnoses for mediastinal mass in children?

The mediastinum is that region of the thorax that lies between the two pleural cavities bounded:
- Superiorly—by thoracic inlet
- Inferiorly—by diaphragm
- Anteriorly—by sternum
- Posteriorly—by vertebral bodies and paravertebral muscles.

The mediastinum is divided as:
- Superior mediastinum
- Inferior mediastinum:
  - Anterior
  - Middle
  - Posterior

The differential diagnosis for mediastinal mass in children is given in **Table 12**.[28]

TABLE 12: Differential diagnosis of mediastinal mass in children.

Mediastinal compartment	Malignant causes	Nonmalignant causes
Anterior and superior mediastinum	• Lymphoma/leukemia • Germ cell tumor • Thyroid tumors • Thymoma	• Thymic cyst, thymic hyperplasia • Retrosternal goiter • Parathyroid adenoma • Lipoma, lymphangioma, hemangioma, aortic aneurysm, infectious lymphadenopathy (TB, fungal)

Contd...

Contd...

Mediastinal compartment	Malignant causes	Nonmalignant causes
Middle mediastinum	Lymphoma	• Pericardial cyst, foregut duplication cysts • Lipoma, lymphangioma, hemangioma, aortic aneurysm, infectious lymphadenopathy (TB, fungal)
Posterior mediastinum	Neurogenic tumors—neuroblastoma (including GN, GNB), paraganglioma, schwannoma, neurofibroma, meningioma, MPNST	Neuroenteric cyst, lipoma, lymphangioma, hemangioma, aortic aneurysm, infectious lymphadenopathy (TB, fungal)

(GN: ganglioneuromas; GNB: ganglioneuroblastoma; MPNST: malignant peripheral nerve sheath tumor; TB: tuberculosis)

21. What is superior mediastinal syndrome and SVCS?

The terms SMS and SVCS are sometimes used interchangeably, as they coexist together for most of the times in children.

Superior vena cava syndrome refers to the signs and symptoms arising out of compression, obstruction or thrombosis of superior vena cava. The term SMS is used when SVCS is associated with obstruction of tracheobronchial tree.

22. What are the clinical features which suggest the diagnosis of SMS/SVCS?

As mediastinum is a closed space, any rapidly growing mass can lead to compression of the anatomical structures contained in it **(Table 13)**.[29]

TABLE 13: Clinical features of SMS/SVC syndrome.

Structure compressed	Signs and symptoms
Tracheobronchial tree	Cough, dyspnea, orthopnea, stridor, wheezing, suprasternal/subcostal retractions
Esophagus	Dysphagia
Recurrent laryngeal nerve	Hoarseness of voice
Superior vena cava	Edema of head, neck and upper limb, plethora, cyanosis, conjunctival congestion, neck engorgement, and dilated veins over neck and chest

(SMS: superior mediastinal syndrome; SVC: superior vena cava syndrome)

The children with mediastinal mass and SMS/SVCS may also develop other complications as follows:
- *CNS symptoms:* Headache, confusion, lethargy, irritability, blurring of vision, syncope etc.—due to carbon dioxide retention and central venous stasis
- Pleural and pericardial effusion—due to impaired lymphatic drainage, obstruction of thoracic duct, and direct involvement by the underlying malignancy.
- Other oncological emergencies like TLS, hyperleukocytosis, compressive myelopathy, etc.

23. What are the possible etiologies that can present with SMS/SVCS in children?

Not all patients with mediastinal masses as listed above presents with features of SMS/SVCS. The severity of symptoms depends on:
- Degree of airway and vascular obstruction
- Rapidity with which the obstruction developed

Compared to adults, children are prone to develop severe symptoms as their airways are of smaller caliber and also more compressible.[29]

The most common causes for SMS/SVCS in children include:
- Compression by malignant mediastinal mass, viz., leukemia/lymphoma, germ cell tumor (GCT), neuroblastoma, sarcoma [Ewings sarcoma (EWS), rhabdomyosarcoma (RMS)]
- Venous thrombosis caused by central venous catheter or cardiac surgery

CASE (Continued)

The child C who presented to emergency with respiratory dysfunction due to SMS was identified to have generalized lymphadenopathy and hepatosplenomegaly without any features of cytopenias. Such presentation in an adolescent boy is commonly seen with non-Hodgkin's lymphoma—probably T-lymphoblastic lymphoma.

24. What are the precautions needed while subjecting the child C to further diagnostic evaluation?

The children with SVCS/SMS are at an increased risk of cardiorespiratory compromise following the administration of anesthetics, anxiolytics, or sedatives. These drugs cause:
- Decreased respiratory drive
- Relaxation of tracheobronchial smooth muscles leading to airway collapse
- Reduced lung volumes
- Negative inotropic effect and peripheral vasodilation leading to decreased venous return

All of these factors may precipitate cardiorespiratory collapse which may require resuscitation with intubation and mechanical ventilation. Tracheal intubation may be difficult and once intubated, these children may require prolonged ventilation till resolution of mediastinal mass. Mechanical ventilation may not be effective when the airway obstruction is distal to trachea. Therefore, the diagnostic evaluation of the child with SMS/SVCS should be performed with least invasive procedure possible.[29,30]

25. Can we predict adverse cardiorespiratory event in a child with SMS/SVCS?

The challenging aspect in the management of a child with SMS/SVCS is that definitive diagnosis is often precluded by high anesthetic risk associated with the mediastinal mass. There are no standard risk criteria to predict the risk and complications of anesthesia in children with SMS/SVCS. Studies have identified certain clinical factors that can predict the anesthetic risk in children with SMS/SVCS as follows:[30]
- *Clinical:* There is a poor correlation between clinical signs and symptoms and subsequent anesthetic complications. Still, stridor, wheezing, and orthopnea are some of the ominous signs that can predict the anesthetic complications.

- *Mediastinal mass ratio:* The children with mediastinal mass occupying >45% of transthoracic diameter were found to be associated with increased risk of respiratory collapse compared to those with mass occupying <30% of transthoracic diameter (33.3 vs. 2.1%)
- *Tracheal cross section area:* Tracheal cross-sectional area calculated using CT scanner <50% of normal predicted value for the age and gender is associated with significantly increased risk of anesthetic complications.
- *Peak expiratory flow rate:* Peak expiratory flow rate (PEFR) of <50% of expected is associated with poor anesthetic risk.

Shamberger et al. developed a risk model by combining tracheal cross-sectional area and PEFR, that can predict the anesthetic risk for children with mediastinal mass as given in **Table 14**.[30]

TABLE 14: Anesthetic risk of children with mediastinal mass.

Tracheal cross-sectional area (% of predicted)	PEFR (% of predicted)	Anesthetic risk
>50%	>50%	Low risk
<50%	>50%	Moderate risk
>50%	<50%	Moderate risk
<50%	<50%	High risk

(PEFR: peak expiratory flow rate)

CASE *(Continued)*

Child C, in view of significant respiratory distress with stridor, the child A could not be shifted for CT scan, which could provide the diagnostic clue as well as predict the anesthetic risk. He underwent bedside ultrasound and echocardiography whose reports as follows:
- *Ultrasonography (USG) chest:* Right-sided mass lesion with moderate to massive pleural effusion. No calcification. Doppler: No evidence of thrombosis
- *Echo:* No e/o pericardial effusion.

26. How will you further evaluate the child C, with unstable respiratory status due to SMS/SVCS?

The child C with SMS probably due non-Hodgkin's lymphoma requires further investigations for confirmation. But he is having significant airway compromise, which suggests that he is at high risk for adverse cardiorespiratory event. We should try to confirm the diagnosis using a least invasive procedure rather than resorting to tissue biopsy **(Flowchart 3)**.

The following ancillary investigations play a vital role in establishing the diagnosis and prompt initiation of definitive therapy in a child with SMS/SVCS:[29]
- *Complete blood count with peripheral smear and flow cytometry:* To look for any blasts, which will confirm the diagnosis of acute leukemia, thereby obviating the need for any other invasive investigations. In addition, presence of cytopenia would indicate possible bone marrow involvement, which would provide an opportunity for diagnosis with bone marrow examination itself, while avoiding more risk involved with tissue biopsy.

Flowchart 3: Approach to a child with SMS/SVC syndrome.

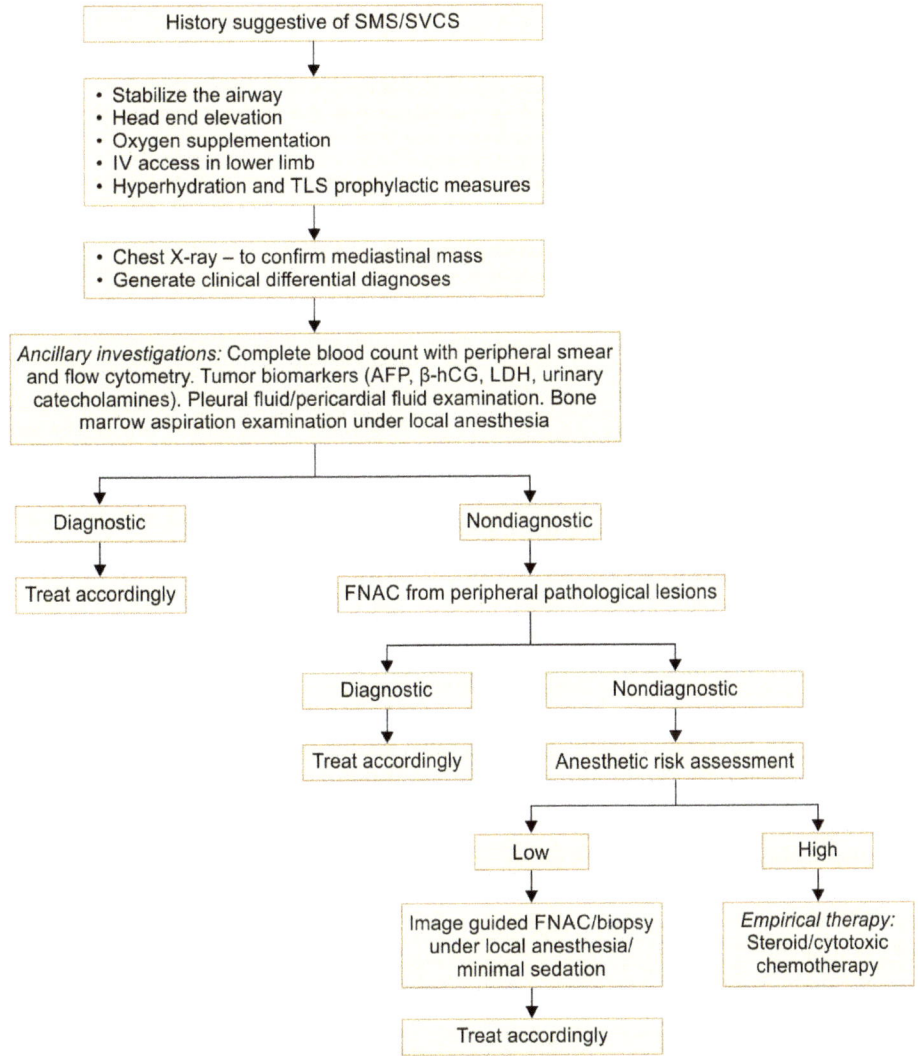

(AFP: α-fetoprotein; β-hCG: β-human chorionic gonadotropin; FNAC: fine needle aspiration cytology; IV: Intravenous; LDH; lactate dehydrogenase; SMS: superior mediastinal syndrome; SVC: superior vena cava syndrome; TLS: tumor lysis syndrome)

- *Bone marrow aspiration examination under local anesthesia:* In situations, where the bone marrow is involved, this may be a useful sample for establishing the diagnosis and may avert the need for more invasive procedures.
- *Tumor biomarkers:* Beta subunit of beta-human chorionic gonadotropin (β-hCG) and α-fetoprotein (AFP), LDH, and urinary catecholamines.
- *Pleural fluid/pericardial fluid examination:* This is often done for therapeutic purposes but may provide diagnostic clues particularly when the child is sick and invasive biopsy is

not possible. In addition to routine analysis, fluid should also be submitted for malignant cytology, flow cytometry, and immunocytochemistry in order to yield a definitive diagnosis.

If none of the above investigations are informative, tissue diagnosis with least invasive procedure is desirable, before starting definitive therapy. Whenever feasible, biopsy/fine needle aspiration from peripheral pathological lesion is preferred over mediastinal mass due to less risk associated.

Though tissue diagnosis is preferable before starting therapy, it may not be always feasible especially when the child has poor anesthetic risk. In such situations, empirical management of SMS/SVCS should be initiated without any delay.

CASE (Continued)

The child C who presented to emergency with respiratory dysfunction due to SMS had normal counts and elevated LDH. In addition, he was identified to have moderate to massive pleural effusion. He underwent therapeutic pleural tap and pleural fluid cytology showed blasts. Pleural fluid flow cytometry confirmed the diagnosis of T-lymphoblastic lymphoma.

27. How will you further manage the child C?

Though definitive diagnosis is desirable, it is not mandatory before starting chemotherapy, as delay in starting chemotherapy may be life-threatening. The empirical therapy should be initiated without any delay based on differential diagnoses generated with the help of clinical, radiological, and other ancillary investigations.

- *Steroids:* Steroids are the first-line agents to be initiated for initial stabilization of children presenting with SMS/SVCS. The steroids reduce the airway edema and reduce the tumor burden in leukemic and lymphomatous masses **(Table 15)**.[31]

TABLE 15: Steroids used for stabilization of children with SMS/SVC syndrome.

Formulation	Dose
Dexamethasone	5–10 mg/m^2/day
Methylprednisolone	1 mg/kg/dose Q6H
Hydrocortisone	5 mg/kg/dose Q6H

(SMS: superior mediastinal syndrome; SVC: superior vena cava syndrome)

- *Cytotoxic chemotherapy:* At times, the steroids alone may not be effective in stabilizing the child with SMS/SVCS, warranting additional therapy. The other cytotoxic chemotherapeutic agents commonly used along with steroids include cyclophosphamide (200 mg/m^2), vincristine (1–1.5 mg/m^2), and anthracyclines (doxorubicin/daunorubicin: 25–50 mg/m^2).[31]

    Both steroids and other cytotoxic chemotherapy may worsen tumor lysis and occasionally precipitate acute renal failure. The main limitation of empirical chemotherapy is their interference with histologic diagnosis. Studies have shown that prebiopsy steroids beyond 24–48 hours have resulted in diagnostic difficulties. So, the children should be reassessed for the anesthetic fitness after 48 hours of empirical therapy for the possibility of tissue diagnosis.[31]

- *Radiotherapy:* The role of emergent radiotherapy for SMS/SVCS is obsolete nowadays due to rapid response rates with steroids and cytotoxic chemotherapy with decreased toxicity.[29]

- *Anticoagulation:* The role of anticoagulants in malignant SVCS is unclear. The systematic review of 101 case series and reports of pediatric SVCS by Nossair et al. have documented that three out of five children with tumor-related SVC thrombosis improved without any need for anticoagulation. Retrospective analysis of the role of anticoagulation among the adults with malignant SVCS reported an inconsistent practice pattern of anticoagulation prescription, 70% (21/30) of patients with thrombosis, and 52% (49/97) of those without thrombosis received anticoagulation. They also documented similar rates of thrombosis with and without anticoagulation.[32]

As the increased risk of bleeding associated with the use of anticoagulants adds to the challenges of establishing a definitive diagnosis, they are often initiated only when the symptoms of SVCS do not resolve after initiation of steroids and cytotoxic chemotherapy.

If SVCS is secondary to central venous line (CVL)-associated thrombosis, the line should be removed and anticoagulation with low molecular heparin (1 mg/kg/dose Q12H) must be started and continued for a minimum period of 6 weeks. The role of direct oral anticoagulants is upcoming in this setting.

CASE *(Continued)*

The child C who presented to emergency with respiratory dysfunction due to SMS was diagnosed as a case of T-lymphoblastic lymphoma by flow cytometry of pleural fluid. He was started on dexamethasone at 10 mg/m2/day along with hyperhydration and allopurinol.

28. How will you monitor the child C, following the stabilization and initial management of SMS?

Continuous monitoring of clinical and laboratory parameters is of prime importance while managing a child with SMS/SVCS. Vigilant monitoring of vital signs, pulmonary, and hemodynamic status is mandatory. Close monitoring of urine output, CBC, serum electrolytes (sodium, potassium, calcium, and phosphorus), urea, creatinine, and uric acid every 6–8 hours should be done.

CASE *(Continued)*

After the initiation of dexamethasone, the child A developed with laboratory TLS with hyperphosphatemia and hyperuricemia, which was managed with single dose of rasburicase without any need for RRT. His respiratory distress gradually resolved over next 36 hours and then he was weaned off O_2 support and his facial puffiness gradually improved. As his respiratory status improved, he underwent CT neck, chest and abdomen for staging along with bone marrow examination. He continued to receive the induction chemotherapy as per unit protocol.

CASE VIGNETTE 4

Febrile Neutropenia

D, a 9-year-old boy, recently diagnosed case of AML received his first induction chemotherapy [Cytarabine, Daunorubicin, Etoposide (ADE)—10 + 3 + 5] till 4 days back, presented to pediatric emergency with fever for the past 1 hour without any other complaints.
- *Vitals:* HR—92/min, RR—24/, BP—102/68 mm Hg, temperature—101.2°F, CFT—3 seconds, and SpO_2: 97% with room air

- *GPE:* Pallor and petechial spots, no significant lymphadenopathy. Oral cavity—grade 2 mucositis, no paranasal sinus (PNS) tenderness, B/L ear—normal, perianal region—normal, right cubital peripherally inserted central catheter (PICC) line in situ
- *System examination:* WNL
- *Presumptive diagnosis:* AML—postinduction course 1—with acute febrile illness with grade 2 mucositis—possibly FN

The resident in ER suspected that the child D could be having neutropenia and he was started immediately on IV piperacillin-tazobactam and teicoplanin, after sending baseline investigations along with blood C/S. The reports of baseline investigations are as follows:
- *CBC:* Hb—7.2 g/dL, TLC—800/mm^3, ANC—150/mm^3, platelets—12,000/mm^3
- *Serum electrolytes:* Na—132 mEq/dL and K—4.2 mEq/dL
- *RFT:* Urea—22 mg/dL and serum creatinine—0.5 mg/dL.

29. What is FN?

Febrile neutropenia is defined as single oral temperature of ≥38.3°C (101°F) or oral temperature of ≥38°C (100.4°F) for 1 hour in a child with ANC <500/mm^3 or ANC >500/mm^3, but expected to fall below 500/mm^3 within next 48 hours.
- Profound neutropenia is defined as ANC <100/mm^3
- Prolonged neutropenia is defined as neutropenia lasting >7 days.

The incidence of febrile episodes during chemotherapy-induced neutropenia is higher with hematological malignancy to the tune of >80% compared to that of solid tumors which ranges between 10 and 50%.[33] The microbiological etiology of FN varies from time to time and from region to region. The knowledge of microbial spectrum as well as its susceptibility data is crucial to frame and periodically modify the guidelines for the choice of empirical antimicrobials.[34]

According to Indian data, bacterial infections are the most common cause for pediatric FN with 60–80% of isolates being gram-negative organisms such as *Escherichia coli*, *Pseudomonas*, and *Klebsiella*. Gram-positive bacterial infections are also on the rise in the recent years with increased use of central venous catheters and other vascular access.[35]

CASE (Continued)

The child D with AML—postinduction course 1, who presented to emergency with acute febrile illness, was identified to have FN.

30. How will you assess the child D with FN?

Though fever in a cancer patient may be caused by noninfectious etiology (pyrogenic drug, transfusion reactions, etc.) also, it is more often caused by infective etiology. Fever is often the only manifestation of severe infection in neutropenic children, as other inflammatory signs might be suppressed. Therefore, all children who are receiving cancer chemotherapy and present with fever, are considered to have FN and managed appropriately, in order to avoid serious complications resulting from delay.

First step in evaluation of child presenting with FN is stabilization. The patient may deceptively appear stable despite being in a state of hemodynamic compromise. Vital signs (temperature, heart/pulse rate, respiratory rate, capillary refill time, blood pressure, and saturation) should be meticulously documented in every child with suspected FN.

Once stabilized, focused history, and examination should be done which can provide the clues to the infective etiology. A systematic approach is required for further assessment and evaluation of a child with FN.

- *History:* The history about underlying malignancy, phase of chemotherapy, and last received chemotherapy should be recorded along with history regarding the current febrile episode including:
  - *Fever:* Onset, duration, and degree of fever
  - *Associated localizing symptoms:* Pulmonary, ENT, cardiovascular, gastrointestinal, genitourinary, neurological, and musculoskeletal system.
  - Oral acceptance
  - Potential exposures
  - History of previous FN episodes, recent hospitalization, antibiotic exposure, and other medications [granulocyte colony-stimulating factor (G-CSF), antimicrobial prophylaxis, etc.] should also be documented.
- *Physical examination:* A detailed physical examination is mandatory to identify the focus of infection and to direct further evaluation. The sites that require specific attention include oral cavity, ear, paranasal sinuses, skin, nails, perianal area, intravascular catheter insertion site, and the site of bone marrow aspiration.

CASE *(Continued)*

The child D with AML—postinduction course 1, who presented to emergency with FN, was hemodynamically stable. He was identified to have no focus of infection other than grade 2 mucositis. Studies have documented that only 20–30% of FN episodes were documented to have clinical focus.

31. What laboratory investigations will you send for the child D?

The following investigations are done for all patients:
- Complete blood count with differentials
- Serum electrolytes and RFTs
- Blood culture and sensitivity.

Blood culture: Blood cultures should be mandatorily sent before starting empirical antibiotics. Adequate amount of PB should be collected by strict aseptic venepuncture. For those children with indwelling CVL, adequate volume of blood should be collected from all lumens of CVL. Repeat samples for blood culture should be sent for children with persistent fever.[36]

Urinalysis and urine culture: Routine urinalysis and culture at the initial evaluation of FN in children is controversial. Studies have shown that both localizing symptoms and pyuria poorly predicted the urinary tract infection (UTI) in children with FN. Because of the concerns associated with invasive methods of urine collection, American Society of Clinical Oncology (ASCO) guidelines, 2017 recommends urinalysis and urine culture in patients in whom a clean-catch, midstream specimen is readily available. But it should not delay the initiation of empirical antibiotics.[36]

Chest X-ray: ASCO guidelines, 2017 recommends CXR only with children with respiratory signs and symptoms, as studies have documented that incidence of pneumonia among asymptomatic children as <3%.[36] In an observational study conducted in author's unit, abnormal CXR at presentation was identified to have significantly associated with adverse outcome. Initial chest radiograph may be noninformative but is indicated as it forms a baseline for comparison with later films, subtle differences in pneumonic process may become apparent on serial radiographs, may provide an indication for tubercular work-up, CT chest, bronchoscopy, and investigations for unusual organisms like *Pneumocystis jiroveci* or other atypical organisms.[35]

Further diagnostic investigations are done to establish the infectious etiology are usually directed by clinical history and examination, which includes stool culture, ear swab for culture, pus culture, nasopharyngeal aspirate for viral polymerase chain reaction (PCR), ultrasound abdomen, cerebrospinal fluid (CSF) analysis, etc.

CASE *(Continued)*

The child D with AML—postinduction course 1, who presented to emergency with FN without any focus other than grade 2 mucositis, was evaluated further as follows:
- Blood culture from peripheral as well as central line
- CXR: Normal study.

32. How will you risk stratify child D?

First step in the management of FN after its identification is risk stratification. Risk stratification helps in deciding the intensity with which further management should take place. Unlike in adults, there is no universally accepted and well validated risk stratification model for pediatric FN. Majority of risk stratification methods are based on patient or disease-related risk factors and episode-specific risk factors **(Table 16)**. Any risk stratification model should be validated for use in a similar setting before adopting and incorporating into routine practice.[36]

TABLE 16: Risk factors utilized for risk stratification of children with febrile neutropenia.

	Risk factors
Patient/disease specific	Age, nutrition status, type of malignancy, remission status
Treatment specific	Intensity of chemotherapy, timing of chemotherapy
Episode specific	Grade of fever, oral acceptance, hemodynamic instability, mucositis, blood counts, CRP, etc.

The risk stratification used in the author's unit is given in **Table 17**.

TABLE 17: Risk stratification of children with FN.

Low risk	High risk
They were receiving: • Minimally myelosuppressive chemotherapy—not expected to induce severe neutropenia such as ALL maintenance phase, chemotherapy for Hodgkin lymphoma, Wilms tumor	They were receiving: • Strongly myelosuppressive chemotherapy—expected duration of severe neutropenia >7 days such as AML, ALL high-risk induction, consolidation, interim maintenance, ALL relapse

Contd...

Contd...

Low risk	High risk
• Briefly myelosuppressive chemotherapy—expected duration of severe neutropenia <7 days such as ALL standard and intermediate risk induction, consolidation, interim maintenance, delayed intensification, RB, Ewing sarcoma, RMS, osteosarcoma, GCT, and LCH	• Myeloablative chemotherapy—requires HSCT to reconstitute bone marrow function
When their malignancy was in remission	When their malignancy was not in remission
Not undergoing hematopoietic stem cell transplantation (HSCT)	Undergoing HSCT
Without any clinical focus of infection that would require prolonged systemic antibiotics—osteomyelitis, septic arthritis, meningitis, endocarditis, pneumonia, neutropenic enterocolitis, etc.	With any clinical focus of infection that would require prolonged systemic antibiotics—osteomyelitis, septic arthritis, meningitis, endocarditis, pneumonia, neutropenic enterocolitis, etc.
Without any oral mucositis grade 3 and grade 4	With oral mucositis grade 3 and grade 4
Without any evidence of organ dysfunction—oxygen requirement >50% FiO_2, mechanical ventilation, without hemodynamic compromise requiring inotropes/vasoactives, serum creatinine ≥2 × ULN for age or twofold increase from baseline, SGOT/SGPT2 × ULN for age, total bilirubin ≥4 mg/dL, GCS ≤11 or acute deterioration of GCS ≥3 points from baseline	With any evidence of organ dysfunction—oxygen requirement >50% FiO_2, mechanical ventilation, hemodynamic compromise requiring inotropes/vasoactives, serum creatinine ≥2 × ULN for age or twofold increase from baseline, SGOT/SGPT2 × ULN for age, total bilirubin ≥4 mg/dL, GCS ≤11 or acute deterioration of GCS ≥3 points from baseline
Without any profound neutropenia—ANC <100 mm³	With profound neutropenia—ANC <100/mm³

(ALL: acute lymphoblastic leukemia; AML: acute myeloid leukemia; ANC: absolute neutrophil count; FN: febrile neutropenia; GCS: Glasgow coma scale; GCT: germ cell tumor; LCH: Langerhans cell histiocytosis; RB: retinoblastoma; RMS: rhabdomyosarcoma; SGOT/SGPT2: serum glutamic oxaloacetic transaminase/serum glutamic pyruvic transaminase; ULN: upper limit of normal)

CASE *(Continued)*

The child D with AML—postinduction course 1 who presented to emergency with FN without any focus or hemodynamic instability will be classified as high FN as per the abovementioned risk stratification criteria.

33. How will you further manage child D?

Early initiation of antimicrobials along with adequate supportive care is the two vital components of the management of pediatric FN. The choice of empirical antimicrobials is guided by the institutional protocol which should be based locally prevailing bacteriological profile and antimicrobial resistance pattern. The choice of inpatient versus outpatient administration of antimicrobials and route of administration is usually dictated by adopting a validated risk stratification strategy which classifies children into low risk and high risk based on clinical and laboratory findings.

Low-risk FN: Despite the lack of validated risk stratification criteria for pediatric FN, there is an increased trend to utilize outpatient oral or parenteral therapy as either initial management or as step-down to outpatient treatment after initial inpatient management. The evidence for this approach is as follows:
- *Outpatient versus inpatient management:* The safety of initial or step-down outpatient management of low-risk FN was established by the two meta-analyses on the subject is given in **Table 18**.

TABLE 18: Safety of outpatient management of low-risk febrile neutropenia.

	Treatment failure	Mortality	Remark
Rivas-Ruiz et al., 2019[37]	RR (95% CI): 1.04 (0.55–1.99)	RR (95% CI): 0.63 (0.15–2.70)	• Systematic review of four pediatric RCT • Inconsistent definition of low risk and regimens used
Manji et al., 2012[38]	• Including modification: Incidence—14.93% versus 27.5 (0.04) • Excluding modification: Incidence—5.41% versus 0% (0.11)	• Overall mortality: 0% versus 1.28% (0.48) • Infection related mortality: 0% versus 1.28% (0.49)	• Systematic review of 16 pediatric prospective studies • Inconsistent definition of low risk and regimens used

(CI: confidence interval; RCT: randomized controlled trial; RR: relative risk)

The additional benefits of this approach include:
- *Improved quality of life:* Both child and parent reported health-related quality of life were higher when managed on outpatient basis compared with inpatient management.[39]
- *Cost-effectiveness:* The cost utility analysis done by Teuffel et al. comparing inpatient and outpatient management of low-risk FN suggests that ambulatory management with either parental or oral antibiotics were more cost-effective than in patient as well as early step-down outpatient management.[40]

American Society of Clinical Oncology guidelines suggest initial or step-down outpatient management of low-risk FN can be considered provided that the careful monitoring and follow-up can be ensured, as a weak recommendation due to moderate quality of evidence.[36]
- *Oral versus parenteral antibiotics:* The safety of initial or step-down oral antibiotics for low-risk FN was established **(Table 19)**.

American Society of Clinical Oncology guidelines suggest that initial or step-down oral antibiotics of low-risk FN can be considered provided that the children are tolerating and are compliant to the oral route of administration of antibiotics, as a weak recommendation based on moderate quality evidence.[36]

TABLE 19: Safety of oral antibiotics for children with low risk febrile neutropenia.

	Treatment failure	Mortality	Remark
Robinson et al., 2018[41]	• Including modification: RR (95% CI): 0.95 (0.72–1.24) • Including modification: RR (95% CI): 0.65 (0.28–1.52) • Readmission: RR (95% CI): 0.50 (0.23–1.08)	NA	• Systematic review of eight pediatric RCT • Inconsistent definition of low risk and regimens used
Manji et al., 2012[38]	• Including modification: Incidence—19.63% versus 22.26 (0.68) • Excluding modification: Incidence—4.69% versus 5.99% (0.66)	• Overall mortality: 0% versus 0.93% (0.70) • Infection-related mortality: 0% versus 0.92% (0.71)	• Systematic review of 16 pediatric prospective studies • Inconsistent definition of low risk and regimens used

(CI: confidence interval; RCT: randomized controlled trial; RR: relative risk)

The most commonly utilized oral antibiotics in pediatric low-risk FN include fluoroquinolones (ciprofloxacin, levofloxacin), amoxicillin-clavulanic acid, cefixime or a combination of the above.

High risk: The prompt initiation of empirical broad-spectrum antibiotics is the cornerstone in management of FN. An ideal empirical antibiotic should have broad antibacterial spectrum, be bactericidal even with neutropenia and less adverse effects. The choice of the empirical antibiotics depends on multiple factors such as:
1. Clinical presentation—clinically stable/unstable
2. Previous infection/colonization with multidrug resistant (MDR) microorganism
3. Bacteriological profile, antimicrobial susceptibility data, and experience of the treating hospital

- *Clinically stable:* Low risk of resistant infections—8th European Conference on Infections in Leukemia (ECIL-8) recommends an antipseudomonal noncarbapenem β-lactam plus β-lactamase inhibitor combination or fourth-generation cephalosporin for clinically stable patients at low risk of resistant infections (without previous colonization or infection with resistant bacteria, or patients treated in institutions with a low rate of resistant pathogens).[42]
    • *Monotherapy versus combination therapy:* Robinson et al. documented no significant differences in failure rates, infection-related mortality, or overall mortality, in their systematic review of nine pediatric RCTs comparing monotherapy versus aminoglycoside-containing combination regimen. This study confirmed the efficacy and safety of monotherapy without the addition of aminoglycosides for clinically stable patients at low risk of resistant infections.[41]
    • *Choice of monotherapy:* Robinson et al. reported that antipseudomonal penicillin plus β-lactamase inhibitor and fourth-generation cephalosporin monotherapy (cefepime) were associated with similar treatment failure, infection-related mortality, and duration of fever.[41]

Karaman et al. documented that monotherapy with cefoperazone-sulbactam or piperacillin-tazobactam monotherapy was equally effective and safe as empirical therapy for febrile neutropenic children.[43]

Meta-analyses of pediatric trials have shown similar efficacy between antipseudomonal cephalosporins, antipseudomonal penicillins, and carbapenems. Paul et al. documented that carbapenems resulted in similar all-cause mortality and a lower rate of clinical failure and antibiotic modifications as compared to other anti-pseudomonal β-lactams as monotherapy in the treatment of FN, but with higher rate of *Clostridium difficile* associated diarrhea.[44]

Due to lack of pediatric safety and efficacy data, novel β-lactam plus β-lactamase combinations, such as ceftazidime-avibactam or ceftolozane-tazobactam, should not be routinely used as empirical antibacterial therapy.[42]

- *Anti-gram-positive cover:* In their meta-analysis of 13 RCTs, Paul et al. documented that addition of upfront empirical anti-gram-positive antibiotics did not reduce the mortality and treatment failure.[45] Current clinical indications for empiric gram-positive cover include:[34]
  - Skin/soft-tissue infection
  - Catheter-related infection
  - Hemodynamic instability
  - Severe mucositis
  - Radiographically confirmed pneumonia
  - Previous colonization with methicillin-resistant *Staphylococcus aureus* (MRSA)/vancomycin-resistant *Enterococcus* (VRE)
  - For those on fluoroquinolone prophylaxis.

  Traditionally, vancomycin is the most commonly used gram-positive cover but recent meta-analysis has showed that vancomycin and teicoplanin were comparable in terms of therapeutic success rates among adult patients with FN.[46]

- *High risk of resistant infections:* Multiple studies have shown that previous colonization or infection with a resistant microorganism is associated with increased risk of multidrug-resistant infections subsequently. ECIL-8 guidelines suggest that the initial empirical antibacterial treatment in these patients should be adjusted on the basis of the susceptibility pattern of the microorganism isolated earlier.[42]

  In centers with a high rate of multidrug-resistant infections, the ECIL-8 guidelines recommended that initial empirical antibacterial treatment should be tailored to the local bacteriological profile and antimicrobial susceptibility data. The ECIL-8 panel recommended periodical local microbiological surveillance to frame and modify the choice of empirical antimicrobial therapy.[42]

  Monotherapy may not be appropriate in centers with a high rate of resistant infections and for patients with high risk of resistant infections, requiring addition of a second gram-negative agent or glycopeptide.

- *Clinically unstable:* With the background of increasing incidence of multi-drug resistant gram-negative bacilli infection, Nadal et al. documented that among adult oncohematological patients with high-risk FN, those presenting with MDR gram negative bacilli (GNB) infection receiving inappropriate empirical antimicrobials had increased risk mortality. They also reported that hemodynamic instability at the time of presentation is an independent risk factor for mortality. In view of this, the ECIL-8 panel recommends a de-escalation strategy (start with broad-spectrum antibiotics and switch to narrow-spectrum antibiotics when safe) for clinically unstable patients. These patients should initially be started preferably with a carbapenem, along with a second anti-gram-negative agent, a glycopeptide, or both.[42]

CASE *(Continued)*

The child D with AML—postinduction course 1 who presented to emergency with high-risk FN without any focus or hemodynamic instability was started on IV piperacillin-tazobactam and teicoplanin after sending baseline investigations along with blood C/S from central and peripheral line.

34. How will you monitor child D started on empirical antibiotics for response?

The child with FN who was started on empirical antibiotics should be reviewed periodically for the response to the antibiotics, evolution of new signs and symptoms, and other complications **(Flowchart 4)**. Careful monitoring of vitals can help in timely identification of clinical deterioration and appropriate management like PICU transfer which can improve the outcomes.[47]

Flowchart 4: Approach to a child with febrile neutropenia.

```
                        Febrile neutropenia
                                │
                                ▼
                    Initiate empirical IV antibiotics
                                │
                                ▼
                        Reassess at 48 hours
                          │              │
              ┌───────────┘              └───────────┐
              ▼                                      ▼
         Responding                            Not responding
              │                                      │
              ▼                                      ▼
  • Discontinuation of empirical           Upgrade to second-line antibiotics
    antibiotics at 72 hours if negative                │
    blood culture at 48 hours along                    ▼
    with evidence of marrow recovery           Reassess at 96 hours
    and afebrile for at least 24 hours           │            │
  • Continue empirical antibiotics till   ┌──────┘            └──────┐
    ANC >500/mm³                          ▼                          ▼
                                      Responding              Not responding
                                          │                          │
                                          ▼                          ▼
                                 Continue empirical        Start empirical antifungal
                                    antibiotics            therapy and screen for
                                 till ANC >500/mm³         invasive fungal infection
```

(ANC: absolute neutrophil count)

Treatment modification in 24–72 hours (Table 20):[36]

TABLE 20: Treatment modification of children with febrile neutropenia on empirical antibiotics.

Clinical condition	Recommendation
Responding to initial empirical antibiotics	• Discontinue dual coverage for gram-negative infection, if started • Discontinue empirical gram-positive coverage, if there is no microbiological indication to continue
Persistent fever but clinically stable	No need to modify the initial empirical antibiotics solely based on the persistence of fever
Persistent fever and clinically unstable	Escalate the initial empirical antibiotics to include coverage for resistant gram-negative, gram-positive, and anaerobic bacteria

Discontinuation of antibiotics:
- *Without clinically or microbiologically defined infection:* There are no clear-cut guidelines among pediatric as well as adult literature regarding the optimal duration of empirical antibiotics and no recommendations were available to guide the timing of safe discontinuation of empirical antibiotics. Majority of available literature recommends discontinuation of empirical antibiotics in patients who have negative blood culture at 48 hours along with evidence of marrow recovery and remain afebrile for at least 24 hours. But this remains low-quality evidence as there is no well-established cut off for defining marrow recovery. Even though there is some evidence supporting early discontinuation of empirical antibiotics in low-risk FN, the safety of such early discontinuation without marrow recovery is not explored at present.

Currently available recommendations for de-escalation of empirical antibiotics are as follows:
- *ASCO guidelines, 2017:*[36]
    - In all patients, discontinue empirical antibiotics in patients who have negative blood cultures at 48 hours, who have been afebrile for at least 24 hours, and who have evidence of marrow recovery (strong recommendation, low-quality evidence).
    - In patients with low-risk FN, consider discontinuation of empirical antibiotics at 72 hours in patients who have negative blood cultures and who have been afebrile for at least 24 hours, irrespective of marrow recovery status, as long as careful follow-up is ensured (weak recommendation, moderate-quality evidence).
- *ECIL-8 guidelines:*[42]
    - Consider a de-escalation strategy in patients with fever of unknown origin (without clinically or microbiologically documented infection) who presented with clinically stable condition and no previous colonization or infection with resistant pathogens, after ≥72 hours of IV antibiotics
        - If patients have been hemodynamically stable since presentation
        - Have been afebrile for 24–48 hours, even before signs of hematological recovery, provided careful patient monitoring is available.
    - Follow-up can be performed on an inpatient or an outpatient basis according to local infrastructure and ability to return quickly to the hospital.

- Step-down strategies in patients with fever without focus
  - Switch to oral antibiotics
    ▷ In low-risk FN—(BIIr—moderate recommendation)
    ▷ In selected high-risk patients—(CIItu—marginal recommendation)
  - Discontinuation of all empiric antibiotics
    ▷ In low-risk FN—(BII—moderate recommendation)
    ▷ In selected high-risk patients—(CIIt—marginal recommendation)
- *With clinically or microbiologically documented infections:* The children with any clinical focus of infection that would require prolonged systemic antibiotics—osteomyelitis, septic arthritis, meningitis, endocarditis, pneumonia, neutropenic enterocolitis—should be continued on appropriate antibiotics for the recommended duration.

The empirical antibiotics should be modified according to the susceptibility pattern for those children with positive blood culture and should be continued for 10–14 days.[36]

CASE *(Continued)*

The child D with AML—postinduction course 1 with high-risk FN who was started on empirical IV antibiotics continued to have fever spikes even after 48 hours. His central as well as PB cultures were sterile after 48 hours of incubation. He developed new onset cough and respiratory distress requiring oxygen supplementation, following which his antibiotics were upgraded to IV meropenem and teicoplanin. However, his fever persisted even after 96 hours of IV antibiotics.

35. How will you further manage child D, who has now developed new onset respiratory symptoms along with prolonged FN?

The child D continued to have high spiking fever despite 96 hours of IV antibiotics. Also, he is now clinically unstable with new onset respiratory symptoms requiring oxygen supplementation.

The children with persistent fever beyond 96 hours of broad-spectrum empirical antibiotics should be screened for invasive fungal infections. Those patients with prolonged and profound neutropenia and those receiving corticosteroids are at high risk of developing invasive fungal infections. This will include children with AML, high-risk ALL, or relapsed acute leukemia, and children undergoing allogeneic HSCT.[36,48]

Screening work up:
- *Mycological evaluation:* Whenever feasible, all appropriate efforts should be made to isolate the causative pathogen and to do resistance testing. This includes blood cultures for yeasts and some molds, cultures and microscopic examination of appropriate liquid, and solid specimens.[48]
- *Biomarkers:*
  - *Galactomannan:* Galactomannan, a cell wall component released by all *Aspergillus* species, detected in serum, bronchoalveolar lavage fluid, and CSF is accepted as a mycological criterion for the diagnosis of invasive aspergillosis in the EORTC/MSGERC definition of invasive fungal diseases. Galactomannan assay is strongly recommended as a diagnostic tool in pediatric patients with prolonged FN (pooled sensitivity: 81% and pooled specificity: 88%) **(Table 21)**.[48,49]

TABLE 21: Threshold for positive galactomannan assay.

Sample	Threshold for positive result (OD)
Blood	≥0.5
BAL	≥1
CSF	≥1

(BAL: bronchoalveolar lavage; CSF: cerebrospinal fluid)

- *β-d-glucan:* According to revised EORTC/MSGERC invasive fungal disease definitions, detection of β-d-glucan in the serum is a mycological criterion for probable invasive candidiasis and probable pneumocystosis (but not for aspergillosis). Due to poor positive predictive value, β-d-glucan testing in serum, BAL, and CSF is not recommended for diagnostic use.[48,49]
- *Fungal PCR:* Standardized PCR-based detection of fungal nucleic acids are now included in the EORTC/MSGERC consensus group criteria for mycological evidence of invasive fungal infection. Fungal PCR can be used for the diagnosis of invasive fungal infection but with less sensitivity and specificity compared with galactomannan assay (pooled sensitivity: 76% and pooled specificity: 58%).[48,49]
- *Imaging:* High-resolution CT-chest is strongly recommended in children at high risk of invasive fungal disease presenting with prolonged FN or in those with focal clinical findings. Compared with adults, children often show nonspecific radiological features such as multiple nodules or fluffy masses and mass-like lesions. Routine CT of the paranasal sinuses should be avoided and should only be performed in patients with localizing signs or symptoms. Other imaging studies should be done as dictated by the clinical features.[49]

CASE (Continued)

The child D with AML—postinduction course 1 with high-risk prolonged FN with new onset respiratory symptoms was evaluated for invasive fungal infection as follows:
- Serum galactomannan: 1.2
- CT chest: s/o aspergillosis.

Antifungal therapy:
Preemptive versus empirical antifungal strategy: The multicenter, randomized clinical trial comparing the efficacy of preemptive versus empirical antifungal therapy in 149 children with prolonged FN reported a significant reduction in the duration of antifungal therapy in favor of preemptive strategy, without any differences in overall mortality, invasive fungal disease-related mortality, and the incidence of proven or probable invasive fungal diseases.[50]

Preemptive antifungal strategy warrants rapid and round the clock availability of pulmonary CT imaging and of galactomannan-assay results, as well as expertise to perform diagnostic bronchoscopies with bronchoalveolar lavage. Because of these limitations, empirical antifungal therapy has been a common practice in children with prolonged FN.[49]

Choice of empirical anti-fungal therapy **(Table 22)**:[49]

TABLE 22: Choice of empirical antifungal agents.

Agent	Dose	Remarks
Liposomal amphotericin B	3–5 mg/kg/dose— once daily	• Liposomal amphotericin B was less nephrotoxic than amphotericin B deoxycholate • Efficacy of liposomal amphotericin B was slightly better than that of amphotericin B deoxycholate
Caspofungin	70 mg/m²/dose followed by 50 mg/m²/dose—once daily	No difference in efficacy was observed between caspofungin and liposomal amphotericin B. Caspofungin was better tolerated than liposomal amphotericin B

Despite the lack of supporting evidence, switching to a different class of mold-active antifungal agents seems reasonable for patients already receiving mold-active antifungal prophylaxis.

CASE *(Continued)*

The child D with AML—postinduction course 1 with high-risk prolonged FN with new onset respiratory symptoms was started on empirical and IV liposomal amphotericin B. He was later diagnosed to have invasive pulmonary aspergillosis and his antifungal therapy was switched to IV voriconazole, following which he stabilized. He became afebrile after 48 hours of antifungal therapy and his respiratory distress became passive. His antibiotics were stopped after 14 days and he continued to receive antifungal therapy for a total duration of 6 weeks.

36. **How will you prevent subsequent infectious complications in further chemotherapy cycles for child D?**

Hygiene measures:
- Hand hygiene
- Personal hygiene
- Central line care
- Oral care
- Perianal care
- Respiratory hygiene
- Environmental hygiene
- Avoiding crowded places, construction sites
- Barrier precautions
- Food hygiene

Antibacterial prophylaxis: Multiple RCTs and meta-analyses have documented that antibiotic prophylaxis reduced the rate of bloodstream infections and FN without any significant effect on overall survival. They also reported an inconsistent association between quinolone prophylaxis and emergence of resistant infections and *C. difficile*-associated diarrhea. In view of these factors, ECIL8 recommends against routine antibacterial prophylaxis.[42]

Antifungal prophylaxis: Primary antifungal prophylaxis is recommended for children with high risk (≥10% estimated natural incidence) of invasive fungal infection. This includes children with acute myeloid leukemia, high-risk acute lymphoblastic leukemia, relapsed acute lymphoblastic leukemia, and those undergoing allogeneic hematopoietic cell transplantation (HCT) in the pre-engraftment and in the postengraftment phase until immune reconstitution, or in patients receiving immunosuppressive treatment for graft-versus-host disease **(Table 23)**.[49]

TABLE 23: Choice of prophylactic antifungal agents.

Agent	Dose	Remarks
Fluconazole	8–12 mg/kg/dose—once daily	Fluconazole is active only against yeasts and should only be used if the institutional incidence of invasive mold infections is low. Recommended for patients undergoing allogeneic HSCT in the pre-engraftment period but not postengraftment period
Voriconazole	9 mg/kg/dose twice daily	• Spectrum includes both yeasts and molds • TDM is suggested (dosing target: trough concentration of 1.0–5.0 mg/L) • Interactions with other drugs are of major concern
Posaconazole	4 mg/kg/dose—thrice daily	• Spectrum includes both yeasts and molds • TDM is suggested (dosing target: trough concentration of ≥0.7 mg/L) • Lesser interaction with other drugs—compared with voriconazole
Liposomal amphotericin B	• 1 mg/kg/dose—every other day • 2.5 mg/kg/dose—twice a week	• Spectrum includes both yeasts and molds • Alternative option for patients who do not tolerate or have contraindications to triazoles

(HSCT: hematopoietic stem cell transplant)

Antipneumocystis prophylaxis: Trimethoprim-sulfamethoxazole (TMP-SMZ) is the standard antipneumocystis prophylactic agent utilized for children receiving chemotherapy. Other agents include dapsone, atovaquone, and pentamidine. The optimal duration of antipneumocystis prophylaxis is unknown.[51]

Antiviral prophylaxis: There is paucity of evidence to recommend routine antiviral prophylaxis for children receiving cancer chemotherapy.

Granulocyte colony-stimulating factor: ASCO guidelines recommend the prophylactic use of G-CSF following chemotherapeutic regimen with estimated FN incidence of >20%.

American Society of Clinical Oncology guidelines recommend secondary prophylaxis with G-CSF for children who developed FN following previous cycle of chemotherapy, during subsequent cycles, especially when dose reduction may compromise the outcome.

Use of G-CSF as an adjunct along with antimicrobial therapy has resulted in shorter duration of neutropenia, shorter hospital stays, and antibiotic usage and thereby reduced cost of treatment. But this did not translate into reduced infection related mortality.[51]

Granulocyte transfusion: Although the currently available evidence for granulocyte transfusion (GTX) is limited, the early use of GTX can be considered for children with profound neutropenia, especially for patients with bacterial and invasive fungal infections.[52]

REFERENCES

1. Feusner JH, Hastings CA, Agrawal AK (Eds). Supportive Care in Pediatric Oncology: A Practical Evidence-Based Approach. Berlin, Heidelberg: Springer Berlin Heidelberg; 2015.
2. Howard SC, Jones DP, Pui CH. The tumor lysis syndrome. N Engl J Med. 2011;364(19):1844-54.
3. Sury K. Update on the prevention and treatment of tumor lysis syndrome. J Onco-Nephrol. 2019;3(1):19-30.
4. Russell TB, Kram DE. Tumor lysis syndrome. Pediatr Rev. 2020;41(1):20-6.
5. Cairo MS, Coiffier B, Reiter A Younes A; TLS Expert Panel. Recommendations for the evaluation of risk and prophylaxis of tumour lysis syndrome (TLS) in adults and children with malignant diseases: an expert TLS panel consensus. Br J Haematol. 2010;149(4):578-86.
6. Keane S, Butler E. A study of the effect of hypotonic hyper-hydration fluids on sodium balance in paediatric haematology/oncology patients receiving chemotherapy. Arch Dis Child. 2016;101(9):e2.
7. Heinz AT, Eichholz T, Queudeville M, Hartmann U, Ott A, Heinzel O, et al. Introducing isotonic fluids into pediatric oncology. Pediatr Hematol Oncol. 2022;39(4):357-64.
8. Rajendran A, Bansal D, Marwaha RK, Singhi SC. Tumor lysis syndrome. Indian J Pediatr. 2013;80(1):50-4.
9. Coiffier B, Altman A, Pui CH, Younes A, Cairo MS. Guidelines for the management of pediatric and adult tumor lysis syndrome: an evidence-based review. J Clin Oncol. 2008;26(16):2767-78.
10. Spina M, Nagy Z, Ribera JM, Federico M, Aurer I, Jordan K, et al. FLORENCE: a randomized, double-blind, phase III pivotal study of febuxostat versus allopurinol for the prevention of tumor lysis syndrome (TLS) in patients with hematologic malignancies at intermediate to high TLS risk. Ann Oncol. 2015;26(10):2155-61.
11. Cochrane. (2017). Urate oxidase for the prevention and treatment of complications from massive lysis (breakdown) of tumour cells in children with cancer. [online] Available from https://www.cochrane.org/CD006945/CHILDCA_urate-oxidase-prevention-and-treatment-complications-massive-lysis-breakdown-tumour-cells-children [Last accessed October, 2022].
12. Philips A, Radhakrishnan V, Ganesan P, Ganesan TS, Ramamurthy J, Dhanushkodi M, et al. Efficacy of single dose rasburicase (1.5 mg) for prophylaxis and management of laboratory tumor lysis syndrome. Indian J Hematol Blood Transfus. 2018;34(4):618-22.
13. Tosi P, Barosi G, Lazzaro C, Liso V, Marchetti M, Morra E, et al. Consensus conference on the management of tumor lysis syndrome. Haematologica. 2008;93(12):1877-85.
14. Edeani A, Shirali A. Chapter 4: Tumor Lysis Syndrome. In: Perazella MA (Ed). Onco-Nephrology Curriculum. Washington, DC: American Society of Nephrology; 2017.
15. Röllig C, Ehninger G. How I treat hyperleukocytosis in acute myeloid leukemia. Blood. 2015;125(21):3246-52.
16. Novotny JR, Muller-Beissenhirtz H, Herget-Rosenthal S, Kribben A, Duhrsen U. Grading of symptoms in hyperleukocytic leukaemia: a clinical model for the role of different blast types and promyelocytes in the development of leukostasis syndrome. Eur J Haematol. 2005;74(6):501-10.
17. Piccirillo N, Laurenti L, Chiusolo P, Sorà F, Bianchi M, De Matteis S, et al. Reliability of leukostasis grading score to identify high risk patients with hyperleukocytic leukemia. Blood. 2008;112(11):2979-9.
18. Jain R, Bansal D, Marwaha RK. Hyperleukocytosis: emergency management. Indian J Pediatr. 2013;80(2):144-8.

19. Ruggiero A, Rizzo D, Amato M, Riccardi R. Management of hyperleukocytosis. Curr Treat Options Oncol. 2016;17(2):7.
20. Bertoli S, Picard M, Bérard E, Griessinger E, Larrue C, Mouchel PL, et al. Dexamethasone in hyperleukocytic acute myeloid leukemia. Haematologica. 2018;103(6):988-98.
21. Azoulay E, Canet E, Raffoux E, Lengline E, Lemiale V, Vincent F, et al. Dexamethasone in patients with acute lung injury from acute monocytic leukaemia. Eur Respir J. 2012;39(3):648-53.
22. Cuvelier GDE, Vitali AM, Ford JC, Dix DB. Multiple intracranial tumors in Philadelphia chromosome positive acute lymphoblastic leukemia: successful treatment following aggressive supportive care, early cranial radiation, high dose chemotherapy and imatinib. Pediatr Blood Cancer. 2008;51(1):135-7.
23. Chen KH, Liu HC, Liang DC, Hou JY, Huang TH, Chang CY, et al. Minimally early morbidity in children with acute myeloid leukemia and hyperleukocytosis treated with prompt chemotherapy without leukapheresis. J Formos Med Assoc. 2014;113(11):833-8.
24. Oberoi S, Lehrnbecher T, Phillips B, Hitzler J, Ethier MC, Beyene J, et al. Leukapheresis and low-dose chemotherapy do not reduce early mortality in acute myeloid leukemia hyperleukocytosis: a systematic review and meta-analysis. Leuk Res. 2014;38(4):460-8.
25. Korkmaz S. The management of hyperleukocytosis in 2017: Do we still need leukapheresis? Transfus Apher Sci. 2018;57(1):4-7.
26. Padmanabhan A, Connelly-Smith L, Aqui N, Balogun RA, Klingel R, Meyer E, et al. Guidelines on the use of therapeutic apheresis in clinical practice—evidence-based approach from the Writing Committee of the American Society for Apheresis: The Eighth Special Issue. J Clin Apheresis. 2019;34(3):171-354.
27. Bewersdorf JP, Giri S, Tallman MS, Zeidan AM, Stahl M. Leukapheresis for the management of hyperleukocytosis in acute myeloid leukemia—a systematic review and meta-analysis. Transfusion (Paris). 2020;60(10):2360-9.
28. Duwe BV, Sterman DH, Musani AI. Tumors of the mediastinum. Chest. 2005;128(4):2893-909.
29. Jain R, Bansal D, Marwaha RK, Singhi S. Superior mediastinal syndrome: emergency management. Indian J Pediatr. 2013;80(1):55-9.
30. Shamberger RC. Preanesthetic evaluation of children with anterior mediastinal masses. Semin Pediatr Surg. 1999;8(2):61-8.
31. Pizzo PA, Poplack DG. Principles and practice of pediatric oncology. Philadelphia: Wolters Kluwer; 2016.
32. Nossair F, Schoettler P, Starr J, Chan AKC, Kirov I, Paes B, et al. Pediatric superior vena cava syndrome: an evidence-based systematic review of the literature. Pediatr Blood Cancer. 2018;65(9):e27225.
33. Freifeld AG, Bow EJ, Sepkowitz KA, Boeckh MJ, Ito JI, Mullen CA, et al. Clinical practice guideline for the use of antimicrobial agents in neutropenic patients with cancer: 2010 update by the Infectious Diseases Society of America. Clin Infect Dis. 2011;52(4):e56-93.
34. Oberoi S, Suthar R, Bansal D, Marwaha RK. Febrile neutropenia: outline of management. Indian J Pediatr. 2013;80(2):138-43.
35. Bothra M, Seth R, Kapil A, Dwivedi SN, Bhatnagar S, Xess I. Evaluation of predictors of adverse outcome in febrile neutropenic episodes in pediatric oncology patients. Indian J Pediatr. 2013;80(4):297-302.
36. Lehrnbecher T, Phillips R, Alexander S, Alvaro F, Carlesse F, Fisher B, et al. Guideline for the management of fever and neutropenia in children with cancer and/or undergoing hematopoietic stem-cell transplantation. J Clin Oncol. 2012;30(35):4427-38.
37. Rivas-Ruiz R, Villasis-Keever M, Miranda-Novales G, Castelán-Martínez OD, Rivas-Contreras S. Outpatient treatment for people with cancer who develop a low-risk febrile neutropaenic event. Cochrane Gynaecological, Neuro-oncology and Orphan Cancer Group, editor. Cochrane Database Syst Rev. 2019;3(3):CD009031.

38. Manji A, Beyene J, Dupuis LL, Phillips R, Lehrnbecher T, Sung L. Outpatient and oral antibiotic management of low-risk febrile neutropenia are effective in children—a systematic review of prospective trials. Support Care Cancer. 2012;20(6):1135-45.
39. Speyer E, Herbinet A, Vuillemin A, Chastagner P, Briançon S. Agreement between children with cancer and their parents in reporting the child's health-related quality of life during a stay at the hospital and at home. Child Care Health Dev. 2009;35(4):489-95.
40. Teuffel O, Amir E, Alibhai SMH, Beyene J, Sung L. Cost-effectiveness of outpatient management for febrile neutropenia in children with cancer. Pediatrics. 2011;127(2):e279-86.
41. Robinson PD, Lehrnbecher T, Phillips R, Dupuis LL, Sung L. Strategies for empiric management of pediatric fever and neutropenia in patients with cancer and hematopoietic stem-cell transplantation recipients: a systematic review of randomized trials. J Clin Oncol. 2016;34(17):2054-60.
42. Lehrnbecher T, Averbuch D, Castagnola E, Cesaro S, Ammann RA, Garcia-Vidal C, et al. 8th European Conference on Infections in Leukaemia: 2020 guidelines for the use of antibiotics in paediatric patients with cancer or post-haematopoietic cell transplantation. Lancet Oncol. 2021;22(6):e270-80.
43. Karaman S, Vural S, Yildirmak Y, Emecen M, Erdem E, Kebudi R. Comparison of piperacillin tazobactam and cefoperazone sulbactam monotherapy in treatment of febrile neutropenia: monotherapy of febrile neutropenic children. Pediatr Blood Cancer. 2012;58(4):579-83.
44. Paul M, Yahav D, Bivas A, Fraser A, Leibovici L. Anti-pseudomonal beta-lactams for the initial, empirical, treatment of febrile neutropenia: comparison of beta-lactams. Cochrane Database Syst Rev. 2010;2010(11):CD005197.
45. Paul M, Borok S, Fraser A, Vidal L, Cohen M, Leibovici L. Additional anti-gram-positive antibiotic treatment for febrile neutropenic cancer patients. Cochrane Database Syst Rev. 2005 Jul 20;(3):CD003914.
46. Kaur J, Mir T, Dixit P, Uddin M, Kadari S, Lee Y, et al. The use of vancomycin versus teicoplanin in treating febrile neutropenia: a meta-analysis and systematic review. Cureus. 2021;13(5):e15269.
47. Agulnik A, Gossett J, Carrillo AK, Kang G, Morrison RR. Abnormal vital signs predict critical deterioration in hospitalized pediatric hematology-oncology and post-hematopoietic cell transplant patients. Front Oncol. 2020;10:354.
48. Donnelly JP, Chen SC, Kauffman CA, Steinbach WJ, Baddley JW, Verweij PE, et al. Revision and update of the consensus definitions of invasive fungal disease from the european organization for research and treatment of cancer and the Mycoses Study Group Education and Research Consortium. Clin Infect Dis. 2020;71(6):1367-76.
49. Groll AH, Pana D, Lanternier F, Mesini A, Ammann RA, Averbuch D, et al. 8th European Conference on Infections in Leukaemia: 2020 guidelines for the diagnosis, prevention, and treatment of invasive fungal diseases in paediatric patients with cancer or post-haematopoietic cell transplantation. Lancet Oncol. 2021;22(6):e254-69.
50. Santolaya ME, Alvarez AM, Acuña M, Avilés CL, Salgado C, Tordecilla J, et al. Efficacy of pre-emptive versus empirical antifungal therapy in children with cancer and high-risk febrile neutropenia: a randomized clinical trial. J Antimicrob Chemother. 2018;73(10):2860-6.
51. Lanzkowsky P. Lanzkowsky's manual of pediatric hematology and oncology. Boston, MA: Elsevier; 2016.
52. Gurlek Gokcebay D, Akpinar Tekgunduz S. Granulocyte transfusions in the management of neutropenic fever: a pediatric perspective. Transfus Apher Sci. 2018;57(1):16-9.

EXPERT OPINION

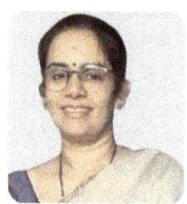

Nita Radhakrishnan
Associate Professor and Head, Department of Pediatric Hematology-Oncology
Post Graduate Institute of Child Health Autonomous Institute
Government of Uttar Pradesh Noida, India.

Case 1: Tumor Lysis Syndrome

1. What is the approach for management of TLS?

Tumor lysis is characterized by metabolic derangements caused by release of intracellular contents into the blood upon lysis of malignant cells either spontaneously or following treatment (chemo-/radio-/immunotherapy). Tumor lysis is expected in patients who present with hematolymphoid malignancies such as ALL, Burkitt leukemia, high-grade NHL, AML as well as in certain solid tumors such as neuroblastoma. It is always better to anticipate and prevent tumor lysis rather than to treat it. In all children who present with symptoms suggestive of leukemia, double maintenance fluids (without potassium or calcium) should be started with diuresis. Biochemical evaluation for tumor lysis (blood urea, serum creatinine, electrolytes, calcium, phosphorus, and uric acid) must be done at the initial suspicion of leukemia/lymphoma as well as repeated periodically. In case the patient presents with tumor lysis, hydration, specific medications such as rasburicase as well as dialysis may need to be instituted along with treatment of the malignancy. Patients are counseled to avoid food with high potassium such as fruits and coconut water till the TLS settles down or the at-risk period (usually the first week of treatment) is over.

2. What risk stratification for TLS do you follow?

The risk stratification is based on disease-specific as well as patient-specific characteristics. Disease-specific characteristics include the type of malignancy (ALL, AML, high-grade NHL being most commonly associated), elevated white cell count (>50,000 cells/μL), advanced stage (in case of lymphomas and solid tumors), high proliferation rate (as in the case of T cell ALL, T cell NHL, Burkitt lymphoma), and high sensitivity to cytotoxic therapy (e.g., response to steroids in case of leukemias/lymphoma). The patient-dependent factors include dehydration, preexisting kidney disease, use of nephrotoxic agents, etc. Patients with low risk have <1% chance and those with high risk have >5% chance of developing TLS. TLS is defined based on the Cairo–Bishop classification. Laboratory TLS consists of hyperuricemia, hyperkalemia, hyperphosphatemia, and hypocalcemia and clinical TLS consists of end-organ involvement in the form of renal failure, seizures, cardiac arrhythmias, and death. The samples for tumor lysis are sent at the time of suspicion of the malignancy and then again as per the clinical status. Children are monitored for urine output, bradycardia, sensorium, development of seizures, and renal failure.

3. When do you consider rasburicase and how many doses are used at your unit?

All patients are admitted and started on double maintenance fluids with furosemide at 0.5 mg/kg/dose twice a day along with oral allopurinol at a dose of 100 mg/m^2/dose thrice a day. As discussed earlier clinical and laboratory monitoring is done at least once in a day for most children and at times 2–3 times a day for children with TLS. Chemotherapy for underlying malignancy is initiated without further delay. Urinary alkalinization is avoided.

Upfront rasburicase is used in:
- Children who present with hyperuricemia with AKI
- Children at high risk of TLS (Burkitt, hyperleukocytosis in T cell ALL)

Children not responding to the hydration with allopurinol are also given rasburicase at the earliest. A dose of 0.15–0.2 mg/kg of rasburicase rounded to the nearest vial size (1.5 mg) is used as a short infusion over 30 minutes. Often a single dose is needed to help reduce very high uric acid levels. Even a lower dose/kg has been found to be effective. In children with a high risk of TLS or those presenting with established AKI, often one dose per day for 5 days is recommended. Glucose-6-phosphate dehydrogenase (G6PD) screening is done prior to its use.

When rasburicase is started, allopurinol is stopped in order to provide substrate for rasburicase to act on. Samples for biochemical testing are to be sent over ice packs, to reduce the ex-vivo breakdown of uric acid resulting in falsely low levels.

4. When do you consider dialysis?

The use of any modality of renal replacement has reduced since the availability of affordable rasburicase in our country. In children who do not respond to double-maintenance fluids, hydration may be increased to triple maintenance with the increase in the dose of furosemide to 1.5–2 mg/kg/day. Additional causes of renal dysfunction such as hyperphosphatemia with calcium phosphate nephropathy, and drug or sepsis-induced nephropathy are also ruled out in nonresponding patients.

Dialysis (hemodialysis) is initiated in patients who present with AKI with anuria, not responding to hydration, hyperklemia/hyperphosphatemia not responding to medical measures, bulky disease in the pelvis (lymphoma usually) presenting with ureteric obstruction where hyperhydration may not be effective. Continuous renal replacement therapy is preferred when available. Peritoneal dialysis is discouraged due to concerns of intra-abdominal disease, thrombocytopenia, coagulopathy, sepsis, etc. that may be coexisting in most patients with TLS.

5. How do you monitor ALL patients on an outpatient basis who are at risk of TLS?

In children who are initiated on ALL induction on an outpatient basis, addition of allopurinol, and oral hydration is advised. They are monitored once in 3–4 days for urine output, biochemical markers (renal function with electrolytes including calcium and phosphorus), and sensorium. Only those at low risk of TLS are initiated on this regimen.

Case 2: Hyperleukocytosis

6. How are cases of hyperleukocytosis managed at your center?

Hyperleukocytosis is defined as leukemia with a white blood count of >100,000/µL. In the case of AML, a lower white cell count of >50,000/µL is considered in view of the larger and stickier blast cells. Symptomatic hyperleukocytosis with evidence of reduced tissue perfusion due to white cell plugs in microvasculature typically in lungs and brain is termed leukostasis.

Children who present with leukostasis are at risk for both tumor lysis as well as leukostasis as in this case. They are initiated on an induction regimen for leukemia with hyperhydration with allopurinol as mentioned in the earlier case of TLS. Those who do not respond are switched to rasburicase and early RRT is considered. Most patients respond by days 2-3 of initiation of therapy. In those who present with leukostasis, organ-specific supportive measures such as ventilation may be needed. Red cell transfusions are avoided in view of the increased risk of hypercoagulopathy that can worsen leukostasis.

Therapeutic leukapheresis although a possibility is not usually performed in view of rebound increase in counts, associated coagulopathy, and logistical issues such as securing a central line in a sick patient.

7. How the approach different if the diagnosis is ALL/AML with hyperleukocytosis?

In ALL, with the initiation of induction chemotherapy (prednisolone only at my center for the first 7 days along with intrathecal methotrexate), improvement is noted over the next 24–48 hours. Often those who do not respond to prednisolone would respond after the intrathecal methotrexate is initiated, probably as a result of its systemic absorption. At times, nonresponding or refractory patients with progressive increase in white cell counts are observed. In these cases, changing of steroid to dexamethasone, addition of cyclophosphamide (T cell disease), addition of day 8 chemotherapy (vincristine, daunorubicin, L-asparaginase), etc. are measures that are adopted.

In the case of AML with hyperleukocytosis, hydroxyurea is often initiated along with induction chemotherapy (3 + 7 regimen). Hydroxyurea is initiated to lower the tumor burden and reduce the risk of complications. Patients would need very close monitoring for coagulopathy (thrombocytopenia, platelet dysfunction, acquired von Willebrand disease, etc.) and tumor lysis. In AML with hyperleukocytosis, DIC is often observed as a result of high levels of tissue factor which triggers coagulation. The risk of mortality is high especially in AML-related hyperleukocytosis and treatment should be initiated immediately. Platelet count is usually maintained above 20,000/µL in this situation in order to prevent CNS bleed. FFP is indicated in patients with deranged coagulation. Patients with acute promyelocytic leukemia (APL) are started on all trans retinoic acid (ATRA) with or without arsenic immediately on the first suspicion without waiting for molecular confirmation. Those with APL and hyperleukocytosis would need cytoreductive treatment in the form of anthracyclines in addition to differentiating agents.

8. What are the indications of using steroids in hyperleukocytosis?

Steroids are used as mentioned above in ALL as part of induction regimen.

9. When do you consider definitive chemotherapy?

Chemotherapy is initiated at the outset is most cases after admitting the child and providing appropriate supportive care. Initiation of definitive treatment is the best modality to reduce high white cell counts in leukemia and prevent end-organ damage. Delaying chemotherapy can result in progression of the disease and its complications. In many centers in India, stabilization of the patient by the addition of oral/low-dose chemotherapy is attempted especially if there are constraints of providing an inpatient bed.

10. Is TLS a contraindication to definitive chemotherapy?

No. On the contrary, definitive chemotherapy is often the best way to reduce tumor load and improve the risk of tumor lysis. In established AKI, the dose of chemotherapy may be modified.

11. What is your opinion regarding leukapheresis and exchange management as modalities to manage hyperleukocytosis?

As mentioned above, although these are therapeutic modalities, they are not preferred due to the temporary improvement provided and additional challenges of coagulopathy, thrombosis, worsening of thrombocytopenia, need for a central line for this purpose, etc. Leukapheresis is also debated as the majority of the disease burden is still inside the bone marrow and is mobilized to the periphery shortly after apheresis. It has not been found to improve clinical outcomes in patients with hyperleukocytosis.

Case 3: Superior Mediastinal Syndrome/Superior Vena Cava Syndrome

12. What is emergency management of SMS?

Superior mediastinal syndrome is defined as the presence of compression of the airway in patients who present with disease in the mediastinum. In children since the thoracic inlet is small, vena caval and airway compression often coexist thus leading to the interchangeable use of superior mediastinal/vena caval syndrome. The emergency management of SMS could consist of head-end elevation, lateral or prone positioning, initiation of oxygen, and other ventilatory strategies as needed. Supine position is discouraged in view of the worsening of tracheal compression due to compression from the disease. For the same reason, a CT scan is often discouraged or performed cautiously under the supervision of a physician capable of intubating the child if need be. IV cannula is secured in the lower limb to reduce the congestion in the superior mediastinum and worsening of intracranial pressure.

The definitive management would consist of achieving a diagnosis of the disease through the least invasive route and initiation of definitive treatment. In cases of leukemia and lymphoma with spill, this can be achieved through PB flow cytometry or bone marrow aspiration. Bone marrow if performed may be done in sitting/lateral position with only local anesthesia. Procedural sedation should be avoided at all costs as it can lead to respiratory depression with fatal consequences. In the case of lymphoma and other causes of a mediastinal mass, a close look for peripheral lymph nodes that may be evaluated is looked for. In the case of germ cell tumors and neuroblastoma, often noninvasive testing in the form of tumor markers may be used. Peripheral lymph nodes or extrathoracic extension of the mediastinal disease may be aspirated under local anesthesia for cytological evaluation or biopsied under local anesthesia if possible. In the absence of such a disease, ultrasound-guided core biopsy, or fine needle aspiration (FNA) may be performed by an experienced radiologist or surgeon.

In a dire emergency where there is a risk of impending respiratory failure and no chance of a noninvasive route of testing, steroids may be initiated as a lifesaving measure with appropriate measures for tumor lysis prevention/treatment. Tissue diagnosis may be reattempted after 24–48 hours of initiation of steroids without alteration of the histological findings. Steroids not only help by reducing tumor volume but also by decreasing airway edema. However, they also pose an additional risk of tumor lysis and even a single dose of steroids used during anesthesia or as premedication for blood transfusion can worsen tumor lysis.

13. How is anesthesia risk assessed for performing a biopsy?

General anesthesia is associated with high morbidity and mortality rates. There are concerns of difficult intubation as a result of compression of the airway due to the mass, edema of vocal cords, and tracheal lumen due to venous congestion and often a risk of bleeding due to coexisting thrombocytopenia. The hemodynamic instability may be further exacerbated by positive pressure ventilation by the increase in intrathoracic pressure and a further reduction in venous return. Extubation is also difficult due to the collapse of tracheal walls leading to the need for reintubation which may often be more challenging. Thus avoidance of general anesthesia and maintenance of spontaneous breathing should be favored as much as possible.

A full assessment of the patient by a competent pediatric anesthesiologist is preferred prior to making a decision on this matter. History, examination, and CXR are mandatory and if possible echocardiography may be performed. The presence of orthopnea, upper body edema, stridor, and wheeze are associated with a high risk of cardiorespiratory collapse. Evidence of compression of tracheal diameter ≤70% of normal with carinal/bronchial compression, presence of SVC obstruction, pericardial effusion, ventricular dysfunction, and supine peak expiratory flow rate (PEFR) of ≤50% are predictors of high anesthetic risk. The main risk of anesthesia is that of subglottic collapse and immediate airway compromise. Due to loss of muscle tone, extubation is often difficult. Hence, as far as possible, an awake state with local anesthesia for procedures may be preferred in such cases.

14. What other drugs besides steroids are considered in the emergency management of SMS due to lymphoma?

In non-Hodgkin lymphoma (especially T lymphoblastic) that presents with SMS, initiation of induction chemotherapy may be considered. In patients with high-risk mature NHL, the use of cyclophosphamide and vincristine also has been found to be beneficial. Tumor lysis should be anticipated and managed appropriately. In case of Hodgkin lymphoma, the initiation of definitive chemotherapy as per the regimen followed adriamycin, bleomycin, vinblastin, dacarbazine (ABVD), vincristine, procarbazine, prednisolone, doxorubicin (OPPA), vincristine, etoposide, prednisolone, doxorubicin (OEPA) will help reduce the tumor burden.

15. How does this treatment affect the definitive chemotherapy?

The use of steroids or other sensitive drugs can affect the histological diagnosis. So also, since in most cases, staging investigations such as positron emission tomography-computed tomography (PET-CT) may be performed after stabilizing the patient, it can result in the downgrading of the disease stage due to partial treatment response.

Case 4: Febrile Neutropenia

16. How is antibiotic selected to manage a case of FN?

The choice of antibiotics in febrile neutropenic setting is usually based on the local antibiogram based on the unit's experience. Since gram-negative infections are more common in our settings, it is preferable to use a third-generation cephalosporin or higher broad-spectrum agent with adequate pseudomonal cover. Gram-positive cover is added upfront in case of children with high risk of mucositis (post high-dose cytarabine), prior MRSA colonization, clinical evidence of skin, soft tissue, and respiratory involvement and in those with hemodynamic instability.

17. Can cases of FN be managed on ambulatory care in our country? If so which patients should be managed in ambulatory care?

Children at low risk of FN (solid tumor, maintenance phase of leukemia, etc.) may be managed on an outpatient basis. The decision is individualized based on the type of disease, the intensity of chemotherapy used, anticipated recovery of neutropenia, prior infections, and the level of understanding and access to care for the family.

18. When do you consider using a gram-positive and antifungal cover for cases of FN at your center?

Gram-positive cover is added upfront in case of children with high risk of mucositis [post high-dose cytarabine, bone marrow transplant (BMT) conditioning], prior MRSA colonization, clinical evidence of skin, soft tissue and respiratory involvement, and in those with hemodynamic instability. Children with central line in situ should have paired blood cultures sent to identify central line-associated bloodstream infection. Preemptive treatment using antifungals with mold cover (voriconazole/posaconazole) is added after 72–96 hours of fever with no improvement. Antifungals are added prophylactically in children at high risk such as BMT recipients, and children undergoing AML and high-risk ALL chemotherapy.

19. What are the indications for use of growth factors and GTXs in the management of FN?

Granulocyte colony-stimulating factor is used prophylactically in patients undergoing chemotherapy with high risk of FN. However, in most induction chemotherapy as well as AML treatment the use of G-CSF is discouraged. G-CSF helps in reducing the period of neutropenia only by around 1 day, which may not be clinically very beneficial. It is useful in solid tumors where intensive chemotherapy is to be given in short intervals.

Granulocyte transfusions, on the other hand, have been found to be highly beneficial in the management of multidrug-resistant infections in FN settings. Regular granulocyte infusion offers protection against bacterial and fungal infections and helps bridge the gap till neutrophil count improves.

20. How does an episode of FN affect the subsequent chemotherapy in hematological malignancy and solid tumors?

The development of FN affects subsequent chemotherapy in the following ways:
- Delay in the initiation of the next cycle of treatment resulting in an adverse impact on final outcomes
- Need for secondary prophylaxis with antimicrobials especially antifungals in further cycles
- Reduction of the intensity of chemotherapy in further cycles in patients who develop grade 3 or 4 neutropenia. This too will impact the overall outcome.
- Increase in cost of treatment
- In persistent colonization of the central line, the line may have to be removed in a few cases, thus increasing the morbidity for the child in future cycles.

Index

Page numbers followed by *f* refer to figure, *fc* refer to flowchart, and *t* refer to table.

A

Abelson murine leukemia virus 161
Absolute neutrophil count 211, 280, 319
Activated partial thromboplastin time 127, 256
Acute lymphoblastic leukemia 1
 relapse 19, 20*t*, 21*t*
Acute myeloid leukemia 40, 41, 43*fc*, 46, 49, 58, 60, 68, 74, 90, 91, 165, 295, 301, 302, 305, 307, 319, 328
 management of 57, 72
 prognostic factors in 59*t*
 relapse 58
Acute promyelocytic leukemia 126*f*, 127, 127*f*, 130
 morphology of 124*f*
Adrenal hypoplasia 244
Adriamycin 222, 230, 279, 336
Advanced myelodysplastic syndrome 246
Alanine aminotransferase 153
Alkalinization 296
Allogeneic hematopoietic cell 328
Allogeneic transplantation 229
Allopurinol 296
All-trans-retinoic acid 127*f*
 dose of 131
Amphotericin B deoxycholate 327
Amsacrine cytarabine etoposide 46, 60
Anakinra 272
Anaplastic large cell lymphoma 171, 177, 179, 181, 182, 185, 295
 pathogenesis of 175
Anaplastic lymphoma kinase 174, 177, 178*f*
Anemia 242
 aplastic 245
 hemolytic 281
 refractory 243
 severe 306
 aplastic 241
 sideroblastic 241
Anesthesia 336
 local 313
Angiotensin converting enzyme 67
Ann Arbor staging classification 221*f*, 221*t*
Anthracyclines 27, 314
 antibiotics 64
 free regimen 136
Anti-anaplastic lymphoma kinase antibodies 179
Antibacterial prophylaxis 327
 role of 48
 use of 48
Antibiotic
 discontinuation of 324
 empirical 323
 prophylaxis 327
Antibody drug conjugates 47
Anticytokine 272
Antifungal prophylaxis 48, 328
 role of 48
Antifungal therapy 326
Antipneumocystis prophylaxis 328
Antithymocyte globulin 246
Antiviral prophylaxis 328
Aortic aneurysm 309, 310
Apple core appearance 124*f*
Arrhythmias, cardiac 332
Ascites 254
Asparaginase 27
Aspergillosis 48
Aspergillus flavus 297
Autoimmune lymphoproliferative disorders 280
Autoimmune lymphoproliferative syndrome 249, 275, 280, 283, 285
 management of 285, 286*fc*
Autoimmunity 281
Autologous stem cell transplant 228, 229
Azacitidine, role of 164

B

Basophilia 102, 138*f*, 140
Basophils 102
B-cell 22
 lymphomas 196
 receptor 207, 214
Bendamustine 232
Berlin-Frankfurt-Münster 23, 46, 60, 91, 93, 206
Beta-D-glucan 326
Bilineage cytopenia 242
Biopsy 336
 abdominal 205*f*
Birbeck granule 268
Blast crisis 102, 142
Blastic transformation 163
Bleomycin 222, 230, 336
Blinatumomab 11, 30, 34, 82
 role of 32
Blood 317
 cell 139
 component therapy 304
 culture 317
Bone 255
 health 223
Bone marrow 4, 21, 46, 89, 142, 156, 160, 161, 242, 244, 245, 245*f*
 aspirate cytology 20*f*
 aspiration 24*f*
 examination 313
 transplant 220, 337
 trephine biopsy 139*f*
Bony lesions 16
Bradycardia 333
BRAF-v600e mutation 275, 277

Brentuximab vedotin 177, 182, 229, 230
Bronchoalveolar lavage 172*f*, 256, 326
Bruton's tyrosine kinase 214
Bulky disease 333
  role of 6
Burkitt's leukemia 332
Burkitt's lymphoma 205, 208*f*, 214*f*, 217
  management of 217
  pathogenesis of 207*f*
Burkitt's pathogenesis 207

C

Cairo-Bishop classification 332
Calcium 298, 315
Calycectasia, diffuse 272
Carbon
  dioxide 310
  monoxide 65
Carboplatin 220, 228, 229
Cardiac dysfunction 50, 67, 234
Cardiomyocytes, death of 67
Cardiorespiratory collapse, high risk of 336
Cardiotoxicity 66, 234
  prevention of 65
Cardiovascular disease 66
Carmustine 232
Castleman disease 280
Cefepime 321
Central nervous system 20, 21, 24, 32, 75, 77, 93, 102, 140, 160, 174, 206, 210, 252, 259, 271, 274, 301
  prophylaxis 78, 131
Cephalosporin monotherapy 321
Cerebral parenchyma 25
Cerebral venous thrombosis 128*f*
Cerebrospinal fluid 21, 22, 194, 211, 318, 326
Ceritinib 178
Chemorefractory, prognosis of 229
Chemotherapy 11, 17, 57, 63, 131, 136, 148*f*, 169, 335, 337
  agents 25
  completion of 234
  cycles 229, 327
  drugs 222
  free approach 132
  low-dose 335
  maintenance 30*f*, 261
  metronomic 72

  myeloablative 319
  postreinduction 30
  postsalvage 213*f*
  post-transplant 164
  pre-transplant 164
  reinduction 28, 224
  role of 57, 163
  standard-dose 226
Chest X-ray 256, 309*f*, 318
Children's cancer group 78
Children's oncology group 47, 63, 77, 93
Chimeric antigen receptor 11, 31, 82
Cholesterol efflux 274
Chromosomal microarray analysis 56
Chromosome abnormalities 146
Chronic cervical lymphadenopathy, differential diagnosis of 188*t*
Cisplatin 212, 230
Cladribine 261, 261*f*, 272
Coagulopathy, mechanism of 125
Colony-stimulating factor 78, 274
Combination therapy 321
Complete blood count 69, 312
Complex inflammatory response 270
Computed tomography 254, 260, 261, 266
  scan image 172*f*
Consolidation chemotherapy 30*f*
Continuous arteriovenous hemofiltration 299
Continuous venovenous hemofiltration 299
Core needle biopsy 173*f*
Corticosteroids 285
Cranial nerve palsy 211
Crizotinib 178, 186
Cyclin dependent kinases 207
Cyclophosphamide 62, 78, 210, 222, 233, 234, 279
  addition of 334
Cyst
  duplication 310
  pericardial 310
  thymic 309
Cytarabine 24, 46, 47, 50, 52, 60, 80, 212, 230, 232, 258, 260, 261, 261*f*, 337
  high-dose 46, 60, 64, 91, 93, 230, 239

Cytogenetic abnormalities 76, 163
Cytogenetic profile 148
Cytogenetic response 145, 150, 151
Cytokine
  receptor-like factor 115, 116
  release syndrome 11, 33
Cytomegalovirus 13, 161, 241, 280
Cytopenia 244, 255, 281
  chronic 287
  refractory 243
Cytoplasmic clusters 41
Cytoreduction 304
  nonspecific 304, 306
Cytoreductive treatment 334
Cytosine arabinoside 57
  high-dose 233
Cytotoxic chemotherapy 293, 314

D

Dacarbazine 222, 230, 336
Dasatinib 152
Daunorubicin 46, 52, 57, 66, 67, 93, 314
Decitabine 82
Dendritic cell 253
  neoplasms 277
Deoxyribonucleic acid 305
Dexamethasone 27, 212, 230, 233, 305, 306, 314, 334
Dexrazoxane 67
Diabetes insipidus 277
Dialysis 333
Diffuse large B cell lymphoma 188, 295
  management of 199
Disseminated intravascular coagulation 126, 127, 301, 302
Diuresis 296
Dizziness 139
Double hit lymphoma 209, 218
Down's syndrome 91, 93, 94, 249
Doxorubicin 25, 66, 222, 230, 314, 336
Drug toxicity 49, 241
Dysplasia, morphological 241

E

Ebstein-Barr virus 161, 280
Electrocardiogram 298
Electrolyte
  abnormality 298
  serum 298

Emperipolesis 273
Empirical anti-fungal therapy 327
Encephalopathy 33
Endobronchial mass 173
Endocrine 223, 271
　abnormality 255
Endothelium thrombogenicity 127f
Enzymes, lysosomal 273
Eosinophilia 140
Epithelial mesenchymal transition 274
Epstein-Barr virus 208, 219, 241
　role of 208
Erdheim-Chester disease 262, 268, 269f, 270f, 274
　diagnosis of 270
　pathogenesis of 274fc
Erythrocyte sedimentation rate 256
Erythroid 241
Etoposide 46, 52, 57, 212, 220, 222, 228-230, 232, 233, 336
Exophthalmos 277

F

Familial platelet disorder 243
Febrile neutropenia 48, 292, 319, 323fc
Febuxostat 296, 297
Fertility 223
　preservation 152f, 158
Fibrin degradation products 126f
Fibrinogen degradation product 127
Fibrinolysis, activation of 126f
Fine needle aspiration 336
　cytology 4, 178f
Flow cytometry 21, 22, 75, 312
Fluconazole 328
Fludarabine 13, 24
　cytarabine 60
Fludeoxyglucose 254, 260
Fludrabine cytarabine 46
Fluorescence in situ hybridization 2fc, 7, 21, 22, 102, 115, 141, 244
Fluorodeoxyglucose 173f, 266
　qualitative 285
　quantitative 285
Fluoroquinolones 48
Fungal infections 49, 338

G

Galactomannan 325
Ganglioneuroblastoma 310
Ganglioneuromas 310
Gemcitabine 228, 229, 234
Gemtuzumab 47
　ozogamicin 46, 63
Germ cell tumor 309, 319
Giant cell 253
Glasgow coma scale 319
Glucose-6-phosphate dehydrogenase 297
Glycogen synthase kinase 274
Goiter, retrosternal 309
Gonadotropin 253
Graft versus host disease 13, 246
　chronic 62, 65
Graham's patch repair 219
Gram-negative
　bacilli 323
　infection 324
Granulocytes 139f
　colony-stimulating factor 46, 49, 60, 170, 198, 268, 328, 328
　macrophage colony-stimulating factor 161, 162
　monocyte-colony stimulating factor 268
　proliferation of 139
　transfusion 329, 338
Growth factors 253, 337
Growth failure 255
Growth retardation 262
Guillain-Barre syndrome 281

H

Headache 139
Hearing loss 262
Hemangioma 309, 310
Hematological disorders 240
Hematopoietic stem cell 252
　transplantation 46, 47, 60, 63, 65, 73, 146, 150, 151, 162, 181, 198, 213, 247, 258, 259, 262, 328
　indications of 153f
　role of 287
Hemodialysis 333
　intermittent 299
Hemoglobin 242
　fetal 161

Hemoglobinuria, paroxysmal nocturnal 244
Hemorrhage 128
　retinal 303
Hepatic toxicity 65
Hepatitis C virus 141
Herpesvirus 241
High methylation group 163
Histiocytic disorders 274, 278
Histiocytoses 275
　cutaneous 277
　malignant 277
　revised classification of 268f
Histone
　deacetylase 82
　lysine methyltransferase 75
Hodgkin's disease 273
Hodgkin's international prognostic score 223
Hodgkin's lymphoma 182, 188, 219, 223, 226, 228, 229, 284, 336
　refractory 219
Human immunodeficiency virus 208, 241, 280
Human leukocyte antigen 246, 268
Hybrid chemotherapy 79
Hydration 304
Hydrocortisone 314
Hydroureteronephrosis 272
Hydroxyurea 141, 304, 306
Hypercalcemia 16
Hyperdiploidy 15
Hyperhydration 295
Hyperkalemia 293, 294, 298, 332
Hyperleukocytosis 76, 139, 292, 301, 303, 334, 335
　clinical features of 301
　initial management of 305
　pathophysiology of 301, 301fc
　prognostic significance of 308
　risk of 302
Hypernatremia 296
Hyperphosphatemia 293, 294, 298, 332
Hyperplasia, thymic 309
Hypersensitivity reaction 296
Hypertriglyceridemia 64
Hyperuricemia 293, 294, 332
Hypocalcemia 293, 294, 298, 332
Hyponatremia 295
　hospital-acquired 296
Hypoplastic marrow 244
Hypothalamic syndromes 255
Hypothesis 252

I

Idarubicin 24f, 46
Ifosfamide 220, 228-230, 234
Imatinib 145, 154
Immature lymphoid cells 205
Immune
   dysregulation 252
   suppression 285
   thrombocytopenia 280
   thrombocytopenic purpura 284
Immunoglobulin 4, 65, 207, 282
   intravenous 218, 286
Immunohistochemistry 205f, 244
Immunophenotypes, leukemias associated 4
Immunophenotyping markers 41t
Immunotherapy 11
   era of 12
Induction chemotherapy 28f
Infection 49
   bacterial 241, 338
   chronic 219
   severe 316
Inflammatory myeloid neoplasm 270
Inflammatory myofibroblastic tumor 175
Inflammatory neoplastic disorder 252
Infliximab 272
Inherited bone marrow failure syndrome 240, 243, 244
Inotuzumab 11, 33
Intensification 43
   chemotherapy 30f
Interferon-alpha 272
Interim maintenance chemotherapy 30f
Interleukin 116, 274, 282, 305
Intracranial tension 301
Intrathecal therapy 78
Iron accumulation 66

J

Janus kinase enzyme 116
Japanese pediatric leukemia 77
Jaundice 251
Juvenile myelomonocytic leukemia 140, 159-161, 165, 244, 283
   diagnosis of 161fc
   diagnostic criteria of 160
   management of 166
   pathogenesis of 162

K

Karyotype
   interpretation of 90
   normal 245
Kidney
   function tests 143
   injury, acute 296

L

Lactate dehydrogenase 206, 210, 295
Langerhans cell histiocytosis 161, 251, 252, 256, 259, 262, 268, 319
   laboratory evaluation in 255t
   pathogenesis of 252
L-asparaginase 212
Lesions 266
Leukapheresis 140, 306, 335
   indications of 140
   therapeutic 334
Leukemia 74, 102, 140, 159-161, 165, 214, 244, 283, 309, 332
   acute 188
      lymphoblastic 1, 7fc, 19, 23, 44, 69, 74, 75, 77, 79, 81, 93, 102, 115, 116, 139, 295, 302, 307, 319
      lymphoid 125
      megakaryoblastic 91, 94
      myelogenous 47
      myeloid 40, 41, 43fc, 46, 49, 58, 60, 68, 74, 90, 91, 165, 295, 301, 302, 305, 307, 319, 328
      promyelocytic 126f, 127, 127f, 130
   characteristics of 89
   childhood acute lymphoblastic 2fc
   chronic
      myelocytic 243
      myeloid 102, 138, 138f, 139, 146, 151, 273, 295, 302, 303, 305
   infantile 74
   lymphoma group 198
   maintenance phase of 337
   myeloid 79, 91, 93
   phenotypic acute 40
   presentation of 75
   second 25
Leukemic cells 76
Leukemoid reaction 140

Leukocyte
   adhesion defect 161
   count 306
Leukocytosis 138f
Leukoproliferative disease 283
Leukostasis 302, 303
Levofloxacin 48
Lipid-Laden histiocytes 271
Lipoma 309, 310
Liposomal amphotericin B 327, 328
   efficacy of 327
Liposomal daunorubicin 24, 46, 60
Liver 254, 255
   dysfunction 51, 255
      mild to moderate 51
   transplantation 262
Lomustine 233
Lung 255, 272
   bilateral 260f
Lymph node
   abdominal 220f
   enlargement 280
Lymphadenopathy 189fc, 278
   infectious 309, 310
Lymphangioma 309, 310
Lymphohistiocytosis, hemophagocytic 268, 277, 280
Lymphoid cells, autoreactive 280
Lymphoma 209, 209f, 280, 308, 309, 332, 336
   malignant 193
   pediatric 190
   study group 77
Lymphophagocytosis 281
Lymphoproliferative disorder 284
   RAS-associated 284

M

Magnetic resonance imaging 128f, 256
Maintenance therapy 132
Malignancy
   hematological 338
   risk of 284
Malignant peripheral nerve sheath tumor 310
Malnutrition 52
Maximum intensity projection 220f
May-Grunwald Giemsa stained slides 19f
Mechanical cytoreduction 306
   types of 306

Mediastinal mass 309, 311, 312
Megakaryocyte 241
Melphalan 81, 232
Mercaptopurine 297
Metabolic disorders 241
Metabolic response 213, 226, 228, 229
Metamyelocyte 138f, 140
Methotrexate 79, 210, 246
   high-dose 78, 80
Methylation 163
   group 163
Methylprednisolone 230, 239, 285, 314
Micromegakaryocytes 243, 245
Minimal disseminated disease 175-177, 196
Minimal residual disease 1, 3, 7, 21-24, 24f, 81, 93, 145, 176, 196
   detection, methods for 3t
Minimally myelosuppressive chemotherapy 318
Mitogen activated protein kinase 252
Mitoxantrone 46, 47, 60, 80
Mixed lineage leukemia 77, 81, 247
Mixed-phenotype acute leukemia 41
Molecular pathway 100
Molecular remission 20, 43, 47, 154, 157
Molecular response 145
Molecular tests 271
Monocytosis 159f
Monotherapy 321
   choice of 321
Multicolor flow cytometry 4
Multiple lytic lesions 266f
Multi-system disease 271
Myelocyte 140
Myelodysplastic syndrome 240, 242-244, 246, 247, 249, 270
   diagnosis of 245
   low-risk 246
   management of 249
Myeloperoxidase, intracellular 41
Myeloproliferative disorders 273
Myelosuppression 51
Myelosuppressive chemotherapy 318, 319

N

Natural killer cell 244
Neoplasms
   myeloid 270
   myeloproliferative 270
Nephrology, pediatric 299
Nephrotoxic drugs 294
Neuroblastoma 175, 188, 332
Neurodegeneration 253, 262
Neurotoxicity 33
Neutropenia 152, 182, 211, 242, 328
Next-generation sequencing 7, 21, 72
Nonhematological disorders 241
Non-Hodgkin's lymphoma 22, 188, 190, 206, 273, 284, 336
   refractory 197
Non-Langerhans cell histiocytosis 266

O

Oligonucleotides, allele-specific 4
Oral phosphate binders 298
Orthopnea 311
Osteonecrosis 65
Osteopenia 65
Osteoporosis 65
Oxaliplatin 234
Ozogamicin 47

P

Papilledema 140, 303
Parathyroid
   adenoma 309
   hormone 143
Parvovirus 241
Peak expiratory flow rate 312
Pearson syndrome 241
Pericardial fluid examination 313
Peripheral blood 4, 156, 161, 301
   smear 138f, 159f
Peripheral smear 87, 89, 312
Peritoneal dialysis 333
P-glycoprotein 25
Philadelphia chromosome 100, 111
   molecular biology of 99
Phosphoprotein 175
Phosphorus 298, 315
Pleural fluid 313
Pneumocystis jiroveci 318
   prophylaxis 28

Pneumonitis 262
Polydipsia 251, 255
Polyethylene glycol 27
Polymerase chain reaction 1, 4, 21, 141, 196, 253
Polyuria 251, 255
Posaconazole 328, 337
Positron emission tomography 173f, 228, 229, 254, 256, 260, 261, 266
Posterior reversible encephalopathy syndrome 153
Postrituximab 218
Potassium 298, 315
Prednisolone 222, 230, 258, 279, 336
Prednisone 210, 222
Priapism 140
Procarbazine 222, 336
Progressive disease 228, 229
Promyelocytes 138f
   abnormal large 124f
Prophylaxis 48
Prothrombin fragment 126f
Prothrombotic factors, plasma levels of 126f
Proto-oncogene, function of 206
Pulmonary function tests 65

R

Radiotherapy 211, 226, 228, 229
Rapamycin 281
   complex 274
Rasburicase 297
Rat sarcoma 283
Reed-Sternberg cells 231
Refractory disease 11, 176
Renal dysfunction 52, 294
Renal failure 332, 333
Renal replacement therapy 299
   indications of 299
Resistant infections, high risk of 322
Respiratory distress 129, 254
Respiratory status 312
Retinoblastoma 319
Retro-orbital infiltration 271
Retroperitoneal lymph node 219
Reverse transcriptase polymerase chain reaction 7, 181, 115, 116
Rhabdomyolysis 262
Rhabdomyosarcoma 175, 188, 319

Rheumatic disease 241
Ribonucleic acid 115, 116
Rituximab 198, 212, 218, 233, 284
    role of 233
    use of 212
Rosai-Dorfman-Destombes disease 277, 278, 281

S

Salvage chemotherapy 73, 212
Seckel syndrome 240
Seizures 33, 332
    development of 333
Sensorium 333
Serum glutamic
    oxaloacetic transaminase 319
    pyruvic transaminase 319
Sexual maturity rating 254
Short stature 255
Shwachman-Diamond syndrome 240
Sirolimus 282
Skin 255
    rash 277, 296
Sodium 298, 315
Sperm cryopreservation 152
Spleen size 254
Splenectomy, role of 164
Stable disease 228, 229
Standard-dose salvage chemotherapy regimens 230
Staphylococcus aureus 140, 322
Stem cell 198
    mobilization 231
    rescue 221
    transplant 24, 24f, 43, 179, 258
Steroids 284, 305, 314
    high-dose 282
Streptococcus pneumoniae 140
Stridor 311
Sulfamethoxazole 28
Superior mediastinal syndrome 292, 310, 314, 335
Superior mediastinal syndrome, management of 335, 336
Superior vena cava syndrome 310, 314
Switch-tyrosine kinase inhibitor 149fc
Syndrome of inappropriate antidiuretic hormone secretion 295
Systemic lupus erythematosus 281

T

T-cell 3, 82
    accumulate 281
    disease 334
    double-negative 281, 282
    receptor 4, 282
    therapy 33
Testicular leukemia 25
Testis 31
Thioguanine 93
Thiotepa 13
Threonine protein kinase 269
Thrombin antithrombin complex 126f
Thrombocytopenia 152, 159f, 242, 243, 335, 336
Thrombosis 128
Thymoma 309
Thyroid tumors 309
Thyroiditis 281
Thyrotropin 253
Tisagenlecleucel 11
Tissue, immunohistochemistry of 205f
Tocilizumab 272
Total body irradiation 61, 65, 181
Total leukocyte count 102, 115, 162
Total lymphocyte count 142
Touton giant cells 277
Toxicity, hematological 198
Trans-retinoic acid 334
Trimethoprim 28
Triphosphate metabolism 273
Triple hit lymphomas 209, 218
Tuberculosis 310
Tumor
    biomarkers 313
    bronchoscopic images of 172f
    cell lysis 299
    solid 332, 338
Tumor lysis syndrome 292, 293, 301, 302, 305
    diagnosis of 293
    management of 332
    pathophysiology of 293fc
    risk of 210
Tyrosine kinase 63
    domain 148, 150, 151
    gene 130
    inhibitor 26, 116, 139, 146, 150, 151, 153, 272

U

Ultrasonography 256
Ultrasound-guided testicular fine needle aspirate cytology 19f
Umbilical cord blood 165
Uremia 293
Uric acid lowering agents 296
Urinalysis 317
Urinary tract infection 317
Urine
    culture 317
    output, monitoring of 298
Urokinase-type plasminogen activator 126f
Urticarial rash 281
Uveitis 281

V

Valvular disease 272
Varicella virus 241
Vascular cell adhesion molecule 305
Vascular endothelial growth factor 273
Ventricular dysfunction 336
Vinblastine 177, 222, 230, 258, 336
    role of 179
    single-agent 179
Vincristine 27, 78, 210, 222, 279, 336
Vinorelbine 228, 229
Vitamin D 143
Voriconazole 28, 328, 337

W

Weight gain 129
Wheezing 311
White blood
    cell 77, 81, 244, 301, 307
    count 7

X

Xanthelasma 277
Xanthogranuloma, juvenile 268, 277, 278
X-ray absorptiometry, dual energy 65

Z

Zoledronic acid 272

EU GSPR Authorised Reprsentative
Logos Europe, 9 rue Nicolas Poussin
1700, La Rochelle, France
Phone: +33 (0) 6 67 93 73 78
E-mail: contact@logoseurope.eu

www.ingramcontent.com/pod-product-compliance
Ingram Content Group UK Ltd.
Pitfield, Milton Keynes, MK11 3LW, UK
UKHW050429150426
5217IPUK00019B/1311